# Primary Care
# Mental Health

# Primary Care
# Mental Health

Edited by Linda Gask, Helen Lester,
Tony Kendrick and Robert Peveler

RCPsych Publications

RCPsych Publications is an imprint of the Royal College of Psychiatrists,
17 Belgrave Square, London SW1X 8PG
http://www.rcpsych.ac.uk

British Library Cataloguing-in-Publication Data.
A catalogue record for this book is available from the British Library.
ISBN 978 1 904671 77 0

Distributed in North America by Publishers Storage and Shipping Company.

The views presented in this book do not necessarily reflect those of the Royal College of Psychiatrists, and the publishers are not responsible for any error of omission or fact.

The Royal College of Psychiatrists is a charity registered in England and Wales (228636) and in Scotland (SC038369).

Printed in the UK by Bell & Bain Limited, Glasgow.

# Contents

# Figures, tables and boxes

# Contributors

**Ella Arensman**, MSc, PhD, is Director of Research at the National Suicide Research Foundation, and Honorary Senior Lecturer with the Department of Epidemiology and Public Health at University College Cork, Ireland.

**Bruce Arroll**, MB ChB, PhD, FRNZCGP, FNZCPHM, is Head of the Department of General Practice and Primary Health Care, University of Auckland, New Zealand.

**Robert Baldwin** is Consultant in Old Age Psychiatry at Manchester Royal Infirmary and Honorary Professor of Old Age Psychiatry at the University of Manchester.

**Peter Bower**, PhD, is Reader in Health Services Research at the Primary Care Research Group, University of Manchester.

**Angela Burnett**, MBBS, BSc, MSc, MRCGP, DRCOG, is a general practitioner (GP) at the Sanctuary Practice in Hackney, East London, and Lead Doctor at the Medical Foundation for the Care of Victims of Torture, London.

**Carolyn Chew-Graham**, BSc, MB ChB, MD, FRCGP, is Professor of Primary Care in the School of Community Based Medicine, University of Manchester; GP Principal in a small practice in central Manchester; Clinical Advisor, Mental Health, Joint Commissioning Team, Manchester; and Royal College of General Practitioners (RCGP) Clinical Champion, Mental Health.

**Frances Cole**, MBBS, has been a GP since 1983 and is a member of the RCGP. Dr Cole is also a qualified cognitive–behavioural therapist.

**Sandra Dietrich**, MA, is a research fellow at the Department of Psychiatry, Leipzig University, Germany, and a project assistant for the German Research Network on Depression and Suicidality.

**Christopher Dowrick**, MD, FRCGP, is Professor of Primary Medical Care at the University of Liverpool, and a GP in north Liverpool.

**M. Elena Garralda**, MD, MPhil, DPM, FRCPsych, FRCPCH, is Professor of Child and Adolescent Psychiatry at Imperial College London, UK, and Honorary Consultant in Child and Adolescent Psychiatry with Central and North West London Foundation Trust.

**Linda Gask**, MB ChB, MSc, PhD, FRCPsych, is Professor of Primary Care Psychiatry at the University of Manchester, and Honorary Consultant Psychiatrist at Salford Primary Care Trust, Greater Manchester.

**Clare Gerada**, MBE, FRCP, FRCGP, MRCPsych, is Medical Director of the Practitioner Health Programme and Vice Chair of the Royal College of General Practitioners. She is a GP in South London with a specialist interest in substance misuse.

**Simon Gilbody**, DPhil, MRCPsych, is Professor of Psychological Medicine and Health Services Research at the University of York, and Hull York Medical School.

**David Goldberg**, DM, MA, MSc, FRCP, FRCPsych, is Professor Emeritus, Institute of Psychiatry, King's College London.

**Oye Gureje**, DSc, FRCPsych, FRANZCP, is Professor and Head of the Department of Psychiatry at the University of Ibadan, and an Honorary Consultant Psychiatrist at the University College Hospital, Ibadan, Nigeria.

**Mark Haddad**, PhD, MSc, BSc (Hons), RGN/RMN, is Clinical Research Fellow at the Institute of Psychiatry, King's College London, and a member of the Royal College of Nursing Mental Health Nursing Forum Committee.

**Ulrich Hegerl**, MD, PhD, is Head and Medical Director of the Clinic of Psychiatry at Leipzig University, Germany, Head of the German Research Network on Depression and Suicidality, Principal Investigator for the European Alliance Against Depression (EAAD) and the 7th Framework Programme 'Optimised Suicide Prevention Intervention' (OSPI), and a member of the European Union Commission of Experts.

**Richard Holt**, PhD, FRCP, is Professor and Honorary Consultant in Diabetes and Endocrinology at the University of Southampton.

**Mohan Isaac**, MD, DPM, FRCPsych, is Professor of Psychiatry at the School of Psychiatry and Clinical Neurosciences, The University of Western Australia, Perth, Australia. Formerly, he was Professor and Head of the Department of Psychiatry at the National Institute of Mental Health and Neuro Sciences, Bangalore, India.

**Tony Kendrick**, BSc, MD, FRCGP, FRCPsych, is Professor of Primary Medical Care at the University of Southampton, School of Medicine, and a practising GP.

**Michael King**, MD, PhD, FRCP, FRCGP, FRCPsych, is a psychiatric epidemiologist whose clinical work is in sexual medicine. He is Professor of Primary Care Psychiatry and Co-Director of PRIMENT Clinical Trials Unit at the Department of Mental Health Sciences, University College London Medical School.

**Michael Klinkman**, MD, MS, is Associate Professor, Departments of Family Medicine and Psychiatry, University of Michigan Medical School; Director of Primary Care Programs, University of Michigan Depression Center; and Chair, Wonca International Classification Committee.

**Tami Kramer,** MBBCh, MRCPsych, is Consultant Child and Adolescent Psychiatrist and Senior Clinical Research Fellow at Central and North West London NHS Foundation Trust, and Imperial College London.

**Helen Lester,** MBBCh, MA, MD, FRCGP, is a GP and Professor of Primary Care at the University of Manchester.

**Barry Lewis,** MB ChB, DRCOG, Dip Occ Health, FRCGP, is Director of Postgraduate GP Education for North West Deanery within NHS NW. Dr Lewis is still in part-time clinical practice in a training practice in Rochdale, north-west England.

**Glyn Lewis,** PhD, FRCPsych, is Professor of Psychiatric Epidemiology, University of Bristol, and Honourable Consultant Psychiatrist in Avon & Wiltshire Partnership Trust.

**Karina Lovell,** PhD, MSc, RN, BA, is Professor of Mental Health, and Mental Health Research Lead in the School of Nursing, Midwifery and Social Work at the University of Manchester.

**Robert Peveler,** MA, DPhil, BM, BCh, MRCPsych, is Professor of Liaison Psychiatry and Head of the Mental Health Clinical Group, University of Southamptom.

**David Pilgrim,** BSc (Hons), MPsychol (Clin), Dip Psychother, MSc, is Professor of Mental Health Policy at the University of Central Lancashire and Honorary Professor at the University of Liverpool.

**Sue Plummer,** BA, MSc, PhD, is a Registered General Nurse and Registered Mental Nurse. She is a Senior Lecturer and Professional Lead for Mental Health at Canterbury Christ Church University.

**David Richards,** PhD, is Professor of Mental Health Services Research, University of Exeter, UK, and is at the heart of the UK's Improving Access to Psychological Therapies Programme (IAPT).

**Anne Rogers,** BA (Hons), MSc Econ, PhD, is Professor of the Sociology of Health Care and Head of the Primary Care Research group at the University of Manchester.

**Marianne Rosendal,** PhD, is Senior Researcher, Research Unit for general Practice, Aarhus University, Denmark, and is the Danish representative of Wonca's International Classification Committee.

**Norman Sartorius,** MD, PhD, FRCPsych, is President of the Association for the Improvement of Mental Health Programmes in Geneva. He is past Director of the Mental Health Programme of the WHO, President of the World Psychiatric Association and of the European Psychiatric Association.

**Debbie Sharp,** FRCGP, is Head of Academic Unit and Professor of Primary Health Care at the University of Bristol.

**Laura Thomas,** MPhil, is a research associate at the University of Bristol currently working in the Academic Unit of Psychiatry on randomised controlled trials investigating depression.

**Andre Tylee,** MD, FRCGP, MRCPsych (Hon), is Head of the Section of Primary Care Mental Health in the Department of Health Services and

Population Research at the Institute of Psychiatry, King's Health Partners Academic Health Sciences Centre, King's College London.

**Airi Värnik**, MD, PhD, is Professor of Mental Health at Tallinn University, Estonia. She is a member of the International Academy for Suicide Research, as well as expert and principal investigator of numerous WHO and European Commission projects.

**Waquas Waheed**, MRCPsych, is Consultant Psychiatrist at Lancashire NHS Foundation Trust, Accrington.

**Annie Wallace**, MSc, is Project Director for Public Health Curriculum Development for the North East Teaching Public Health Network, hosted by the University of Sunderland.

**Lisa Wittenburg**, MSW, is a project manager for the European Alliance Against Depression at the Department of Psychiatry, University of Leipzig, Germany.

**Geoffrey Wolff**, BSc (Hons), MB, ChB, MRCPsych, MD, Dip CBT, is Consultant Psychiatrist in Eating Disorders, South London & Maudsley NHS Foundation Trust, and Visiting Senior Lecturer, Institute of Psychiatry, King's College London.

# Preface

We hope this book will prove to be an important resource for anyone interested in mental health in primary care settings, including primary care practitioners with a special interest in mental health, mental health practitioners with a special interest in primary care, health service planners, commissioners and policy-makers. It covers the range of common mental health problems found in primary care, and gives up-to-date guidance on approaches to prevention and treatment, training, research and evidence-based practice.

Part I covers the conceptual basis of primary care mental health and overarching themes, including international policy perspectives, epidemiology, sociology, the patient's perspective and classification. In Part II, individual chapters address well recognised clinical syndromes, including depression, anxiety, psychosis and eating disorders, but also broader areas of practice, such as perinatal health, sexual problems, medically unexplained symptoms, and problems affecting older people, younger people and minority ethnic groups.

Part III addresses issues of policy and practice, including quality improvement, service organisation and multidisciplinary working. Finally Part IV touches on reflective practice, including teaching and learning, the generalist perspective, evidence-based practice, and the mental health of practitioners themselves. The UK context is described in detail, along with a range of international insights into practice and policy.

Each part of the book has a brief introduction written by the editors.

*Linda Gask, Helen Lester, Tony Kendrick and Robert Peveler*

# Part I: Conceptual basis and overarching themes

The seven chapters in Part I cover a range of fundamental concepts and provide the keys to understanding much of the rest of the book. They highlight a series of interesting themes, including the fundamental and growing importance of primary care mental health, but also the problems inherent in its delivery, as well as the importance of context and the tension in encouraging service users to have a choice and a voice within a wider system that tends to exclude people with mental health diagnoses.

We start by asking a fundamental question – what is primary care mental health? This first chapter provides an overview of the concept and describes the range of relevant policy initiatives in this area, the types of mental health problems seen and treated in primary care and strategies that are being used nationally and internationally to improve integration across the interface between primary and secondary care. The international focus is continued with a chapter on primary care mental health in low- and middle-income countries and a thoughtful essay by Sartorius, informed by 40 years of work on the world stage, on the extent to which and manner in which treatment of mental disorders and their prevention differ between settings.

The chapters on the epidemiology and the classification of mental illness in primary care both highlight the complexities of primary care mental health. Describing the rates of disorder within primary care, for example, is difficult, since it is almost impossible to obtain a representative sample of primary care physicians to collaborate with a research team. Patients in primary care are also much less likely to present with clearly identifiable diagnostic syndromes, which affects both the classification process and the epidemiological evidence base. Understanding these issues sheds light on the apparent under-diagnosis of many mental health problems by primary care practitioners.

Perhaps above all, Rogers and Pilgrim in Chapter 4, looking through a critical sociological lens, capture the spirit of many chapters in Part I by suggesting that primary care has moved from the margins to the mainstream and now represents a new and central field of the management of mental health in society.

# CHAPTER 1

# What is primary care mental health?

Linda Gask, Helen Lester, Tony Kendrick and Robert Peveler

Summary

This chapter provides an overview of the concept of primary care and of primary care mental health. It describes the range of relevant policy initiatives in this area, the types of mental health problems seen and treated in primary care and strategies that are being used nationally and internationally to improve integration across the interface between primary and secondary care.

## Primary care mental health

This book is about *primary care mental health*, a concept that has emerged relatively recently in the history of healthcare.

The World Health Organization (WHO) has defined 'primary care mental health' to incorporate two aspects (WHO & Wonca, 2008):

- first-line interventions that are provided as an integral part of general healthcare
- mental healthcare that is provided by primary care workers who are skilled, able and supported to provide mental healthcare services.

Doctors have provided emotional care in the form of support, advice and comfort for their patients for centuries, alongside other professional, spiritual and lay workers, friends and families. However, in the past 40 years or more in the UK, since the pioneering research carried out by first by the husband and wife team of Watts & Watts (1952) and later by John Fry (Fry, 1960), within their own practices, and by Michael Shepherd and his colleagues at the General Practice Research Unit in London (Wilkinson, 1989), there has been a particular interest in the mental healthcare that is provided within primary and general healthcare settings by a range of professionals who are not specialists in mental health. In that time, the focus of both research and development has shifted and changed in a number of different ways: from an emphasis on detection of disorders, towards better 'chronic disease' management; from the general practitioner (GP) working alone to the partnership between the doctor, the extended primary care team and the local community; from the narrow focus of research on the behaviour of the doctor towards an exploration of the view of the patient; and, in policy terms, a shift from viewing the GP as an 'independent' agent towards increasing attempts to influence the decisions that he or she makes in the assessment and management of mental health problems and the promotion of good mental health.

Many of these changes are encapsulated in the change of terminology from 'psychiatry and general practice', the title of the forerunner to this publication, which was jointly published by the Royal Colleges of Psychiatry and General Practice over a decade ago (Pullen *et al*, 1994), to a broader view of 'primary care mental health' (from the title of this publication now commissioned by the Royal College of Psychiatrists) reflecting the wider involvement of a range of health professionals in primary and specialist settings.

## Definitions

We recognise that there is enormous international variation in what is meant by the term 'primary care'. According to the Institute of Medicine (1996) in the USA, primary care is the:

> provision of integrated, accessible healthcare services by clinicians who are accountable for addressing a large majority of personal health needs, developing a sustained partnership with patients, and practicing in the context of the family and community.

Primary care systems can be categorised according to whether they act as gatekeepers to specialist services (as in the UK), provide free-market services in parallel to specialist services, or function in a complex system containing both free-market and gatekeeper functionality (as in the USA); whether they are free to patients at the point of care delivery; whether they are led by doctors or non-medical personnel; and the degree to which they provide continuity of care.

How can we define mental health? According to the WHO (2007), it is:

> a state of well-being in which the individual realises his or her own abilities, can cope with the normal stresses of life, can work productively and fruitfully, and is able to make a contribution to his or her community.

That is, it is not merely the absence of illness. Cultural differences, subjective assessments, and competing professional theories all affect how 'mental health' is defined.

The concept of mental illness is more highly contested. Unlike in physical healthcare, the underlying pathology of most mental 'illness' is far from clear, so, except in rare cases like Alzheimer's 'disease', we cannot apply this term.

Instead, psychiatry recognises symptoms which commonly occur together, and such a constellation is given the name of a 'syndrome'. 'Illness' is the term applied when the presence of symptoms leads to loss of functioning or impairment. 'Disability' can occur in the context of mental and physical illness as a result of society's actions and reactions to the impairment (Lester & Tritter, 2005). But inability to function is largely a subjective experience, particularly with the common mental health problems that are treated in primary care. A further complication is that the classification systems used throughout the world for the diagnosis and treatment of mental disorders have evolved from research in specialist settings (see Chapter 7), where fewer than 10% of those with mental health problems in the community are actually seen and treated. We favour a patient-centred rather than a disease-based approach, so that, even though we do have chapters based on disorders, and we do discuss epidemiology, we recognise the need to treat symptoms which do not meet the criteria for particular disorders, adopt an integrated, individually tailored approach, and take the lead from the patient (Tinetti & Fried, 2004; Johnston *et al*, 2007).

## Mental health problems in the primary care setting

The setting of primary care has, in the past two decades, assumed a considerable international importance for both the recognition and the treatment of mental health problems (WHO & Wonca, 2008). There is increasing international recognition of the economic and social burden of mental illness (Murray & Lopez, 1997; Layard, 2006). In high-income countries, the majority of mental health problems seen in the primary care setting fall into the category of 'common mental disorders', such as anxiety and depression, while more severe and enduring mental health problems, such as schizophrenia and other psychoses, are treated, at least initially, by specialist mental health services. Although 'common mental disorders' are, on average, less severe than those disorders seen in secondary care, the total public health burden that they pose in terms of disability and economic consequences is considerably greater (Andrews & Henderson, 2000). Mental health issues are the second most common reason for consultations in primary care in the UK (McCormick *et al*, 1995) and GPs spend on average approximately 30% of their time on mental health problems (Mental Health Aftercare Association, 1999). It is of course perfectly possible for one individual to have both a common mental health problem and a more severe and enduring mental illness.

However, even in countries where specialist mental health services are well developed, such as the UK and USA (Department of Health and Human Services, 1999), many people with more severe and enduring mental illness receive their ongoing mental healthcare primarily within primary care, for reasons of choice or lack of access to specialist care. In low- and middle-income countries, specialist mental healthcare may be poorly developed or even non-existent, such that, by default, primary care will be the primary provider of mental healthcare (Patel, 2003).

There is considerable international variation in the way in which primary care practitioners are engaged in providing mental healthcare (for an excellent and detailed comparison of practices in European countries see WHO Europe, 2008). For example, in some European countries GPs cannot prescribe psychotropic medication without agreement from a psychiatrist and in others no role is seen for primary care in the management of people with severe and enduring mental health problems.

There are important differences in the way that people with mental health problems present in primary care compared with secondary care. There is often comorbidity with physical illness and a common mode of presentation of emotional problems in the primary care setting is that of medically unexplained symptoms, which may or may not be recognised by the physician as indicative of underlying emotional distress, even in the presence of expressed verbal and non-verbal cues of distress (Ring *et al*, 2005). The critical point here, however, is that primary care clinicians will often encounter undifferentiated, unfiltered and unrecognised symptoms, concerns, worries and problems (Balint, 1964), which may or may not be identifiable as mental health syndromes. Specialist mental health clinicians, in contrast, are far more likely to encounter filtered symptoms that are recognised and understood as representative of a mental health problem.

## Providing mental healthcare

From the perspective of both the patient and the healthcare system, there are numerous advantages to providing mental healthcare in the primary care setting. Care can be provided closer to the patient's home, in a setting that is free from the stigma that is still inevitably associated with mental healthcare facilities, by a healthcare worker who will ideally have pre-existing knowledge of the patient and his or her family, who is able to provide holistic treatment and continuity of care for the full range of the patient's problems, including physical problems, and good links to local resources for assistance with associated social problems. Primary care is also best placed to manage those problems, such as medically unexplained symptoms, that straddle the artificial interface between 'mind' and 'body'. Research into the views of people with serious mental illness has revealed the importance that they place on the care provided in the primary care setting from their own GP (Lester *et al*, 2005). From the perspective of the healthcare system, effective primary care is cost-effective (Starfield, 1991). Specialist mental healthcare resources can then be directed towards those most in need and likely to benefit from more intensive care.

Disadvantages of treatment in the primary care setting, however, are that primary care workers may lack the time, the specific interest, a positive attitude and the skills or knowledge to recognise and manage mental health problems optimally. There is considerable variation, both between and within countries, in how mental health problems are managed in primary care (Üstün & Sartorius, 1995) and in rates of referral to specialist services. GPs in the UK, for example, have been criticised for a perceived failure to diagnose mental illness (particularly depression) (Docherty, 1997) and their inability to provide good physical healthcare for people with severe and enduring mental illness. However, as described above, primary care is a complex environment – a 'messy swamp' of experiences and interpretations that rarely conform to textbook definitions (Schon, 1983). Many GPs have little formal training in mental health. One survey found that only a third of GPs had had mental health training in the previous 5 years, while 10% expressed concerns about their training or skills needs in mental health (Mental Health Aftercare Association, 1999).

## The primary care team

Across the world, many GPs still work as single-handed practitioners. Fig. 1.1 shows a typical primary care team structure in the UK. However, in many countries primary care has increasingly been provided by a team of professionals working together: doctors, practice nurses and the extended team of healthcare assistants, receptionists and other workers who visit the practice. They may include not only a range of specialised nurses (health visitors, community nurses, midwives) but also mental health professionals, such as community mental health (psychiatric) nurses, psychologists, graduate mental health workers (see below) and psychiatrists. The role of the extended practice team in providing mental healthcare has been acknowledged and in recent years there have been specific initiatives aimed at members of the team, such as training health visitors in the recognition and management of postnatal depression (Holden *et al*, 1989) or practice

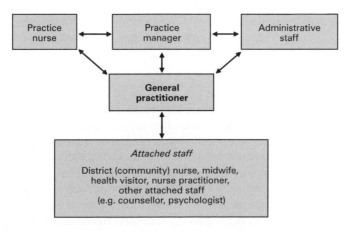

**Fig. 1.1** Typical primary healthcare team structure in the UK.

nurses in the management of people on depot neuroleptic treatment (Gray *et al*, 1999).

In some places, mental health professionals are closely linked with the team. In the UK, counsellors have become increasingly common in primary care over the past two decades and more recently a new group of 'graduate mental health workers', usually graduate psychologists with a training in brief psychological interventions to diploma level, have come into post in some areas. GPs have been encouraged to develop special interests ('GPs with a special interest', or GPwSI) in mental health (as have nurses). Some of these doctors have developed their interest within their own practice, while others have been working with new 'primary care mental health teams' at an intermediate level between primary and specialist care.

## Organising care

The primary care organisation needs not only to provide primary mental healthcare to its patients or service users, but also to have clearly defined pathways of care and protocols for the delivery of treatment and for referral to other services (primary care mental health services, specialist mental health services, social care and voluntary agencies). It also needs effective means of data collection and management and record-keeping to ensure that people with mental health problems, especially those with more severe disorders, who are vulnerable or at risk or who are in receipt of repeat medication, receive effective and timely mental and physical healthcare. It also has to ensure that the team of staff is properly trained and up to date and that the mental health needs of the workforce are adequately catered for in what can be a very stressful job.

# Mental health policy and primary care

As far back as the 1960s, when GPs in the UK were beginning to work in group practices, Michael Shepherd (1966) suggested:

> the cardinal requirement for improvement of mental health services ... is not a large expansion of and proliferation of psychiatric agencies, but rather a strengthening of the family doctor in his/her therapeutic role.

The WHO echoed this belief in 1978, in its Alma-Ata Declaration, which stated that 'the primary medical care team is the cornerstone of community psychiatry' (WHO, 1978). However, as indicated by Norman Sartorius in the next chapter, the key role of primary care in the provision of mental healthcare was *not* formally acknowledged in the Alma-Ata Declaration. Throughout next two decades, the emphasis in both international research and policy was on documenting the extent of morbidity of mental health problems in primary care and the quality of care provided by primary care workers, with a strong theme of increasing recognition and treatment of depression in the community. This work included the development of guidelines for depression and numerous 'initiatives' on depression such as the Defeat Depression Campaign in the UK (Wright, 1995), the DART (Depression Awareness, Recognition and Treatment Programme) (Regier *et al*, 1988) in the USA, the Beyond Blue project in Australia (http://www.beyondblue.org.au) and the Nuremburg (now European) Alliance Against Depression in Germany (http://www.eaad.net/enu/general-population.php).

In addition to public education, the focus of many of these campaigns has been on educating primary care workers. In later chapters we critically discuss this and other approaches to quality improvement in primary care mental health, such as 'quality improvement breakthrough collaboratives' in the USA (Katzelnick *et al*, 2005) and the recent introduction of financial incentives in the UK (under the Quality and Outcomes Framework).

Mental health policy on the role of primary care has developed considerably over the past two decades, with increasing interest in the configuration and delivery of evidence-based mental healthcare in the post-institutional era (Department of Health, 1999). Primary care in the UK, for example, has specific responsibility for delivering standards 2 and 3 of the National Service Framework (NSF) for Mental Health and is also integrally involved in the delivery of the other five standards. The *NHS Plan* (Department of Health, 2000) further underpinned the NSF with over £300 million of investment to help implementation, included specific pledges to create 1000 new graduate mental health workers to work in primary care and encourage a shared care approach. Guidelines for improving the quality of mental health have also emphasised the role played by primary care (e.g. those produced by the National Institute for Health and Clinical Excellence in the UK). Specific references are provided in the appropriate chapters.

## The interface between primary care and specialist care

A significant area of international policy interest has been developing the interface between primary and specialist care (WHO & Wonca, 2008). The 'pathways to psychiatric care' were first described by Goldberg & Huxley (1980) (Table 1.1) and their model delineates the filters through which people with mental health problems must pass from community to specialist care. This work is discussed further in Chapter 3, in relation to epidemiology. In many countries, newly developed primary care services are taking over the care of people with mental illness who were previously either institutionalised or under the care of mental health services. This process began in the USA and the UK 40 years ago and ever since there has been ongoing debate about who should be referred to specialist mental services (or behavioural health services in the USA), who should receive care in a primary setting and how the interface should be most efficiently configured to promote joint working between professionals and optimal outcomes for patients (Gask, 2005).

Health policy in the UK has been particularly concerned, not just in mental health but across the field of healthcare, in shifting the care of many people

9

**Table 1.1** Pathways to psychiatric care

| Levels and filters | Factors operating |
|---|---|
| Level 1: Psychiatric morbidity in the community | |
| First filter: decision to consult | Severity/type of problems<br>Learned behaviour<br>Stress<br>Availability of services<br>Money |
| Level 2: Total primary care morbidity | |
| Second filter: GP recognition | GP interviewing skills<br>Personality<br>Training<br>Attitudes<br>Presenting symptoms of the patient<br>Demographics |
| Level 3: Conspicuous primary care morbidity | |
| Third filter: Referral | Confidence<br>Attitudes<br>Symptoms/attitudes of patient and family<br>Services available |
| Level 4: Patients in formal mental health services | |
| Fourth filter: Decision to admit | Availability of beds<br>Community services<br>Symptoms/risk to self or others<br>Attitudes of patient/family |
| Level 5: In-patient care | |

From Goldberg & Huxley (1980).

who would previously have received specialist care in the hospital setting into both primary care and, more recently, new 'intermediate care' services, at the interface between primary and specialist care (Department of Health, 2006). Despite the universal healthcare funding provided by the National Health Service (NHS), problems still exist at the interface because of the different funding mechanisms for primary care services and hospital services in England and Wales. Similar problems exist in integrating care across the 'divide' in other countries, where, for example, funding for primary care and hospital care may be provided by different parts of government, or state or nationally (as in Australia), or different types of organisation or professional may be funded to provide only particular types of healthcare by insurers, as may be the case with behavioural health in the USA.

## Integrating mental health into primary care

From an international policy perspective (WHO & Wonca, 2008), integrating mental health services into primary care is the most viable way of closing the treatment gap and ensuring that people get the mental healthcare they need (Box 1.1).

Primary care for mental health is affordable, and investments can bring important benefits; however, certain skills and competencies are required to effectively assess, diagnose, treat, support and refer people with mental disorders; it is essential that primary care workers are adequately trained and supported in their mental health work. It is also clear that, with the considerable international variation in the way that both primary and specialist services are provided, there is no single best practice model that can be followed by all countries. Rather, successes have been achieved through sensible local application of broad principles. Integration is most successful when mental health is incorporated into health policy and legislative frameworks, and supported by senior leadership, adequate resources and ongoing governance. To be fully effective and efficient, primary care for mental health must be coordinated with a network of services at different levels of care and complemented by broader health system development.

Numerous models exist that attempt to address the problems at the interface between primary and specialist care in order to provide truly 'shared care' (Craven & Bland, 2002; Bower & Gilbody, 2005). Much of the research has focused on attempting to improve outcomes for people with common mental health problems by integrating new staff such as counsellors or psychologists into the primary care team (Bower & Sibbald, 2000). However, work on the model of 'collaborative' care, which was developed in the USA (Katon & Unutzer, 2006) and which builds on earlier work on the redesign of delivery systems for people with chronic health problems such as diabetes (e.g. http://www.improvingchroniccare.org),

---

**Box 1.1** Seven good reasons for integrating mental health into primary care

1   The burden of mental disorders is great.
2   Mental and physical health problems are interwoven.
3   The treatment gap for mental disorders is enormous.
4   Primary care for mental health enhances access.
5   Primary care for mental health promotes respect of human rights.
6   Primary care for mental health is affordable and cost-effective.
7   Primary care for mental health generates good health outcomes.

From WHO & Wonca (2008).

is now generating a great deal of interest. Recent guidelines for the care of depression in the UK (see http://www.nice.org.uk/CG023) have also highlighted the concept of 'stepped care' in service delivery, with differing levels of intensity of care from primary to specialist care provided seamlessly, with decision-making about 'stepping up' or 'stepping down' according to severity, progress and patient choice. These models are described in more detail in later chapters.

## People, patients and service users

There has also, more latterly, been increasing interest from both the research and policy perspective in understanding not only the views and wishes of the primary care professionals but also those of the patient. A new strand of qualitative work in primary care mental health over the past decade has focused both on patients' experiences of mental health and illness and help-seeking behaviour and on their experiences of mental healthcare from their primary care providers. This has included studies on depression (Gask *et al*, 2003; Lawrence *et al*, 2006), severe and enduring mental illness (Lester *et al*, 2005) and the experiences of such diverse groups as African–Caribbean women in Manchester (Edge *et al*, 2004) and Caucasian Scottish women in Edinburgh (Maxwell, 2005) with postnatal depression.

At this point we should consider terminology. Mental health policy in the UK uses the term 'service users' for people with mental health problems. While this is a commonly used term in specialist settings, it is not widely used for people with mental health problems who receive their care only in the primary care setting (where most people are happy to be called 'patients') and it is not universally used across the world. In this book, we use the terms 'patient', 'service user' and 'people with mental health problems' as appropriate to the setting that is being described.

## The focus of this book

We have written this book with the needs in mind of people working in primary care who provide first-line treatment for a range of mental health problems. We adopt an international perspective in our discussion of primary care mental health, recognising the different ways in which health and social care, particularly primary care, is delivered in different countries (and indeed within some countries) and how this influences the way in which mental healthcare is delivered. However, it is inevitable, given our own backgrounds, that our starting point will be the care provided by GPs and the wider primary care team in the UK. Nevertheless, our guiding principle throughout is that 'holistic care will never be achieved until mental health is integrated into primary care' (WHO & Wonca, 2008).

---

Key points

- Primary care mental health is a relatively recent concept in the history of healthcare.
- There are important differences in the way that people present with mental health problems in primary and specialist settings.
- There is increasing interest in the role of primary care in the delivery of mental healthcare across the world.
- However, integrating primary and specialist care effectively remains a challenge.

---

# Further reading and e-resources

WHO & Wonca (2008) *Integrating Mental Health into Primary Care: A Global Perspective.* Downloadable from http://www.who.int/mental_health/policy/services/ mentalhealthintoprimarycare/en/index.html

WHO Europe (2008) *Policies and Practices for Mental Health in Europe: Meeting the Challenge.* Downloadable from http://www.euro.who.int/eprise/main/WHO/Progs/MNH/ baseline/20080602_1?language=

http://www.improvingchroniccare.org – introduces the 'chronic care model' for depression and a range of other common disorders in primary care.

http://www.mentalneurologicalprimarycare.org – UK version of the WHO guide to mental and neurological health in primary care, partly done as an online textbook resource for primary care mental health.

http://www.mind.org.uk – an information-packed website from a leading mental health charity in England and Wales.

http://www.rethink.org – website of a leading UK mental health charity which focuses on severe mental illness.

# References

Andrews, G. & Henderson, S. (2000) *Unmet Need in Psychiatry.* Cambridge University Press.

Balint, M. (1964) *The Doctor, His Patient and the Illness.* Churchill Livingstone.

Bower, P. & Gilbody, S. (2005) Managing common mental health disorders in primary care: conceptual models and evidence base. *BMJ*, **330**, 839–842.

Bower, P. & Sibbald, B. (2000) On-site mental health workers in primary care: effects on professional practice. *Cochrane Database of Systematic Reviews*, **(3)**, CD000532.

Craven, M. A. & Bland, R. (2002) Shared mental health care: a bibliography and overview. *Canadian Journal of Psychiatry*, **47(2 Suppl. 1)**, iS–viiiS, 1S–103S.

Department of Health (1999) *A National Service Framework for Mental Health.* Department of Health.

Department of Health (2000) *The NHS Plan: A Plan for Investment, a Plan for Reform.* Department of Health.

Department of Health (2006) *Our Health, Our Care, Our Say: A New Direction for Community Services.* Department of Health.

Department of Health and Human Services (1999) *Mental Health: A Report of the Surgeon General – Executive Summary.* Department of Health and Human Services, Substance

Abuse and Mental Health Services Administration, Center for Mental Health Services, National Institutes of Health, National Institute of Mental Health.

Docherty, J. D. (1997) Barriers to the diagnosis of depression in primary care. *Journal of Clinical Psychology*, **58**, 5–10.

Edge, D., Baker, D. & Rogers, A. (2004) Perinatal depression among black Caribbean women. *Health and Social Care in the Community*, **12**, 430–438.

Fry, J. (1960) What happens to our neurotic patients? *Mayo Clinic Proceedings*, **185**, 85–89.

Gask, L. (2005) Overt and covert barriers to the integration of primary and specialist mental health care. *Social Science and Medicine*, **61**, 1785–1794.

Gask, L., Rogers, A., Oliver, D., *et al* (2003) Qualitative study of patients' views of the quality of care for depression in general practice. *British Journal of General Practice*, **53**, 278–283.

Goldberg, D. & Huxley, P. (1980) *Mental Illness in the Community*. Tavistock.

Gray, R., Parr, A. M., Plummer, S., *et al* (1999) A national survey of practice nurse involvement in mental health interventions. *Journal of Advanced Nursing*, **30**, 901–906.

Holden, J. M., Sagovsky, R. & Cox, J. L. (1989) Counselling in a general practice setting: controlled study of health visitor intervention in treatment of postnatal depression *BMJ*, **298**, 223–226.

Institute of Medicine (1996) *Primary Care: America's Health in a New Era*. Institute of Medicine.

Johnston, O., Kumar, S., Kendall, K., *et al* (2007) A qualitative study of depression management in primary care: GP and patient goals, and the value of listening. *British Journal of General Practice*, **57**, 892–899.

Katon, W. & Unutzer, J. (2006) Collaborative care models for depression: time to move from evidence to practice. *Archives of Internal Medicine*, **66**, 2304–2306.

Katzelnick, D. J., Von Korff, M., Chung, H., *et al* (2005) Applying depression-specific change concepts in a collaborative breakthrough series. *Joint Commission Journal on Quality and Patient Safety*, **31**, 386–397.

Lawrence, V., Banerjee, S., Bhugra, D., *et al* (2006) Coping with depression in later life: a qualitative study of help-seeking in three ethnic groups. *Psychological Medicine*, **36**, 1375–1383.

Layard, R. (2006) The case for psychological treatment centres. *BMJ*, **332**, 1030–1032.

Lester, H. E. & Tritter, J. Q. (2005) Listen to my madness. Exploring the views of people with serious mental illness using a disability framework. *Sociology of Health and Illness*, **27**, 649–669.

Lester, H., Tritter, J. Q. & Sorohan, H. (2005) Patients' and health professionals' views on primary care for people with serious mental illness: focus group study. *BMJ*, **330**, 1122.

Maxwell, M. (2005) Women's and doctors' accounts of their experiences of depression in primary care: the influence of social and moral reasoning on patients' and doctors' decisions. *Chronic Illness*, **1**, 61–71.

McCormick, A., Fleming, D. & Charlton, J. (1995) *Morbidity Statistics from General Practice: Fourth National Morbidity Study 1991–1992*. HMSO.

Mental Health Aftercare Association (1999) *First National GP Survey of Mental Health in Primary Care*. MACA.

Murray, C. J.& Lopez, A. D. (1997) Alternative projections of mortality and disability by cause 1990–2020: Global Burden of Disease Study. *Lancet*, **349**, 1498–1504.

Patel, V. (2003) *Where There Is No Psychiatrist: A Mental Health Care Manual*. Gaskell.

Pullen, I., Wilkinson, I., Wright, A., *et al* (1994) *Psychiatry and General Practice Today*. Gaskell (Royal College of Psychiatrists & Royal College of General Practitioners).

Regier, D. A., Hirschfield, R. M. A., Goodwin, F. K., *et al* (1988) The NIMH Depression Awareness, Recognition, and Treatment Program: structure, aims, and scientific basis. *American Journal of Psychiatry*, **145**, 1351–1357.

Ring, A., Dowrick, C. F., Humphris, G. M., *et al* (2005) The somatising effect of clinical consultation: what patients and doctors say and do not say when patients present medically unexplained physical symptoms. *Social Science and Medicine*, **61**, 1505–1515.

Schon, D. (1983) *The Reflective Practitioner: How Professionals Think in Action.* Temple Smith.

Shepherd, M., Cooper, B., Brown, A., *et al* (1966) *Psychiatric Illness in General Practice.* Oxford University Press.

Starfield, B. (1991) Primary care and health. A cross-national comparison. *JAMA*, **266**, 2268–2271.

Tinetti, M. T. & Fried, T. (2004) The end of the disease era. *American Journal of Medicine*, **116**, 180–185.

Üstün, T. B. & Sartorius, N. (1995) *Mental Illness in General Health Care.* Wiley.

Watts, C. A. H. & Watts, B. (1952) *Psychiatry in General Practice.* Churchill.

WHO (1978) *Declaration of Alma-Ata.* WHO. Downloadable from http://www.who.int/hpr/NPH/docs/declaration_almaata.pdf.

WHO (2007) *Mental Health: Strengthening Mental Health Promotion.* Fact sheet no. 220. WHO. At http://www.who.int/mediacentre/factsheets/fs220/en.

WHO Europe (2008) *Policies and Practices for Mental Health in Europe: Meeting the Challenge.* Downloadable from http://www.euro.who.int/eprise/main/WHO/Progs/MNH/baseline/20080602_1?language=

Wilkinson, G. (1989) The General Practice Research Unit at the Institute of Psychiatry. *Psychological Medicine*, **19**, 787–790.

Wright, A. F. (1995) Continuing to defeat depression. *British Journal of General Practice*, **45**, 170–171.

# CHAPTER 2

# Mental health and primary healthcare: an international policy perspective

Norman Sartorius

### Summary

This chapter describes how the Alma-Ata conference on primary healthcare defined primary healthcare, and discusses what needs to be considered today in planning, developing and evaluating mental health components of primary healthcare.

It is impossible to imagine that the officials who proposed Alma-Ata[1] as the venue for the International Conference on Primary Health Care, a ministerial meeting held under the auspices of the World Health Organization (WHO) in September 1978, did so because of the symbolism of the apple. Yet, in many ways this would have been a good choice. It is the apple[2] from the tree of knowledge that was involved in the eviction of Adam and Eve from the paradise of ignorance; and primary healthcare has been seen by many as the knowledge-based answer to health problems – that led, however, to a rude awakening in the paradise of thinking that the health problems of the world can be resolved by relying on specialists. It was an apple that Paris was to give to the most beautiful goddess. By choosing Aphrodite, who promised him the most beautiful woman, Paris voted against wisdom, represented by Athena, and against becoming the ruler of a kingdom, offered to him by Hera, thus triggering the Trojan War; primary healthcare has been described as an emotional rather than rational choice and its promotion led to discord in the field of health and wars between its partisans and opponents. The apple was a symbol of fertility offered to Hera by Gaia when Hera was to marry Zeus; and primary healthcare was to be

---

1  Alma-Ata means the Father of the Apple in the Kazakh language.
2  In the original text of the Bible there is no mention of apples, since they were not known in the Orient at the time, but of 'fruit'. Later Christian paintings show, however, the snake offering an apple, which thus became the forbidden fruit.

the way to a vast improvement in healthcare, enabling many more people to get treatment than would any other system. And even more than that, the island of the apple trees (Avalon) was the place to which the select could come to enjoy heavenly delights.

The conference which, in the town of the Father of the Apple – Alma-Ata – formally defined primary healthcare, had consequences that were condensed in the symbolic meanings of the apple. Primary healthcare summarised the essence of experience and evidence about the improvement of health conditions and was a true step forward in our knowledge about healthcare. The introduction of primary healthcare created discord at all levels of the healthcare system in many countries. It was seen as a foolish pseudo-humanitarian choice of a strategy by some and as a plan that contained a real promise for the health of the world by others. It was interpreted as a recipe for the provision of care that would achieve much and cost little; others said that the whole idea of loading primary healthcare with all the tasks related to the improvement of health was ludicrous.

The fact that all the countries participating in the Alma-Ata conference agreed to the definition of primary healthcare and adopted the report of the meeting did not seem to prevent the signatories from ascribing to the term 'primary healthcare' a variety of meanings, ranging from 'medical care at the point of first contact with the health services' to 'the care provided by simply trained health workers'. In addition to these definitions – based on where care is given and who provides it – primary healthcare has also been used to indicate the provision of care by a system in which general practitioners serve as the entry point to the health system, as well as the package of care interventions that are essential and should be covered by any government's health insurance system.

## Definition of primary healthcare

The definition adopted at the Alma-Ata conference – and later quoted as if it were a citation from the Bible – was complex and showed that those who drafted it had to negotiate the wording to arrive at a consensus. It said that primary healthcare is:

> essential health care based on practical, scientifically sound and socially acceptable methods and technology made universally accessible to individuals and families in the community through their full participation and at a cost that the community and country can afford to maintain at every stage of their development in a spirit of self-reliance and self-determination. (WHO, 1978a)

This definition does not describe a particular system of care and is much closer to an ethical credo than to a listing of elements of care provision or to a specification of settings and techniques that should be used to provide care. All the descriptors contained in the definition have value in relation to ethical decisions, not to specific activities. Thus, the words 'essential health care' are not further defined, and it was later assumed that they refer to action that is essential for the survival of the society, which means that primary healthcare should be directed to diseases or conditions of major public health importance. The way to decide on the public health importance of a condition is described in documents produced at about the same time as the Alma-Ata Declaration and the conference report, and suggest that, to be of public health importance, a disease should be frequent, should have grave consequences for the individual and the community, and should be amenable to treatment or prevention. There is no directive about the types of intervention that could be included in primary healthcare; thus, they could be of high cost or of low cost, they could be dependent on high levels of technology or be very simple.[3]

The definition goes on to state that the interventions must use scientifically sound methods. The application of this principle would require that any method proposed for use in primary healthcare should be shown to be both useful and effective through an appropriate array of studies. Many of the methods currently used in healthcare have not been examined in such studies. It is difficult to find references to published papers on the reliability of diagnosis made by percussion of the thorax, on the most effective length of an interview with a patient or on the many other methods of clinical investigation. What is more, the fact that the soundness of a method has been established in one setting does not necessarily mean that the method will be reliable in a different setting. The corollary of the requirement to establish the scientific soundness of methods is that an essential element of primary healthcare must be a mechanism to collect data about the usefulness of a particular method over time and across users. Research, and in particular evaluative research, should thus be introduced and financed in the framework of primary healthcare: a requirement that was until now usually met with surprise and rejection by the same health authorities who profess their devotion to the principles of primary healthcare.

But the methods used in primary healthcare must not only be scientifically sound: they must also be practical. It is not quite clear what that means. Should they be easy to use even for persons who did not receive much training? Should their application take little time because of the need to provide care to many? Should they be usable under conditions of fieldwork? All of these interpretations are possible and probably, in some vague way, should be covered by the term 'practical'.

The next requirement is much more difficult to satisfy: it indicates that the methods and technology that should be employed in primary healthcare must be socially acceptable. This might mean that the government, acting on behalf of the people, will have to assess whether a particular method

---

3  At about the same time, the WHO issued statements about the 'appropriate technology' that was both effective and of low cost: all other technologies – no matter how effective – were considered inappropriate if of high cost. Just where 'low cost' to save a human life ends and 'high cost' begins was left unanswered.

may be used or not. But the government, even when elected by the people, does not necessarily act in a manner that is acceptable to the citizens who voted for it. Sometimes for obvious reasons and sometimes for reasons that are not evident to the electorate, governments reject the use of some technological advance or a method that is scientifically sound; and vice versa, sometimes methods that are neither scientifically sound nor acceptable to the population are introduced. A survey of the population to establish what they consider to be an acceptable method of treatment is also not a viable option:[4] two other possible interpretations of the primary healthcare definition 'socially acceptable' therefore remain: either the drafters referred to moral standards about acceptability of a treatment method (which would, for example, disallow therapeutic abortion in some countries) or used the word as a mild warning intended to make governments think about the population's wishes and prejudices.

The next requirement of primary healthcare is that it must be accessible to all people, regardless of gender, race, religion, legal status or age. This further confirms the ethical nature of the definition, by underlining the need for an equitable distribution of resources. There are, however, two possible interpretations of this requirement: the first is that health services must be made *available and accessible* to all; the other is that the services that *exist* must be made *accessible* to all. The latter is difficult but has a chance of being introduced in the foreseeable future; the former requires tough decisions about cuts in the budgets of other sectors because the expense of making healthcare available and accessible to all citizens would mean a transfer of considerably more resources (i.e. cuts of budget in other sectors) than even the most enlightened governments would be willing or able to reserve for healthcare.

The fifth descriptor of primary healthcare – that it must be made accessible through the active participation of individuals and families in the community – can also be interpreted in two ways: the first is that the members of the community should contribute to the cost of care; and the second is that they should be the ones who will participate in the making of decisions about primary healthcare and then take part in the realisation of their decision. The second interpretation would mean a significant redistribution of authority and responsibility for healthcare, which is currently designed by government officials responsible for the health system and implemented by the healthcare system, which is organised, by and large, in a hierarchical fashion, from the ministry of health to the health workers in the community. Although there are examples of excellent decisions concerning healthcare priorities by the community – for example in Thailand – there is no firm evidence about the safety and efficacy of

---

4  On occasion, the population forces the government's hand and asks for the application of a measure that has not yet been scientifically proven to be useful. Such was, for example, the case of medications for the treatment of AIDS, which were released for use by the US Food and Drug Administration under pressure from patient-led groups.

proceeding in this manner. A community may decide to drop certain activities that do not seem very important to its members at a particular time, even if this might carry a considerable risk for that community in the future and for other communities. The answer to the dilemma of leaving the decision to communities or entrusting it to experts and governments might lie in a comprehensive education of all of the world's communities – which would be a task of formidable proportions.

The next part of the definition liberates governments from the obligation to do anything about primary healthcare: it states that all the above should be done at a cost that the community and country can afford. The concept of 'being able to afford' relates to the decisions about priorities in general. Thus, if a government decides to put all its money into the construction of a hotel chain that might (or might not) increase income from tourism, it will not be able to afford any improvement in healthcare. At present, the usual complaint is that too much money is spent on armaments: but the problem is of wider proportions since, until now, there have been no transparent rules about the obligatory minimum standards of government responsibility for the satisfaction of citizens' needs. What is more, there is no clarity about the criteria that should be used to decide which needs deserve priority if the scarcity of resources does not allow the government to deal with all of them at the same time. Thus, even if no funds were expended to buy weapons, there would still be no guarantee that the funding of healthcare would improve.

The final part of the definition clearly reflects the moment when it was written. At the time, and for a short while after, 'self-reliance' and 'self-determination' were put forward as principles partly as a reflection of the cultures of the Protestant West and partly as a reflection of a reluctance within the Third World to continue receiving obtrusive advice and dictates that came with funds from the rich country donors and organisations. Self-reliance soon disappeared and gave way to interdependence (rather than independence) as an ethically more acceptable principle. Self-determination also soon vanished, to be replaced by calls for collaboration in the field of health (particularly among countries of the same political bloc) and by the growing popularity of the concept of non-alignment.

## Mental health components of primary healthcare

The promotion of mental health is listed among the essential elements of primary healthcare in the report of the Alma-Ata conference (WHO, 1978b) but found no place in the text of the Alma-Ata Declaration (WHO, 1978a). This difference – which gave many of those responsible for mental health programmes a considerable disadvantage in the search for funds – was a consequence of the fact that, immediately after the government representatives in Alma-Ata had accepted the text of the Declaration by acclamation, a representative of the government of Panama objected to the fact that mental health was not mentioned in the Declaration, although it was seen as worthy of inclusion among essential elements of care earlier in the course of the conference. The Declaration had already been adopted: to change it would have required another session and time on the last day of the conference was short. So, the WHO's representative in the conference secretariat proposed to include the promotion of mental health in the report of the conference without changing the text of the Declaration that had just been adopted. This was accepted and thus the matter was closed.

Promotion of mental health can mean several things (Sartorius, 1998; and see Chapter 24). The simplest interpretation is that the promotion of mental health equals a reduction in the numbers of people with mental illness in a community. A more comprehensive interpretation considers that the promotion of mental health should include the prevention and treatment of mental illness as well as the enhancement of the coping capacity of individuals and communities. The latter is close to the notion of reaching 'positive' mental health, a vague concept defined in a great variety of ways. A still more comprehensive view could be that the promotion of mental health has to do with the elevation of mental health on the scale of values of individuals and communities.

For the drafters of the primary healthcare documents in Alma-Ata, it was possible to include 'positive' mental health in the report because, although vague, the requirement was harmonious with the general spirit of the definition of the contents of primary healthcare (similar, for example, to the protection of mothers and children). The treatment of mental illness was not a worthy task in their eyes – nor in the eyes of the majority of decision-makers in the field of health – because they did not consider mental disorders as a major public health problem[5] (although they satisfied all the criteria for a problem of major public health importance) (WHO, 1981). Mental health decision-makers and many of the leaders in the field of mental health, however, interpreted the 'promotion of mental health', among the essential elements of primary healthcare, as being an invitation to deal with mental disorders at the level of primary contact between community members and the health service.

To mental health specialists, it seemed clear that the only way to overcome the disproportion between the numbers of highly qualified mental health specialists – psychiatrists, psychiatric nurses, psychiatric social workers, psychologists and others – and the numbers of people with mental illness in low- and middle-income countries was to involve general healthcare workers in mental healthcare. The WHO'S technical report *Organization of Mental Health Services in Developing Countries* (WHO, 1975) is an example of the many documents and papers that were published urging the inclusion of

---

5 The criteria for the designation of a disease as a major public health problem are high prevalence, severe consequences if left untreated and the tendency to remain stable or grow in the future unless prevented or reduced by healthcare interventions.

mental health among the tasks of primary healthcare workers. The experts who wrote that report recommended that countries concentrate on the most serious yet frequent mental and neurological disorders, such as psychotic disorders and epilepsy, and equip health personnel at the first line of the health service with sufficient knowledge to recognise and treat serious mental disorders and with the medications needed to do so. To confirm that the strategy it proposed worked, the WHO carried out a study of the effects of such an extension of mental healthcare (WHO, 1984). The study – and others carried out at the time – showed that it is possible to implement the strategy of extension of mental healthcare by training general healthcare staff working at the point of primary contact and by allowing them to use a limited range of psychotropic medications. However encouraging this finding was, it did not support the prediction that the system introduced would continue to function after the study was completed and serve as a model for other areas in the same country and elsewhere.

Some countries included mental health among the essential components of primary healthcare but many did not. In Thailand, for example, the government decided to do so and defined a mental health component of primary healthcare wider than others. In addition to the treatment of mental disorders, the Thai authorities also indicated that they would pay attention to the psychosocial aspects of healthcare in general and of primary healthcare in particular: this, however, was an exception and different from other countries, which focused 'primary mental healthcare' activities on the treatment of a small number of disorders. With such a definition of the promotion of mental healthcare, the shift of mental health activities from tertiary care facilities to the periphery was successful in a relatively small number of countries, for example in Iran, which has trained a large number of primary healthcare workers to recognise and deal with the mental disorders they encountered in their work. There were notable examples of the successful introduction of mental health into primary healthcare but they nonetheless remained isolated stories rather than models (Cohen *et al*, 2002).

The WHO organised its programme in the field of mental health in a comprehensive manner (e.g. WHO Division of Mental Health, 1992). It argued that mental health programmes must be distinguished from the programmes of provision of services to people with mental disorders, and must include four sets of activities (Box 2.1). These four sets of activities were to be considered integral parts of mental health programmes at all levels of healthcare – from community self-care activities to referral services – in clinical practice, research and education.

The priority of mental health programmes in low- and middle-income countries was and remained low (see Chapter 6). This meant that it was difficult to introduce changes to mental health services, which were in many countries restricted to a few large mental hospitals built in colonial times. The introduction of mental health elements into primary healthcare thus

---

**Box 2.1** Core activities of mental health programmes

Activities are those dealing with:

- the treatment of mental disorders
- the prevention of mental and neurological disorders (specifically including alcohol- and drug-related problems)
- the promotion of mental health
- psychosocial aspects of general health and development programmes.

---

happened only infrequently, and was often restricted to a geographical area defined by a medical school as 'its' territory for demonstration programmes. Demonstration and pilot programmes were in fact quite frequent: it was their generalisation that was the main challenge, and that has still not been overcome in any low- or middle-income country – in part because of a gradual weakening of enthusiasm for the strategy of primary healthcare, which remained an important set of ethical aims but proved unsuccessful as a recipe for the provision of care to the majority of those who need it most.

As time went by, the concept of mental health elements incorporated into primary healthcare became restricted to the recognition and treatment of mental disorders at the primary level of contact between the population and the health system. In countries in which there is a significant cadre of general practitioners, this meant that they were invited to take on the treatment of common mental disorders, such as depression and anxiety. In countries where the role of general practitioners is played by internists or by nursing staff, the same principle prevailed – that is, to place emphasis on the training of primary care personnel so that they can recognise mental disorders and then participate in their treatment, directed by a mental health specialist, or carry it out themselves and consult specialists only if they have difficulties in the process of treatment.

The strategy of providing all staff at primary healthcare level with knowledge about mental disorders and their treatment has also changed over time. While at the beginning the emphasis was on providing knowledge, it soon became clear that it is necessary to pay as much, if not more, attention to the teaching skills that are needed in dealing with mental disorders (see also Chapter 29). Similarly important changes happened with other parts of this strategy. The notion of training all health personnel has gradually been replaced by an emphasis on training primary care personnel who have expressed an interest and wish to learn more about the management of mental disorders at their level. The offer of knowledge about mental disorders has also become more restricted – focusing on the recognition of disorders that need referral and the recognition and treatment of mental disorders that are very frequent and can be handled at the primary healthcare level, such as depression and anxiety states. The teaching staff have also been changing – while, at the beginning, psychiatrists were teaching general practitioners, it became obvious that it is much more effective to organise teaching sessions in which a psychiatrist and a general practitioner share the responsibility for the training sessions. Lectures and systematic presentation of knowledge gave way to the discussion of cases that the primary healthcare workers brought forward. A similar procedure has also gained popularity, particularly in the USA, in teaching medical specialists who were the primary contact personnel – for example, internists and gynaecologists.

# The future

While it is clearly useful that general healthcare staff at any level of healthcare can recognise mental disorders in persons who seek help from them, it is necessary to do much more about the treatment of mental illness in the community. In the countries of western Europe, approximately 6% of the general population suffer from some form of mental illness that needs qualified help: yet only half of them get it. This is not so for other illnesses – only 5% of people with diabetes do not get medical attention in the same countries (Alonso *et al*, 2007). The situation is probably even less favourable in eastern Europe and it is clearly worse in some low-income countries, in which the WHO estimates that only one out of ten people with a serious mental illness gets appropriate treatment (Sartorius, 2001; WHO, 2001).

The steps that would have to be taken to improve mental health service coverage through primary healthcare – in addition to the training of all health workers about psychiatric illness and its treatment – include the five issues set out in Box 2.2.

The definition of primary healthcare adopted by the ministerial conference in Alma-Ata announced some of the principles of providing healthcare. These dealt with issues of equity in the provision of care and with the need to consider the improvement of the health of the population as a whole when constructing the health systems. Over time, two important trends emerged. The first was the growing difference between and within countries in what was named 'primary healthcare'. The second was the realisation that, in the organisation of healthcare in the community, governments must give special attention to matters that were hardly mentioned in the original definition and the accompanying documents on primary healthcare. These included the need to involve the private sector in the planning and evaluation of care, the imperative to provide significant moral and material support to families who are taking care of people with chronic illnesses and the need to consider matters such as stigma and other psychosocial issues in the organisation of health services.

The goals of the mental health component of primary healthcare have, over time, become restricted to the treatment of a small number of

---

**Box 2.2** New areas of action to improve mental health service coverage

1  *A significant and continuing investment into programmes that can reduce the stigma attached to mental illness.* Fear of being stigmatised will stop people coming to ask for help when they have a mental illness. It will also reduce the willingness of healthcare workers to provide services to those who are mentally ill. It reduces the priority given to mental healthcare and the resources that are needed for it. It is possible to fight stigma and reduce it on the condition that the programmes designed to do so are appropriately supported (Sartorius & Schulze, 2005).

2  *The involvement of the private sector in decision-making and in the evaluation of mental health activities incorporated in primary health services.* The documents and recommendations concerning primary healthcare do not discuss the role of private practice, the views and activities of private practitioners, the services provided by privately owned institutions, or the role of the pharmaceutical and other industries – although all of them are involved in most activities concerning healthcare. It is time to face the reality and find ways that will allow the development of a coherent collaboration between stakeholders in the field of mental health and in the provision of primary healthcare.

3  *The involvement of service users with mental disorders in evaluating activities related to mental health in the framework of primary healthcare.* It would be useful to do this for all aspects of primary healthcare: in the field of psychiatry, collaboration with families and patients with mental illness in the design and provision of care is of particular importance.

4  *The development of legislation (and of attitudes) that will allow the families of people who are mentally ill to provide care to their sick members.* Families in most countries of the world have diminished in size yet are still expected to support all of their members, to transmit culture, to bring up children and to help those members who are ill. They can do so for a while but excessive burden will break them. It is therefore urgent to think of significant moral and financial support for the families or other carers who have a person with mental illness in their care.

5  *Provision of materials – such as the classification of mental disorders adjusted to primary healthcare (see Chapter 7) and guidelines for the appropriate use of treatment tools as soon as they become available – that are adjusted to the needs and practices of those working in primary healthcare.* The distribution of these materials should be complemented by opportunities to refine skills necessary for mental health work and by arrangements that will allow primary care personnel to share their experience with their peers and with the mental health specialists who are to develop tools and knowledge necessary for good mental healthcare.

frequent mental disorders by primary care workers. While the treatment of at least some mental disorders is a laudable effort, this restriction of the role that mental health could play at the level of first contact between the population and the health system is harmful. The mental health effort at all levels of care and particularly at the primary care level should be wider and include involvement in dealing with psychosocial aspects of healthcare in general, the prevention of mental illness and the promotion of mental health, understood as an effort to give greater value to mental life and functioning.

---

**Key points**

In the three decades since the Alma-Ata conference many things have changed. It is now necessary to review and revise the way in which mental health components of primary healthcare are developed. Six new areas of action that need to be added to previous requirements are proposed.

1 Fighting stigma related to mental illness and all that is related to it.
2 The involvement of the private health sector.
3 The involvement of users and carers in the planning and the evaluation of mental health activities in primary healthcare.
4 The development of legislation and of other measures that will ensure that families and carers receive sufficient moral and material support to be able to provide care for the person with mental illness.
5 Appropriate technological support for the provision of mental healthcare in the framework of primary healthcare.
6 The consideration of psychosocial aspects of primary healthcare in general.

---

## Further reading and e-resources

WHO & Wonca (2008) *Integrating Mental Health into Primary Care: A Global Perspective* (contains a chapter on primary care). Downloadable from http://www.who.int/mental_health/policy/services/mentalhealthintoprimarycare/en/index.html

WHO Europe (2008) *Policies and Practices for Mental Health in Europe: Meeting the Challenge.* Downloadable from http://www.euro.who.int/eprise/main/WHO/Progs/MNH/baseline/20080602_1?language=

## References

Alonso, J., Condony, M., Kovess, V., *et al* (2007) Population level of unmet need for mental healthcare in Europe. *British Journal of Psychiatry*, **190**, 299–306.

Cohen, A., Kleinman, A. & Saraceno, B. (eds) (2002) *World Mental Health Casebook*. Kluwer Academic/Plenum Publishers.

Sartorius, N. (1998) Universal strategies for the prevention of mental illness and the promotion of mental health. In *Preventing Mental Illness – Mental Health Promotion in Primary Care* (eds R. Jenkins & T. B. Üstün), pp. 61–67. Wiley.

Sartorius, N. (2001) Psychiatry in developing countries. In *Contemporary Psychiatry, Volume 2: Psychiatry in Special Situations* (eds F. Henn, N. Sartorius, H. Helmchen & H. Lauter), pp. 249–258. Springer-Verlag.

Sartorius, N. & Schulze, H. (2005) *Reducing the Stigma of Mental Illness. A Report from a Global Programme of the World Psychiatric Association.* Cambridge University Press.

WHO (1975) *Organization of Mental Health Services in Developing Countries. Sixteenth Report of the WHO Expert Committee on Mental Health.* WHO Technical Report Series No. 564. WHO.

WHO (1978a) *Declaration of Alma-Ata.* WHO. Downloadable from http://www.who.int/hpr/NPH/docs/declaration_almaata.pdf.

WHO (1978b) *Primary Health Care. Report of the International Conference on Primary Health Care, Alma-Ata, 6–12 September 1978.* WHO.

WHO (1981) Health programme evaluation: guiding principles for its application in the managerial process for national health development. In *Health for All Series No. 6,* pp. 34–35. WHO.

WHO (1984) *Mental Health Care in Developing Countries: A Critical Appraisal of Research Findings. Report of a WHO Study Group.* WHO Technical Report Series No. 698. WHO.

WHO (2001) *The World Health Report 2001: Mental Health; New Understanding, New Hope.* WHO.

WHO Division of Mental Health (1992) *Mental Health Programmes: Concepts and Principles.* Document WHO/MNH/92.11. WHO.

# CHAPTER 3

# The epidemiology of mental illness

Laura Thomas and Glyn Lewis

### Summary

Epidemiology has many uses but its main utility in primary care lies in describing rates of disease. It is relatively straightforward to obtain the prevalence of psychiatric disorder in community surveys, although for relatively uncommon conditions such as psychosis the community estimates are rather unreliable. However, describing the rates of disorder within primary care is more difficult, as it is almost impossible to obtain a representative sample of primary care physicians to collaborate with a research team. A large proportion of people with psychiatric disorder do not get diagnosed by their doctor. There are many reasons for this discrepancy, but some relate to the symptoms of psychiatric disorder and the relationship between medically unexplained symptoms and depression and anxiety. Many of the current reports on rates of psychiatric disorder ignore the issue of need and the ability to benefit from an intervention: even though a large proportion of people are not receiving treatment, it is not clear what proportion would benefit from medical or psychological intervention. This chapter reviews the theoretical issues that arise in this topic area, before summarising current knowledge about the prevalence and incidence of common mental disorders.

## What is epidemiology?

Epidemiology is the study of factors affecting the health and illness of populations, of how often diseases occur in different groups of people and why. The uses of epidemiology (Morris, 1957) are therefore quite varied. They range from studies about what might cause a disease to a purely descriptive account of how many people have or develop a condition. From the perspective of primary care, both these aspects could be important. Primary care, at least as provided in countries such as the UK, where almost everyone is registered with a general practitioner (GP), is population-based medicine. Primary care physicians often provide advice about prevention as well as treating people with existing conditions. They are also faced with the whole range of morbidity, and so data from household samples are often of value in helping to understand the population served by primary care. The gradations between normality and abnormality or between health and disease are as obvious to the primary care physician as to the epidemiologist. In this chapter, we restrict our discussion to descriptive aspects of epidemiology and their relevance to mental health in primary care.

'Mental illness' and 'psychiatric disorder' are terms that refer collectively to all of the diagnosable mental disorders (see Chapter 7 for further discussion). 'Mental disorders' are characterised by abnormalities in cognition, emotion or mood or by behavioural impairere in social interactions. A substantial range of conditions is therefore covered by this term, reflected in Chapter 5 of ICD–10 (World Health Organization, 1992). The commonest psychiatric disorders are depression and anxiety and, as a result, much of the research in primary care has focused on them. However, it is important to remember that other conditions, such as schizophrenia, bipolar affective disorder and dementia, also present to primary care physicians and require treatment in primary care. The preoccupation with depression and anxiety reflects the fact that most people with those conditions are treated within primary care, whereas secondary care, at least in the UK, tends to take the lead for psychotic conditions such as schizophrenia and for dementia.

In describing the epidemiology of mental illness in primary care, we have to consider the different organisational and reimbursement arrangements that occur around the world (see Chapter 1). Despite this diversity, the majority of studies have found that patients with a psychiatric disorder are most likely to present to primary care services (Katon & Schulberg, 1992), even in the USA (Regier *et al*, 1978; Wang *et al*, 2007). However, the importance and role of primary care will differ also by diagnostic category. People with psychotic conditions can also present via the legal system and the hospital emergency department, as well as directly to specialist psychiatric services.

## Pathways to psychiatric care

In 1980, David Goldberg and Peter Huxley published an influential book that reported on the current state of the referral process for individuals with mental illness. They described a model for the pathway by which an individual with a psychiatric disorder might travel through the health service (Fig. 3.1). It provides a useful framework for the epidemiology of psychiatric disorder, in relation to the health service (Goldberg & Huxley, 1980). Level 1 refers to all psychiatric disorders in the population. Epidemiological data for this level are usually collected through large cross-sectional surveys of the household population, such as the UK Psychiatric Morbidity Surveys (Jenkins *et al*, 1997*a,b*), the National Comorbidity Survey in the USA (Kessler *et al*, 1994) and the World Health Organization (WHO) World Mental Health Survey Initiative (Demyttenaere *et al*, 2004). For filter 1, the decision to consult a primary care physician, the key individual is the

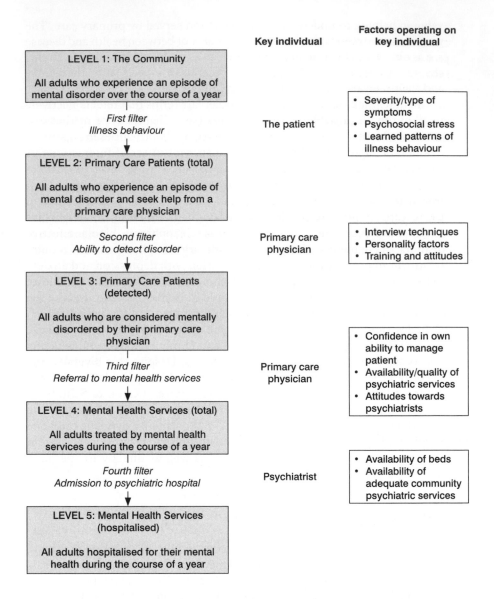

**Fig. 3.1.** The pathway to psychiatric care: five levels and four filters. Reproduced with permission from Goldberg & Huxley (1980).

patient him- or herself. Level 2 refers to all psychiatric disorders in general practice, even if the GP has not diagnosed the disorder. Epidemiological data for this group would be made available through surveys of primary care service attenders. Filter 2 refers to the detection and diagnosis of psychiatric disorder; so, level 3 is 'conspicuous' or diagnosed psychiatric disorder within primary care. Michael Shepherd's influential 1966 survey was effectively a cross-sectional survey at level 3 (Shepherd *et al*, 1966). The third filter is the process of referral to secondary care and level 4 refers to morbidity reaching secondary care.

This framework has proved extremely useful in thinking about primary care. However, its applicability varies according to the exact structure of the health service in a particular country. For example, in the USA and in some European countries, patients can refer themselves directly to a psychiatrist or psychologist, without the need for primary care intervention or referral. This has been termed the 'American bypass' (Goldberg & Huxley, 1980) and will have an impact on epidemiological data from the USA, making it more difficult to draw comparisons with countries that do not have self-referral as part of the mental health system. (It should be noted, though, that the health maintenance organisation movement in the USA has since reduced the scope of individuals to self-refer direct to specialist services.)

The other qualification of this model is that it was designed, primarily, to understand the path taken by people with the common mental disorders of depression and anxiety. The pathways to care for people with psychotic disorders and dementia can differ from this pattern (Gater *et al*, 1991). As mentioned, people with psychotic disorder frequently present directly to psychiatric services as a result of legal or police involvement, or through attendance at hospital emergency departments. Nevertheless, primary care still plays a key role in identifying and referring people with schizophrenia and dementia.

## Assessment and definition of psychiatric disorder

The classification and measurement of psychiatric disorder has attracted interest and controversy for many years (see Chapter 7). The great emphasis that has been given to measurement in psychiatry has often been a distraction, but accurate measurement and clarity about diagnostic issues is a prerequisite for any scientific process. Classifications have to be useful to survive in clinical practice, and will persist if they are used, even if they find little favour in the scientific journals. If these functions of classification are to be effectively fulfilled, psychiatric diagnoses need to be reliable. Although the reliability of diagnosis tends to be largely a concern of the research community, we should not forget that clinicians also need to be able to make diagnoses with sufficient reliability in order to communicate with each other and their patients, and to apply the results of research studies to their clinical work.

There is now an international consensus over almost all the diagnostic categories used in psychiatry and it is reassuring that both the major diagnostic manuals, DSM–IV and ICD–10, are now extremely similar, although there is still considerable disagreement about their applicability to primary care (see Chapter 7). From the perspective of primary care, one important issue is the relationship between categories and continua. Of course, the diagnostic system is in categories, but there is now more emphasis on thinking of many psychiatric disorders along a continuum of severity. This has been the case for some time in relation to depression (Paykel & Priest, 1992; Lewinsohn *et al*, 2000). More recently, there has also been an increasing body of evidence in relation to a continuum of psychotic experiences (van Os *et al*, 2000). This is in tune with a long tradition within medical epidemiology that argues that almost all medical conditions in the community are most accurately viewed along a continuum (Rose & Barker, 1978). For clinicians, categories are useful in order to guide decision-making, but in the real world most illness does not exist in simple categories but along continua. Kendell's (1968) classic study illustrated the continuum between the neurotic and endogenous forms of depression. Likewise, community surveys show that the key symptoms of depression are common in the community and exist across the whole range of severity (Jenkins *et al*, 1997*b*).

It is important to be aware that, in primary care, the whole range of psychiatric syndromes will be seen. Primary care physicians will see a large number of people in a 'grey' area, where treatment decisions are difficult to make and diagnosis is uncertain. One of the major challenges of research in this area is to help primary care physicians rapidly assess patients with psychiatric disorder in order to aid decisions about pharmacological and psychological treatment or referral. For example, there is increasing concern within primary care that patients with very mild depressive symptoms or problems of living are being medicalised and treated with antidepressants (Heath, 1998). Making the diagnosis of depression is at the heart of this controversy and regarding depression along a continuum of severity seems a helpful approach.

## Prevalence of mental illness within the community

Mental illnesses are common, and are found in people of all ages, in all regions, countries and societies. It is estimated that approximately 450 million people worldwide have a mental health problem, with 25% of people suffering from a disorder at some point during their lives. The impact of this is costly to society, with an estimated 14% of the global burden of disease due to neuropsychiatric disorders. There is a great deal of variation between the headline figures given in different surveys. This is often because of differences in the way that psychiatric disorders are assessed, rather than, necessarily, because of differences in actual prevalence. It is also difficult to estimate the prevalence of relatively uncommon conditions such as schizophrenia using cross-sectional surveys. It is more common for the admission rate for schizophrenia to be estimated from statistics collected in secondary care, although more intensive local studies on incidence have also been carried out.

It is useful to use the available prevalence figures in order to estimate the number of individuals with certain conditions for each UK GP with a list size of 2000 individuals. From the Psychiatric Morbidity Survey run by the UK Office of National Statistics (ONS) (Singleton *et al*, 2001), in such a population one would expect, at any one time, a GP to have about 50 people with depression and 10 people with a psychotic illness. Ferri *et al* (2005) estimated that 5.4% of those aged 60 years and over have dementia. For each GP, this corresponds to about 20 people with dementia. There will also be a large number of people with anxiety disorders (about 180) and a further 180 or so with milder degrees of depression and anxiety, not meeting the more specific diagnostic criteria.

## The burden of psychiatric disorder

Psychiatric disorder is extremely disabling: it leads to difficulty in securing employment, and it can deleteriously affect relationships with family, friends and work colleagues. For many years, the public health significance of psychiatric disorder was difficult to quantify, as most international statistics used mortality in order to compare the burden of different medical conditions. The World Bank attempted to change this by adopting a methodology that calculated the 'disability-adjusted life years' (DALYs) lost to various diseases. This approach was designed to enable morbidity and mortality to be compared and therefore allow a rational setting of public health priorities. There are well-discussed limitations of this approach, particularly in the values of disability associated with each condition. Despite such limitations, the World Bank report and associated publications (Murray & Lopez, 1997*a,b,c*) provided the first estimates that have allowed comparison between psychiatric disorders and physical illness leading to death. The report estimated that neuropsychiatric disorders led to 8% of the global burden of disease (GBD) measured in DALYs lost to illness. For adults aged 15–44 years, psychiatric disorders are estimated to account for 12% of the GBD; if 'self-inflicted, intentional injuries' are added, the proportion reaches 15.1% for women and 16.1% for men. In fact, mental disorders are projected to increase to 15% of the GBD, and major depression is expected to become second only to ischaemic heart disease in terms of disease burden by the year 2020.

It is worth noting that even though schizophrenia and dementia are the most disabling conditions for an individual, the larger numbers of people with depression lead to a greater aggregate burden in terms of DALYs in the World Bank study. Similarly, it has been argued that mild depression, below the threshold for meeting diagnostic criteria, leads to more disability, in aggregate, than the disability associated with the more severe depressions meeting diagnostic criteria (Broadhead *et al*, 1990). In this sense, the priorities of public health appear to contrast with those from a clinical perspective, where the priority is those with, individually, a more severe problem.

# Psychiatric disorder among primary care attenders

The WHO Collaborative Study on Psychological Problems in General Health Care was a cross-cultural study that estimated prevalence rates among primary care attenders in 14 different countries (Üstün & Sartorius, 1995). All sites used the same diagnostic criteria and there were marked differences in the prevalence rates of mental disorder at the different sites. Of course, it is important to note that the comparability of primary care studies such as this is poor. It is virtually impossible to select primary care clinics at random, as a proportion of the doctors will refuse to take part. Also, the sites for this study were chosen largely by the location of interested epidemiologists and primary care physicians, who then selected primary care centres in a rather unsystematic way. Nevertheless, this study has provided some important comparative data on primary care attenders throughout the world. Table 3.1 lists the prevalence figures and breaks this down further by listing the most common mental disorder diagnoses in primary care: depression, anxiety and substance misuse (see also Chapters 8 and 10).

# Presentation of psychiatric disorder in primary care

It has been known for some time that primary care physicians in many parts of the world do not identify all those with psychiatric disorders who

**Table 3.1** Worldwide prevalence (%) of major psychiatric disorders in primary healthcare

| Cities | Current depression | Generalised anxiety | Alcohol dependence | All mental disorders |
|---|---|---|---|---|
| Ankara, Turkey | 11.6 | 0.9 | 1.0 | 16.4 |
| Athens, Greece | 6.4 | 14.9 | 1.0 | 19.2 |
| Bangalore, India | 9.1 | 8.5 | 1.4 | 22.4 |
| Berlin, Germany | 6.1 | 9 | 5.3 | 18.3 |
| Groningen, Netherlands | 15.9 | 6.4 | 3.4 | 23.9 |
| Ibadan, Nigeria | 4.2 | 2.9 | 0.4 | 9.5 |
| Mainz, Germany | 11.2 | 7.9 | 7.2 | 23.6 |
| Manchester, UK | 16.9 | 7.1 | 2.2 | 24.8 |
| Nagasaki, Japan | 2.6 | 5 | 3.7 | 9.4 |
| Paris, France | 13.7 | 11.9 | 4.3 | 26.3 |
| Rio de Janeiro, Brazil | 15.8 | 22.6 | 4.1 | 35.5 |
| Santiago, Chile | 29.5 | 18.7 | 2.5 | 52.5 |
| Seattle, USA | 6.3 | 2.1 | 1.5 | 11.9 |
| Shanghai, China | 4 | 1.9 | 1.1 | 7.3 |
| Verona, Italy | 4.7 | 3.7 | 0.5 | 9.8 |
| Mean prevalence | 10.4 | 7.9 | 2.7 | 24.0 |

Source: Goldberg & Lecrubier (1995).

consult them (Goldberg & Huxley, 1980). There is much inter-practice and inter-practitioner variability in the rates of diagnoses of mental illness in primary care. The studies by Goldberg and colleagues have illustrated the characteristics of both the consultation and the doctor that tend to increase identification. For example, a more empathic, patient-led consultation style improves detection (Goldberg et al, 1993), in line with other studies that suggest an 'inhibited emotional tone' and 'authoritarian style' are less likely to lead to a diagnosis of depression (Tylee et al, 1993). Training of GPs can improve detection, but usually by a relatively modest amount, in countries where mental health is included in the basic training of doctors (see Chapters 25 and 29).

The majority of consultations in primary care are initiated by the patient. Patients come to their consultations with their own ideas of what they want to present, and how they choose to present it. In particular, the patient will choose which symptoms to disclose and whether to present somatic rather than psychological symptoms (Weich et al, 1995). Patients' beliefs about the reason behind their symptoms influence whether or not they are likely to consult their doctor, and how they present their problem when they do attend the appointment (King, 1983). Kessler et al (1998) found that the differing attributional styles of patients were strongly associated with whether a patient was diagnosed with a disorder or not. When reporting the prevalence and incidence of psychiatric disorders in primary care, especially for depression and anxiety, it is important therefore to remember that there is a complex interplay between doctor and patient that determines the rates of disclosure and detection. Differences, both within countries and internationally, will depend upon the differences in presentation as well as the doctor's detection of disorder.

Finally, most of the studies of presentation have concentrated on depression or on emotional disorders in general (i.e. common mental disorders). There is little on the detection of anxiety disorders, dementia or psychotic illness in primary care. Even if secondary care takes a leading role for some of these conditions, there is still a key role for primary care and many people will present via primary care (Lester et al, 2005; Lester, 2006).

# Medically unexplained symptoms (MUS)

There are many reasons why patients with psychiatric disorder might present physical symptoms to primary care physicians. A key reason is that many of the symptoms of psychiatric disorder are, in some respects, 'physical', for example the fatigue associated with depression or palpitations associated with anxiety. However, these overlap with the so-called medically unexplained symptoms (MUS). Peveler et al (1997) estimated that 20% of patients who present physical symptoms at primary care facilities do not have a relevant pathological explanation for their condition after a medical evaluation. The most widely examined condition is probably fatigue and associated chronic fatigue syndromes.

There is a strong association between reporting MUS and the presence of psychiatric disorder, although the direction of causality has not been established (Wessely *et al*, 1999). In primary care, it is possible that individuals will have both a MUS and a psychiatric disorder. On the other hand, many people who present with MUS do not have diagnosable psychiatric disorders. There has been more agreement in recent years over the criteria for conditions such as chronic fatigue syndrome and fibromyalgia but there are still quite dramatic changes in diagnostic rates over time, probably due to diagnostic fashion rather than real changes in incidence (Gallagher *et al*, 2004) (see also Chapter 11).

It is often stated that the presentation of physical symptoms is more common in some low- and middle-income countries – although there is probably much variation between the high-income countries of the world as well. There may well be differences in interpretation (Ryder *et al*, 2002), as well as the perception of stigma (Durvasula & Mylvaganam, 1994), or at least in the perceived appropriateness of presenting psychological symptoms to physicians.

## International perspective

A recent set of articles published in the *Lancet* (Patel *et al*, 2007) argue that low- and middle-income countries are still in drastic need of the resources, workforce and infrastructure for an adequate mental health service. Some 85% of the world's population live in these countries. Psychiatric disorder has received little priority in these regions. Demographic transition and improved measures to combat infectious disease are leading to a change in the pattern of disease in many poor countries (Feachem *et al*, 1992). In Chile, for example, life expectancy is now over 70 years and, along with many other areas of the world, the burden of disease is largely produced by non-communicable diseases familiar in higher-income countries. Ferri *et al* (2005) have estimated that, by 2040, 70% of people with dementia in the world will live in low- and middle-income countries. Despite this, there are still important gaps in mental healthcare. Many of these poorer countries lack mental health legislation; a third of the World Health Organization's 191 member countries have no mental health laws. Worldwide, at least two-thirds of those suffering from a mental disorder will receive inadequate or no treatment, even in higher-income countries. In many low- and middle-income countries this treatment 'gap' approaches 90% (see Chapter 6).

## Prevalence versus need

Most of the epidemiological research in primary care has concentrated on identifying people with psychiatric disorders but has ignored the most important issue. There is little point in identifying people if they cannot benefit from treatment, whether medical or psychological. For health services researchers, the 'ability to benefit' from a medical intervention is the key issue. In order to assess needs, we therefore require robust evidence about the cost-effectiveness of interventions.

The recent World Mental Health Survey has reported the proportion of people who receive any mental healthcare in a range of countries around the world (Wang *et al*, 2007). These results again emphasise the critical role that primary care plays in providing mental healthcare. It also documented the large numbers of people with psychiatric disorder who do not receive any care. For people with severe disorders, between 11% and 61% received mental healthcare. But these figures do not take account of whether the individuals concerned would benefit from available interventions. Many may have conditions that have not responded to treatment. Others may have short-lived symptoms that would remit without intervention. Future research in this area will require more attention to the difference between need and prevalence if it is to provide useful information for practitioners and policy-makers.

---

### Key points

- For primary care mental health, the main purpose of epidemiology is to provide a description of the rates of disease.
- The Goldberg and Huxley model provides a framework for thinking about the prevalence of disease in the community and in primary care.
- A large number of people do not consult primary care physicians about their mental health problems.

---

# References

Broadhead, W. E., Blazer, D., George, L., *et al* (1990) Depression, disability days and days lost from work. *JAMA*, **264**, 2524–2528.

Demyttenaere, K., Bruffaerts, R., Posada-Villa, J., *et al* (2004) Prevalence, severity, and unmet need for treatment of mental disorders in the World Health Organization World Mental Health Surveys. *JAMA*, **291**, 2581–2590.

Durvasula, R. & Mylvaganam, G. (1994) Mental health of Asian Indians: relevant issues and community implications. *Journal of Community Psychology*, **22**, 97–107.

Feachem, R. G. A., Kjellstrom, T., Murray, C. J. L., *et al* (1992) *The Health of Adults in the Developing World*. World Bank.

Ferri, C. P., Prince, M., Brayne, C., *et al* (2005) Global prevalence of dementia: a Delphi consensus study. *Lancet*, **366**, 2112–2117.

Gallagher, A. M., Thomas, J. M., Hamilton, W. T., *et al* (2004) Incidence of fatigue symptoms and diagnoses presenting in UK primary care from 1990 to 2001. *Journal of the Royal Society of Medicine*, **97**, 571–575.

Gater, R., de Almeida, S., Barrientos, G., *et al* (1991) The pathways to psychiatric care: a cross-cultural study. *Psychological Medicine*, **21**, 761–774.

Goldberg, D. P. & Huxley, P. (1980) *Mental Illness in the Community – The Pathway to Psychiatric Care*. Tavistock.

Goldberg, D. P. & Lecrubier, Y. (1995). Form and frequency of mental disorders across centres. In *Mental Illness in General Health Care: An International Study* (eds T. B. Üstün & N. Sartorius), pp. 323–334. Wiley, on behalf of WHO.

Goldberg, D. P., Jenkins, L., Millar, T., *et al* (1993) The ability of trainee general practitioners to identify psychological distress among their patients. *Psychological Medicine*, **23**, 185–193.

Heath, I. (1998) Commentary. There must be limits to the medicalisation of human distress. *BMJ*, **318**, 436–440.

Jenkins, R., Bebbington, P., Brugha, T., *et al* (1997a) The National Psychiatric Morbidity Surveys of Great Britain: strategy and methods. *Psychological Medicine*, **27**, 765–774.

Jenkins, R., Lewis, G., Bebbington, P., *et al* (1997b) The National Psychiatric Morbidity Surveys of Great Britain: initial findings from the Household Survey. *Psychological Medicine*, **27**, 775–790.

Katon, W. & Schulberg, H. (1992) Epidemiology of depression in primary care. *General Hospital Psychiatry*, **14**, 237–247.

Kendell, R. E. (1968) *The Classification of Depressive Illness*. Maudsley Monographs 18 (1st edition). Oxford University Press.

Kessler, D., Lloyd, K., Lewis, G., *et al* (1998) Symptom attribution and the recognition of depression and anxiety in general practice. *BMJ*, **318**, 436–440.

Kessler, R. C., McGonagle, K. A., Zhao, S., *et al* (1994) Lifetime and 12-month prevalence of DSM–III–R psychiatric disorders in the United States. Results from the National Comorbidity Survey. *Archives of General Psychiatry*, **51**, 8–19.

King, J. (1983) Attribution theory and the health belief model. In *Attribution Theory: Social and Functional Extensions* (ed. M. Hewstone), pp. 170–186. Blackwell.

Lester, H. (2006) Current issues in providing primary medical care to people with serious mental illness. *International Journal of Psychiatry and Medicine*, **36**, 1–12.

Lester, H., Tritter, J. Q. & Sorohan, H. (2005) Patients' and health professionals' views on primary care for people with serious mental illness: focus group study. *BMJ*, **330**, 1122.

Lewinsohn, P. M., Solomon, A., Seeley, J. R., *et al* (2000) Clinical implications of 'subthreshold' depressive symptoms. *Journal of Abnormal Psychology*, **109**, 345–351.

Morris, J. N. (1957) *Uses of Epidemiology*. Livingstone.

Murray, C. J. & Lopez, A. D. (1997a) Alternative projections of mortality and disability by cause 1990–2020: Global Burden of Disease Study. *Lancet*, **349**, 1498–1504.

Murray, C. J. & Lopez, A. D. (1997b) Global mortality, disability, and the contribution of risk factors: Global Burden of Disease Study. *Lancet*, **349**, 1436–1442.

Murray, C. J. & Lopez, A. D. (1997c) Regional patterns of disability-free life expectancy and disability-adjusted life expectancy: Global Burden of Disease Study. *Lancet*, **349**, 1347–1352.

Patel, V., Araya, R., Chatterjee, S., *et al* (2007) Treatment and prevention of mental disorders in low-income and middle-income countries. *Lancet*, **370**, 991–1005.

Paykel, E. S. & Priest, R. G. (1992) Recognition and management of depression in general practice: consensus statement. *BMJ*, **305**, 1198–1202.

Peveler, R., Kilkenny, L. & Kinmonth, A. L. (1997) Medically unexplained physical symptoms in primary care: a comparison of self-report screening questionnaires and clinical opinion. *Journal of Psychosomatic Research*, **42**, 245–252.

Regier, D. A., Goldberg, I. D. & Taube, C. A. (1978) The de facto United States mental health services system. *Archives of General Psychiatry*, **35**, 685–693.

Rose, G. A. & Barker, D. J. P. (1978) What is a case? Dichotomy or continuum? *BMJ*, *ii*, 873–874.

Ryder, A. G., Yang, J. & Heine, S. J. (2002) Somatisation vs. psychologisation of emotional distress: a paradigmatic example for cultural psychopathology. In *Online Readings in*

*Psychology and Culture* (eds W. J. Lonner, D. L. Dinnel, S. A. Hayes, *et al*), Unit 9, Chapter 3. Centre for Cross-Cultural Research, Western Washington University, Bellingham, Washington, USA.

Shepherd, M., Cooper, B., Brown, A. C., *et al* (1966) *Psychiatric Illness in General Practice*. Oxford University Press.

Singleton, N., Bumpstead, R., O'Brien, M., *et al* (2001) *Psychiatric Morbidity Among Adults Living in Private Households*. The Stationery Office.

Tylee, A. T., Freeling, P. & Kerry, S. (1993) Why do general practitioners recognise major depression in one woman patient yet miss it in another? *British Journal of General Practice*, **43**, 327–330.

Üstün, T. B. & Sartorius, N. (1995) *Mental Illness in General Health Care: An International Study*. Wiley, on behalf of WHO.

van Os, J., Hanssen, M., Bijl, R. V., *et al* (2000) Strauss (1969) revisited: a psychosis continuum in the general population? *Schizophrenia Research*, **45**, 11–20.

Wang, P. S., Guilar-Gaxiola, S., Alonso, J., *et al* (2007) Use of mental health services for anxiety, mood, and substance disorders in 17 countries in the WHO World Mental Health Surveys. *Lancet*, **370**, 841–850.

Weich, S., Lewis, G., Donmall, R., *et al* (1995) Somatic presentation of psychiatric morbidity in general practice. *British Journal of General Practice*, **45**, 143–147.

Wessely, S., Nimnuan, C. & Sharpe, M. (1999) Functional somatic syndromes: one or many? *Lancet*, **354**, 936–939.

World Health Organization (1992) *The ICD-10 Classification of Mental and Behavioural Disorders. Clinical Descriptions and Diagnostic Guidelines*. WHO.

# CHAPTER 4

# A sociological view of mental health and illness

Anne Rogers and David Pilgrim

Summary

Primary care has moved from a marginal setting in relation to mental health to one which represents a new and central field of the management of mental health in society. Central to analysing the operation of primary care are considerations of: the newly emerging patterns of primary care mental health working (e.g. general practitioners as therapists and managers of primary care mental health counselling); the importance of structural inequalities, including class, gender, age and race; help-seeking; and new approaches to management and treatment. Newly legitimate judgements are being made about the nature of mental health problems and their amelioration, and primary care is emerging as a new area of contestation between professionally delivered services and lay people.

This chapter draws on the conceptual framework developed in our previous work (Rogers & Pilgrim, 2005). The aim is bring together a sociological understanding of mental health[1] in the context of primary care mental health (see also Chapter 1). Until recently, such an understanding of mental health in primary care would have simply extended a traditional focus on psychiatry. However, in a post-asylum world in many high-income countries, new service arrangements have placed primary care more centre stage. Moreover, these service arrangements are part of a wider reorientation in Western civil society regarding mental health problems (Pilgrim & Rogers, 1994). Not only are 'common mental health problems' now given greater political salience than in the past, but those previously warehoused in the psychiatric system are, for the bulk of their lives, now 'managed' in primary care. Matters of 'social inclusion' pertaining to the

---

1  This represents a (not the) sociology of mental health and illness, not least because we draw on a range of theoretical and empirical work, including our own and that of colleagues.

latter group are addressed in community, not hospital settings, potentially making primary care workers more pertinent in their role than in the past and maybe even in relation to their secondary care colleagues.

# The newly emergent field of primary care mental health

In this chapter, primary care (as a field of activity) and the individual are viewed as inextricably linked. In referring to the work of Mauss (1934) and Bourdieu (1977), we explore primary care as a new and distinctive 'field' of activity, exchange and 'habitus', a set of dispositions that generate practices and perceptions[2] of the way in which people encounter primary care. Primary care presents technologies and relationships. Patients respond to its ministrations and their actions; thoughts and feelings are thus governed and shaped by these new practices (or they are resisted and rejected). The actions and dispositions of individuals are influenced by material circumstances and their social position within wider society. Their group membership is important, given the variable and unequal relationship that exists between social groups. This complex intersection of individual experience and action with social processes is now explored further.

## The changing status and role of general practitioners and service users

While primary care has managed common distress for a long time, little theoretical attention has been paid to it as a primary provider of mental healthcare in its totality, for all-comers. This is because, until relatively recently, general practice functioned as a referral and support system for the putatively more expert secondary care, or 'specialist', mental healthcare system. General practitioners (GPs) were viewed as non-specialists or far less experienced mental health practitioners. Their generalist role meant, at best, they could only be pale imitations of psychiatrists or their supportive attendants. An example of this role has been in relation to therapeutic law. GPs have traditionally provided a 'second opinion' to that of a fully trained psychiatrist (a role to continue under new mental health legislation in

2 Marcel Mauss used 'habitus' to refer to 'those aspects of culture that are anchored in the body, or, daily practices of individuals, groups, societies and nations. It includes the totality of learned habits, bodily skills, styles, tastes, and other non-discursive knowledges that might be said to "go without saying" for a specific group' (Mauss, 1934). For Bordieu (1977), 'dispositions' refer to forms of know-how and competence, acquired in social contexts and which dispose an individual to continue with particular practices. For him, 'habitus' accounts for what people do and believe on an everyday basis, being so familiar and habitual (and unconscious) that it goes largely unnoticed. Thus it includes the common English notion of 'habits' but also incorporates the active notion of a sediment of past functions, which operate in the present to shape perceptions, thoughts and actions, and therefore mould ongoing social practices.

England and Wales). This has 'put them in their place' as non-experts, an attribution reinforced in the past by psychiatrists complaining that GPs operated the 'wrong' referral thresholds or they referred 'inappropriately' or they 'failed to recognise' or they 'underdiagnosed' mental illnesses such as 'depression'.

The field of primary care also offers up a different setting in which to scrutinise the secondary services, which have elicited particular forms of critique from the mental health users' movement. The co-option of the users' voice by managerialism in specialist services has revealed the socio-political adjustments specialist mental health workers and their management have made in the face of such criticism (Pilgrim, 2005). With its tradition of relative voluntarism (compared with the secondary care sector) and with its users less prone to celebrate or 'come out' about their psychological difference, new socio-political dynamics are appearing about what it means to be a person with a mental health problem in a primary care setting.

Whereas chronic users of specialist services express their views from an oppressed and articulated identity, this is a less obvious scenario in primary care, where patients typically avoid being labelled as mental health service 'users'. Psychiatric patients who have been diagnosed with a more serious illness suffer their 'otherness' or wear it as a badge of honour to reassert their lost agency by declaiming their oppressed identity (Rogers & Pilgrim, 1991). By contrast, those with common mental health problems express a preference for seeing GPs rather than specialists (Pilgrim & Rogers, 1993; Lester *et al*, 2005). They do this precisely to ensure a connection to 'normality' and to distance themselves from the more stigmatising world of the secondary sector.

## New ways of working

The picture above of GPs as ersatz psychiatrists, always playing catch-up in relation to the expertise of 'real psychiatrists', can no longer be squared with the political ambit of primary care as a field of activity. Primary care has now been given a central, not marginal, role in the management of mental disorder in society. Not only does this reorientate the role of the GP, it now necessitates a re-engineering of the primary care workforce (Department of Health, 2007*a*). New ways of working and new types of worker are present in primary care. These reflect two parallel developments noted earlier: patients with severe mental illness are now managed for extensive periods of time in primary care (see Chapter 15) and 'common mental health problems' have taken on new policy and political significance.

The latter shift is linked *both* to the rise in the number of people considered to be suffering from anxiety and depression *and* the heightened legitimacy of providing talking therapies for a wider range of patients. This greater emphasis on talking treatments for common mental health problems reflects the confluence of several processes: increased consumer demand; evidence of inequalities in access to psychological therapies; and a new political sensitivity about the socio-economic burden of common distress. In the UK context, that fiscal burden has found its focus on those who could be shifted from the patient role back into the labour market using psychological technologies. An economic analysis (e.g. Layard, 2005) asserts that psychological technologies can solve the problems of long-term unemployment by the technical fix of a limited number of sessions of cognitive–behavioural therapy (CBT).

Such proposals are consistent with the current British government's aspiration to increase the availability of psychological therapies – the Improving Access for Psychological Therapies Programme (Department of Health, 2007b) – by using computer-delivered CBT. They also coincide with the government's utilisation of the technical fix of CBT to enable people with mental health problems to return to work, thus reducing the fiscal burden of invalidity benefit: the 'Pathways to Work' scheme proposed, note, from the Department of Work and Pensions, not the Department of Health (Stationery Office, 2002). (See also Chapter 26 on psychological therapies.)

There have been shifts, too, in the way in which depression is accepted and managed at a micro level within primary care. These changes are reflected in evidence from a series of studies of British GPs, between 1995 and 2001 (May et al, 2004), which explored the ways in which the medical knowledge and practice are organised and worked out in relation to chronic conditions, including 'depression'. With regard to depression, a comparative analysis was undertaken in relation to: (1) the moral evaluation of the patient (and judgements about the legitimacy of symptom presentation); (2) the possibilities of 'disposal'; and (3) doctors' empathic responses to the patient. The comparison with other categories, such as chronic low-back pain and medically unexplained symptoms, illuminates something of the value placed on the certainty with which GPs are able to frame and manage psychological problems. There is relative congruence in primary care between the clinical and lay people's psychological model of 'depression', which recognises the psychological consequences and the certainty of a variety of aetiological factors, many of which are considered to lie outside the remit of medicine to solve. The term 'depression', and even 'clinical depression', has now entered the vernacular (contrast this with other psychiatric diagnoses, in which such a confident conflation is not possible). Similarly, symptoms are viewed as being relieved by therapeutic intervention but importantly also by existential changes in the life worlds of patients (May et al, 2004).

While the focus of analysis in the relevant literature has typically been on the consultation and management of primary care service users, there has been a move away from the traditional form of participation in primary care, involving consultation with a single GP. Rather than the often idiosyncratic consultation with the family doctor offering up a prescription of antidepressants and perhaps a referral to a lengthy waiting list, to be seen by a clinical psychologist in secondary care, now the primary care user's experience is increasingly characterised by multiple contacts, with a range of new primary care mental health workers, deploying new technologies. This newly re-engineered and resourced workforce, with its current narrow conventional modus operandi of CBT, constitutes mental health work for the majority of those in contact with the National Health Service (NHS) for their troubles. CBT may, for the time being, be the new 'people's therapy' but it has no reflexive conceptual apparatus to understand the origins of distress beyond that of the acquired personal cognitive style of the individual patient. The attributions made by psychological therapists trained in CBT are decontextualised. They beg a sociological question: 'What is the pertinent social context of each patient's presentation?' When accessing talking treatments, the new consumers of NHS primary mental healthcare can now enjoy being treated in a way that may take more account of subjective thoughts and feelings, providing a contrast with a more biomedical model. However, respect for the 'individual psychology' of each patient, as a human right, does not make psychology, as a form of human science, efficient at understanding the emergence of mental health problems. A broader view of the social patterning of mental health presentation in primary care is required. Sociology is needed to contextualise mental health presentations in primary care – psychology tells us little or nothing about context.

# The importance of (easily forgotten) structural inequalities

The social variables of class, gender, age and race are central concepts of enquiry within the sociology of mental health and illness (Rogers & Pilgrim, 2005). Here we summarise some key points in this regard with reference to primary care.

## Class

In primary care settings, professionals undertake moral work in identifying 'good' and 'bad' patients along dimensions of class (Stimson & Webb, 1975). Middle-class patients are more active than working-class patients in presenting their ideas to the doctor and in seeking further explanations, which suggests there is a need to account for social class differences in the outcomes as well as the processes of consultations (Boulton et al, 1986). A social class gradient is well established in relation to mental health problems, with a variety of causes attributed to aetiology (e.g. the social drift and social causation hypotheses). Primary care professionals are seemingly well aware of the social causes of conditions, particularly in relation to conditions such as depression, but may not have the resources or influence to help patients (Chew-Graham *et al*, 2004). With these limited powers over social conditions, workers in primary care have to resort to tactics that bring closure into the immediate consultation (Chew-Graham *et al*, 2004). These tactics include the immediate offer of medication, offers of sympathy and advice, and the use of disposal strategies, such referring on to counselling or CBT.

## Gender

Gender remains an important and contested topic in relation to primary care consultations and is of particular relevance to points we make below about help-seeking. Women are overrepresented in primary care attendances and so will present with all health problems (including mental health problems) more frequently and earlier on average than men. Indeed, this overrepresentation has been one explanation for the higher rate of recorded mental health problems in women. However, other and not mutually exclusive factors also pertain to this phenomenon. For instance, the overrepresentation may be due to the failure of men to access primary care services when they experience similar life crises (Rogers *et al*, 2001). Women live longer than men and because of salary differentials are in lower-paid work than men on average. The first of these factors increases the prevalence of mental health problems in the female population and the second increases their incidence, as low-paid, insecure work is linked to poor mental health.

The pressures of conforming to the standards of hegemonic masculinity might contribute to lack of disclosure and or suicidal behaviour. However, such a generalisation about men, masculinity and mental health comes with caveats. Sociological research has shown that it is possible to find men who are willing to talk about depression and who have the resources to construct identities that resist culturally dominant definitions of masculinity. This, though, may not be sufficient for translation into help-seeking because of countering influences such as an emphasis on control, strength and responsibility to others (Emslie *et al*, 2006).

## Age

The experience and consequences of the presentation of mental health problems change as a result of age and ageing. Positive mental health increases rather than decreases with age (except in the very old). Whether this is an artefact of the reporting of symptoms (with lowering personal expectations of well-being over time) or reflects objective changes in social conditions is a moot point. Certainly the reporting of the experience of older people in primary care seems to suggest that it may be the way in which mental illness is framed, or rather the failure to do so, that may account for these epidemiological findings. Many older people come to regard symptoms of depression as a normal consequence of ageing and do not think it appropriate to mention non-physical problems in a medical consultation. This view is seemingly shared by professionals. Burroughs *et al* (2006) found that GPs conceptualised late-life depression as a problem of their everyday work, rather than as an objective diagnostic category, and described depression in demedicalised terms as part of a spectrum that included loneliness and a lack of social networks, and its causes as 'understandable' and 'justifiable'. This view of the inevitability of depression seems to coalesce with therapeutic nihilism – the feeling that nothing can be done for this group of patients. In turn, this may lower professional expectations about developing the skills and resources needed to manage depression in older patients.

## Race

Service contact and access are characterised by a gradient of coercion. Coercion is particularly salient to the experience of Black people when contacting services, including primary care. Not all service provision is coercive to the same degree but a graduated system of coercion operating in different service sectors is relevant in making judgements about the extent to which services meet expressed (rather than defined) need. Outside of acute in-patient provision and forensic services, the coercive/social control function is lessened and the use of services is more akin to those with physical conditions. Even though primary care can be a route to compulsory detention and a background factor in people's decisions to access primary care, overall, primary care is the least coercive aspect of the health system (Rogers & Pilgrim, 2003).

One explanation for the overrepresentation of Black people in certain parts of the mental health system relates to the type of service contact that is made, including the overrepresentation in forensic and acute psychiatric settings and the purported underrepresentation in primary care. Historically there has been a relatively low level of registration with primary care services on the part of African–Caribbean people (Koffman & Taylor, 1997) and lower rates of treatment for depression compared with other ethnic groups when they are in contact with services (Nazroo *et al*, 1997).

The place where certain behaviours are displayed may also be a factor in explaining lower levels of contact with primary care. For example, if more behaviour is labelled publicly as being perplexing and threatening, this in turn may be linked to the tendency towards more frequent labelling of psychosis by agents of the state (police officers and psychiatrists), thus circumventing the use of primary care (Rogers, 1990).

The way in which people label their own problems is also likely to be implicated in help-seeking for primary care. This is illustrated by a recent study undertaken to illuminate the meaning of perinatal depression held by Black Caribbean women (Edge & Rogers, 2005). This suggested a rejection of 'postnatal depression' as a central construct for understanding responses to psychological distress associated with childbirth and early motherhood. Black Caribbean women's ideas about perinatal depression were linked to coping with personal adversity. There was a rejection of a notion of depression as illness and instead a tendency to normalise distress, within a self-concept which stressed the importance of being 'Strong-Black-Women' for maintaining psychological well-being. This identity served to reinforce notions of resilience, empowerment and coping strategies based on the need to solve problems practically, assertively and materially. These women eschewed service contact (including primary care), thus obviating the attachment of psychiatric labels to emotional and psychological distress experienced around birth. The women underplayed the need for professional support for experiences they did not couch in illness terms – which may explain lower rates of help-seeking and response from primary care.

Differences in the expression of underlying conceptual models of physical and mental health and illness, as well as in representations of distress (e.g. somatic metaphors), are implicated in patterns of help-seeking for other groups. There is evidence in narrative accounts of a strong sense of a notion of depression among South Asian women (Fenton & Sadiq, 1996) but sometimes with a translation of distress into somatic expressions and vice versa. The conceptualisation of musculoskeletal problems of South Asian respondents suggests a lack of demarcation between pain located in specific parts of the body and broader social and personal concerns associated with psychological distress (Rogers & Allison, 2004). The complexities and multifaceted theories of causality and attribution were accompanied by accounts of help-seeking strategies and perceptions of the appropriateness of support from various sources (Rogers & Allison, 2004). Help from family members was referred to more than individual strategies of managing pain and assistance from medical sources, including primary care (Rogers & Allison, 2004). This variegated picture is now part of the postmodern condition in which the social world itself is increasingly uncertain in terms of options and outcomes. However, this postmodern sensibility about different possibilities is not necessarily reflected in medical practice, which still tends towards a modernist discourse of categories (rather than continuities or dimensions) and the duality of mind and body. As a consequence, the ambiguity of the postmodern condition, which we all now share, can create anxiety and irritation in practitioners. For example, when faced with medically unexplained symptoms, GPs tend to show negative attitudes to patients. That irritation and negativism in turn can arouse greater patient anxiety, motivating a further search for medical solutions, further 'somatisation' and greater dependency on services (Nettleton, 2006).

## Help-seeking and access

The primary care system is situated at the interface between the health service and wider society. In the UK, it was intended specifically to fulfil the goal of ensuring universal *access* to healthcare based on 'clinical need' (the original ethos of the NHS in 1948). Thus it was designed mainly to provide a gatekeeper role to regulate appropriate and efficient access to secondary care. But now this singular relationship between primary care and secondary care has become more complex. The emergence of voluntary organisations, the increase of private practice, user-led services and self-management are significant changes in the pattern of service provision, affecting patterns of help-seeking and decisions to access primary care.

Before this complexity emerged, this service arrangement was associated in medical training with a biomedical symptom focus in provisional differential diagnoses in the GP role (although the Balint tradition, of looking for the psychological aspects of symptoms as unconscious communications, was a counter-trend). When a symptom focus is applied narrowly to mental health problems, there is often a mismatch between the patient and medical perspectives about salience. Whereas doctors will be eliciting symptoms of a mental illness (typically in primary care 'depression', 'anxiety' or 'common neurotic misery'), patients are more likely to be reporting functional incapacity, not symptoms *per se*, although they will have been experiencing symptoms for a varying amount of time. Indeed, the 'clinical iceberg' in epidemiological studies indicates that some patients have symptoms but never make contact with a service (Rogers *et al*, 1998a,b).

Decisions to present are context specific and reflect people's judgements about inner and outer resources available to mitigate their distress. Access and utilisation are thus social processes, with subjective, as well as objective, features. They involve a dynamic and recursive relationship with patients' own resources for responding to and managing episodes of illness. These patient-based factors impact constantly on their help-seeking behaviour. Traditional epidemiological approaches to symptom level and need for types of care (e.g. Huxley & Goldberg, 1975) only hint at this complexity. Because they are overly focused on symptoms, at the expense of context, they are problematic, both methodologically and conceptually (Gately *et al*, 2007).

An alternative model of mental health consultations, which includes the social processes involved, is offered by Pescosolido *et al* (1998). This has now influenced the way in which lay contact with services and demand management in primary care is understood. This alternative perspective frames help-seeking and access to mental healthcare as processes that are continually negotiated in a recursive manner between individuals, their social networks[3] and the primary care services they consult. Thus help-seeking and access are subject to many influences arising from individuals and their social domestic and personal contexts, as well as from more

---

3  Social networks and groups modulate access to care through, for example, their involvement in the decision-making process and their use as a therapy group.

macro-level influences. The latter include the ways in which services are configured or resources allocated. In this way, primary care mental health services can be seen as being able, on an ongoing basis, to constitute and redefine the objects of attention and intervention for mental health problems.

Thus the field of local service characteristics shapes what happens in mental health consultation and provides a context for each patient's habitus: individuals with mental health problems are actively engaged in constituting and defining what they understand to be appropriate to present as a mental health problem for attention and intervention. Thus mental health and its presentation and management in primary care reflect a dynamic interplay between several contemporaneous and iterative processes. An example of this point can be given here in a study conducted by the authors and colleagues of access to psychological treatment in primary care in the 1990s, in which the help-seeking concerns of patients and frameworks of understanding of their referrers were compared and contrasted (Pilgrim *et al*, 1997). The patients' accounts revealed a complex process of access, operating in a unique biographical context. The latter included expectations and experience of counselling, the timing of help-seeking, triggers to help-seeking, lay problem formulation, the perceived adequacy of GPs and self-care strategies. Negotiations for help-seeking to ameliorate psychological distress in a primary care setting reflected both objective processes and subjective attributions about these processes from the two parties studied.

## Treatment

Given the complex set of factors we noted above – social structure and the context and recursive nature of help-seeking – in relation to mental health problems, the notion of 'treatment' is rendered problematic. It can be thought of as decontextualised medical or quasi-medical interventions but its more general moral sense is also important. The latter refers to the way in which people with mental health problems are 'treated'. For example, studies of patients with a psychosis show us that they have been devalued and treated poorly by most societies in the past. Since the Second World War, an abiding sensitivity about these outcomes has persuaded policy-makers and service professionals to address the human rights of patients in two senses. The first and most obvious is the sensitivity people have when in distress about being treated as subjects, not objects (one of Kant's 'categorical imperatives'). The second and related aspect is their desire to be treated like fellow citizens. A range of critiques emerged about both of these aspects from critical professionals and the mental health service users' movement.

These more general concerns about the wider notion of 'treatment' have affected its narrower conception. At the same time, the consumerism encouraging this interaction has been linked to the commodification of the welfare state and the prioritisation of market forces in regulating professional and patient behaviour alike. Consumerism may have brought with it a growth in the demand for talking treatments but the market economy has also ensured the continued extensive use of psychotropic medication. The latter is marketed heavily by the pharmaceutical industry and it is often perceived to be cost-effective when deployed by GPs. This particular consultation tactic in overwhelming social and personal circumstances for the doctor and patient was noted earlier and is again below.

Primary care is the setting within which newer, more experimental forms of treatment are introduced, such as facilitated self-help and CBT. These experiments are not without controversy and so primary care, not psychiatry, has now become a new field of both practice and academic debate. Top-down policy experiments to 'roll out' treatments such as CBT have been left to primary care (i.e. not specialist services) to implement. Psychological difference now is about responding to the expressed needs of people as consumers, as well exploiting primary care as a site of social engineering (to get people off welfare and back to work). Primary care has been cast in the role of reversing structural inequalities within society and ameliorating the outcomes of the social processes that generate distress. Thus a new form of medicalisation has emerged, with inequalities and social alienation being reframed as its existential end-points: the distress 'inside' individuals. Social problems are thus being individualised in new ways (Shaw & Taplin, 2007).

The prescribing of medication in primary care has been identified as an area where the legitimacy and moral authority of the doctor are enacted. It is also a healthcare arena where the power and influence of patients can be enhanced (through shared decision-making) or thwarted through the embedded power imbalance between GP prescription preferences and those of recipients (Britten *et al*, 2004). Prescribing by GPs has been identified as an arena that has broad social and political implications that stretch beyond individual outcomes for patients. The pragmatic need to respond to the range of psychosocial features of distress and madness with biomedical treatments connects all types of psychotropic drugs. A biomedical response to distress and madness will inevitably and paradoxically be both inadequate and yet justifiable within a societal norm of *psychosocial problems* being presented for amelioration or resolution to *medical experts*. In these difficult circumstances, prescribers will operate their own version of situated rationality. Because of their clinical autonomy, GPs may both share and constitute clinical norms, on the one hand, and differ from one another at times, on the other.

Nowhere is this more apparent than in relation to the prescribing of psychotropic medication and in particular the dilemmas the legacy of the benzodiazepine controversy has created for recent practitioners. In the

1980s, the prescribing of these drugs was considered to be both a clinical and social problem, which brought medical decision-making under public scrutiny. Current GPs report a number of points when discussing the clinical dilemmas created (Rogers *et al*, 2007). Who should be blamed for iatrogenic addiction to benzodiazepines? Should it be older psychiatrists, who initially advocated their use, or the GPs who gave them out in the past so zealously? What about the drug companies, which privileged profits over evidence about the problems of the drugs? Who should now be given them and who should be denied them? Are there deserving and undeserving patients in this regard?

The unresolved problem of these drugs also highlights broader patterns in the political economy and social norms of drugs used to alter mental states. Today's favoured drug is tomorrow's taboo. Why are recreational drugs a problem but prescribed ones valuable treatments? Another binary opposition in the discourse about psychotropic drugs is between legal and illegal ones. To complicate matters, some drugs, such as diamorphine, are legally prescribed but their purchase and use are illegal outside of medical jurisdiction.

Healy (2004) describes a cycle of legitimacy associated with drugs that are frequently prescribed for symptoms of common distress (be it anxiety, depression or their frequent co-occurrence). For example, the bromides of the 1920s had given way by the 1940s to the barbiturates. Similarly, the benzodiazepines have now given way to the antidepressants. The selective serotonin reuptake inhibitors (SSRIs) were hailed as more effective and less toxic and dependency-forming than the older antidepressants. However, there is now evidence that the drugs are linked to psychological dependency and an increased risk of suicide and homicide at the hands of their recipients (Healy *et al*, 2006). In 2004, the US Food and Drug Administration (FDA) issued a 'black box' warning to all physicians about the use of the drugs for adolescents and children because of the raised risk of suicide amid claims that the FDA had previously suppressed this evidence (Lenzer, 2004). Debates about the SSRIs have consequently opened up controversies about the role of the state in protecting patients and others, the role of the media in exposing or exaggerating risks (Leonard, 2004) and the role of the pharmaceutical industry in generating research to selectively favour its interests at the expense of public safety.

The problems with psychotropic medication such as iatrogenesis and addiction are now well documented. However, these drugs are marketed strongly to GPs and the continued professional development of the latter is enmeshed with drug-industry funding, prompting medical societies to issue cautionary guidance to their members (e.g. Royal College of Psychiatrists, 2003). Also they are cheap and quick to use for prescriber and patient alike (compared with labour-intensive talking treatments). Moreover, the idealisation or preference of various interest groups for talking treatments can be tempered by two other forms of evidence. The first is that they, too, produce iatrogenic effects which weaken their overall cost-effectiveness because incompetent or abusive therapists generate 'deterioration effects' (Pilgrim & Guinan, 1999). The second is that the model of demonstrating the effectiveness of talking treatments (i.e. randomised controlled trials) may overvalue the technocentric aspects of helping interventions for mental health problems, which may divert attention from the ubiquitous importance of the therapeutic alliance (Box 4.1).

These points highlight that relationality, rather than technique, in primary mental healthcare is at the centre of best practice. But what of the advocacy of new technologies that can deliver therapy impersonally, such as computer-based CBT? Research on the use of this technology suggests that the importance of relationality does indeed become clear, when it is removed. Various versions of this shift towards technology-mediated self-help exist, which range from completely computerised versions, such as *Beating the Blues*, to facilitated self-help by a practitioner and a model with minimal intervention from a non-trained or minimally trained professional. What is striking is that, compared with self-help interventions for physical complaints, or at least those with a large somatic component, such as irritable bowel syndrome, self-help using such a model may be relatively ineffective (Mead *et al*, 2005).

One reason for this outcome seems to be the importance, or relevance, given to the role of the therapist. Thus, a study exploring the acceptability

---

**Box 4.1** The importance of the therapeutic alliance

Overall, treatment groups and placebo groups respond more than no-treatment groups in controlled trials. However, most studies show no difference or equivocal results when the treatment and placebo groups are compared. This narrow or absent gap between treatment groups and placebo groups is also found in drug trials, for example of antidepressants, reminding us of the personal dimension to any receipt of treatment (Pilgrim & Dowrick, 2006).

Patients of effective therapists report feeling well understood. Thus empathy and a common understanding between the parties predict outcome. This empathic connection seems to occur very early in successful therapeutic partnerships and constitutes the 'therapeutic alliance'. It includes rapport, hope, trust, common understanding and bonding, and so has linguistic, social and affective dimensions. The upshot is that a supportive, warm, positive attitude of the therapist, who speaks a language that the client understands and is trusted by that client, predicts therapeutic success.

This consistent finding about the therapeutic alliance can be contrasted with the highly equivocal or absent findings about a positive correlation between therapeutic success and the therapist's: preferred model; age or experience; gender; verbal style; professional background; or ethnicity.

of this model for patients in primary care found that while there was, in principle, an acceptance of the manual of CBT, which focuses on symptom resolution, patients were also keen to seek insights into the cause of their difficulties (Macdonald *et al*, 2007). Moreover, subjectively the patients had difficulty in limiting the professional facilitator to that role. Instead, what happened was that the participants in the study made attributions of a therapeutic relationship. The research accounts from them framed the latter by expectations and past history of seeing a therapist and of developing a helping relationship (Rogers *et al*, 2004).

# Conclusions

This chapter has suggested that primary care represents a new and central field of the management of mental health in society. This is evidenced by a newly emerging primary care mental health workforce (GPs as therapists and managers of mental health rather than being merely referral agents, primary care counsellors, primary care mental health workers, etc.), which places GPs, rather than psychiatrists, at the forefront of arbitrating about mental health problems – newly legitimate judgements are being made about their nature and their amelioration. This new arrangement has been accompanied by claims about a new set of drugs and technologies for managing mental health problems which are likely to give rise to major contestability about the nature of employment and the role of primary care as an agent of the state, for the social control of populations. This enlarged and central role played by primary care also brings with it an onus to ameliorate inequalities and adverse circumstances, which are aetiological influences in the generation of mental health problems.

The relocation of the mainstay of mental health provision is likely to give rise to a new field of contestation between lay people and primary care in relation to the principles operating around access to assistance and contact with health professionals and the technologisation and de-professionalisation of key therapeutic approaches (such as computerised CBT). At the same time, self-help for users has always constituted a major aspect of everyday responses to mental health problems (Rogers *et al*, 1998a,b; Hardiman & Segal, 2003).

The type of self-care technology that is fashioned around a set of top-down, traditionally evidenced-based principles may prove to have limited appeal and acceptability if it is implemented in a mechanistic way, according to a fixed set of criteria regarding the type and severity of the problem. While novel and in principle effective interventions may help and be welcomed in providing early-warning signs, ameliorating symptoms and promoting more effective functionality in domestic and work roles, lay people may also soon look back with nostalgia to the days of the ad hoc and relatively open-ended consultation, in which relatively formed the focus, and a problem was openly negotiated.

Key points

- Primary care has moved from a position of marginality to become a primary provider of mental healthcare.
- New roles and ways of working have emerged within primary care over the past decade.
- Sociology is needed to contextualise mental health presentations in primary care.
- The social variables of class, gender, age and race are central concepts of enquiry within the sociology of mental health and illness applied to primary care.
- Primary care constitutes and redefines the objects of attention and intervention for mental health problems.
- Newer experimental forms of treatment have been introduced to primary care, such as facilitated self-help and CBT.
- Primary care has become a new focus of both practice and academic debate and a field of contestation between lay people and primary care in relation to the principles operating around access to assistance and contact with health professionals and the technologisation and deprofessionalisation of key therapeutic approaches (such as computerised CBT).

## Further reading

Khan, N., Bower, P. & Rogers, A. (2007) Guided self-help in primary care mental health – meta-synthesis of qualitative studies of patient experience. *British Journal of Psychiatry*, **191**, 206–211.

## References

Boulton, M., Tuckett, D., Olson, C., *et al* (1986) Social class and the general practice consultation. *Sociology of Health and Illness*, **8**, 325–350.

Bourdieu, P. (1977) *Outline of a Theory of Practice*. Cambridge University Press.

Britten, N., Stevenson, F., Gafaranga, J., *et al* (2004) The expression of aversion to medicines in general practice consultations. *Social Science and Medicine*, **59**, 1495–1503.

Burroughs, H., Lovell, K., Morley, M., *et al* (2006) 'Justifiable depression': how primary care professionals and patients view late-life depression. A qualitative study. *Family Practice*, **23**, 369–377.

Chew-Graham, C., May, C. R. & Roland, M. (2004) The harmful consequences of elevating the doctor–patient relationship to be a primary goal of the general practice consultation. *Family Practice*, **21**, 229–231.

Department of Health (2007a) *New Ways of Working: A Best Practice Implementation Guide*. Department of Health.

Department of Health (2007b) *Improving Access to Psychological Therapies (IAPT) Programme. Computerised Cognitive Behavioural Therapy (CCBT) Implementation Guidance*. Department of Health.

Edge, D. & Rogers, A. (2005) Dealing with it: Black Caribbean women's response to adversity and psychological distress associated with pregnancy, childbirth, and early motherhood. *Social Science and Medicine*, **61**, 15–25.

Emslie, C., Ridge, D., Ziebland, S., *et al* (2006) Men's accounts of depression: reconstructing or resisting hegemonic masculinity? *Social Science and Medicine*, **62**, 2246–2257.

Fenton, S. & Sadiq, S. A. (1996) Culture, relativism and the expression of mental distress: South Asian women in Britain. *Sociology of Health and Illness*, **18**, 66–85.

Gately, C., Rogers, A. & Sanders, C. (2007) Re-thinking the relationship between long-term condition self-management education and the utilisation of health services. *Social Science and Medicine*, **65**, 934–945.

Hardiman E. R. & Segal, S. P. (2003) Community membership and social networks in mental health self-help agencies. *Psychiatric Rehabilitation Journal*, **27**, 25–33.

Healy, D. (2004) Shaping the intimate: influences on the experience of everyday nerves. *Social Studies of Science*, **34**, 219–245.

Healy, D., Herxheimer, A. & Menkes, D. B. (2006) Antidepressants and violence: problems at the interface of medicine and law. *Public Library of Science (Medicine)*, **3**, 372.

Huxley, P. & Goldberg, D. (1975) Social versus clinical prediction in minor psychiatric disorders. *Psychological Medicine*, **5**, 96–100.

Koffman, J. & Taylor, P. (1997) Evidence-based approach to treating depression. *British Journal of General Practice*, **47**, 327–328.

Layard, R. (2005) *Happiness*. Penguin.

Lenzer, J. (2004) Secret US report surfaces on antidepressants in children. *BMJ*, **329**, 307.

Leonard, B. E. (2004) SSRIs, aggression and suicide – a cause for concern or the result of media hype? *Irish Journal of Psychological Medicine*, **21**, 40–42.

Lester, H. E., Tritter, J. Q. & Sorohan, H. (2005) Providing primary care for people with serious mental illness: a focus group study. *BMJ*, **330**, 1122–1128.

Macdonald, W., Mead, N., Bower, P., *et al* (2007) A qualitative study of patients' perceptions of a 'minimal' psychological therapy. *International Journal of Social Psychiatry*, **53**, 23–35.

Mauss, M. (1934) Les techniques du corps. *Journal de Psychologie*, **32** (3–4). Reprinted in Mauss (1936) *Sociologie et anthropologie*. PUF.

May, C., Allison, G., Chapple, A., *et al* (2004) Framing the doctor–patient relationship in chronic illness: a comparative study of general practitioners' accounts. *Sociology of Health and Illness*, **26**, 135–158.

Mead, N., Macdonald, W., Bower, P., *et al* (2005) The clinical effectiveness of guided self-help versus waiting-list control in the management of anxiety and depression: a randomised controlled trial. *Psychological Medicine*, **35**, 1633–1643.

Nazroo, J. Y., Edwards, A. C. & Brown, G. W. (1997) Gender differences in the onset of depression following a shared life event: a study of couples. *Psychological Medicine*, **27**, 9–19.

Nettleton, S. (2006) 'I just want permission to be ill': towards a sociology of medically unexplained symptoms. *Social Science and Medicine*, **62**, 1167–1178.

Pescosolido, B. A., Brooks-Gardner, C. & Lubell, K. M. (1998) How people get into mental health services: stories of choice, coercion and muddling through from first timers. *Social Science and Medicine*, **46**, 275–286.

Pilgrim, D. (2005) Protest and cooption: the voice of mental health service users. In *Beyond the Water Towers: The Unfinished Revolution in Mental Health Services 1985–2005* (eds A. Bell & P. Lindley): pp. 25–45. Sainsbury Centre for Mental Health.

Pilgrim, D. & Dowrick, C. (2006) From a diagnostic–therapeutic to a social–existential response to 'depression'. *Journal of Public Mental Health*, **5**, 6–12.

Pilgrim, D. & Guinan, P. (1999) From mitigation to culpability: rethinking the evidence on therapist sexual abuse. *European Journal of Psychotherapy, Counselling and Health*, **2**, 155–170.

Pilgrim, D. & Rogers, A. (1993) Mental health service users' views of medical practitioners. *Journal of Interprofessional Care*, **3**, 167–176.

Pilgrim, D. & Rogers, A. (1994) Something old, something new…. sociology and the organisation of psychiatry. *Sociology*, **28**, 521–538.

Pilgrim, D., Rogers, A., Clarke, S., *et al* (1997) Entering psychological treatment: decision making factors for general practitioners and service users. *Journal of Interprofessional Care*, **2**, 313–323.

Rogers, A. (1990) Policing mental disorder: controversies, myths and realities. *Social Policy and Administration*, **24**, 226–237.

Rogers, A. & Allison, T. (2004) What if my back breaks? Making sense of musculoskeletal pain among South Asian and African-Caribbean people in the North West of England. *Journal of Psychosomatic Research*, **57**, 79–87.

Rogers, A. & Pilgrim, D. (1991) 'Pulling down churches': accounting for the British mental health users movement. *Sociology of Health and Illness*, **13**, 129–148.

Rogers, A. & Pilgrim, D. (2003) *Mental Health and Inequalities*. Palgrave Macmillan.

Rogers, A. & Pilgrim, D. (2005) *A Sociology of Health and Illness* (3rd edition). Open University Press.

Rogers, A., Day, J. C., Williams, B., *et al* (1998a) The meaning and management of neuroleptic medication: a study of patients with a diagnosis of schizophrenia. *Social Science and Medicine*, **47**, 1313–1323.

Rogers, A., Hassell, K. & Nicolaas, G. (1998b) *Demanding Patients? Analysing Primary Care Use*. Open University Press.

Rogers, A., May, C. & Oliver, D. (2001) Experiencing depression, experiencing the depressed: the separate worlds of patients and doctors. *Journal of Mental Health*, **10**, 317–333.

Rogers, A., Oliver, D., Bower, P., *et al* (2004) People's understanding of a primary care-based mental health self-help clinic. *Patient Education and Counseling*, **53**, 41–46.

Rogers, A., Pilgrim, D., Brennan, S., *et al* (2007) Prescribing benzodiazepines in general practice: a new view of an old problem. *Health*, **11**, 181–198.

Royal College of Psychiatrists (2003) *Interim Guidance on the Relationship Between Psychiatrists and Commercial Sponsors and the Sponsorship of College Activities*. Royal College of Psychiatrists.

Shaw, I. & Taplin, S. (2007) Happiness and mental health policy: a sociological critique. *Journal of Mental Health*, **16**, 3.

Stationery Office (2002) *Pathways to Work: Helping People Into Employment*. Cmd 5690. Stationery Office.

Stimson, G. & Webb, B. (1975) *Going to See the Doctor: The Consultation Process in General Practice*. Routledge and Kegan Paul.

# CHAPTER 5

# The service user perspective

Helen Lester and Linda Gask

Summary

This chapter highlights some key issues from the service user's perspective. We start with an overview of the importance of language, for example the different meanings of the words 'user', 'patient' and 'survivor'. We then examine the views of service users themselves, particularly people experiencing depression and psychosis. The second half of the chapter focuses on services users' experience of primary care mental health, and how this experience can be measured. We conclude by discussing ways in which primary care could increase user involvement in developing and delivering services and positive examples of user involvement.

## The importance of language

The language used to describe 'service users' (our preferred term) is perhaps more varied in mental health than in any other sector of health and social care. Most of the literature on service users comes from the context of specialist psychiatric care rather than primary care. 'User', 'survivor', 'patient', 'customer', 'citizen', 'consumer': all imply different notions of the roles and responsibilities of people with mental health problems and the relationship between services and users. Pilgrim & Rogers (1999) have described a useful four-part typology of users as consumers, survivors, providers or, perhaps most commonly, as patients.

'Consumerism' is a relatively new ideology within the public sector in the UK, linked to the rise of general management principles in the National Health Service in the 1980s and the development of a market economy through the introduction of an internal market. It is also linked to the growing acknowledgement of the importance of customer satisfaction, with users of health and social care as customers who can exercise an informed choice about the services they receive and, if not satisfied, take their 'business' elsewhere. However, as Rogers & Pilgrim point out:

> many psychiatric patients do not ask for what they get – it is imposed on them. Various sections of the 1983 Mental Health Act, like its legal predecessors, are utilised to lawfully impose restraints and treatments on resentful and reluctant recipients. In such circumstances, mental patients could be construed to be consumers if being dragged off the street and force fed was a feature of being a customer in a restaurant. (Rogers & Pilgrim, 2001, p. 169)

Poverty can also limit choice, with private sector mental health services out of bounds, while, at times of crisis, the ability and motivation to obtain information about a range of services and select between them can be difficult (Rogers *et al*, 2001; Lester *et al*, 2004). For many people across the world with mental health problems, simply getting access to any kind of service, not the luxury of choosing between services, is the key issue. Choice also implies a possibility of exit from the system, a notion that is difficult to sustain in a society whose courts recognise the validity of advanced directives only when they prospectively authorise treatment, not when they are used to reject the possibility of treatment (Szasz, 2003). Choice, then, as a central part of consumerism, appears to be a relative concept if you are a mental health service user.

In contrast, the user as 'survivor' is linked to the growth in the early 1970s of collective activities of mental health service users initially in the Netherlands and the USA. Recognising the wisdom of the dominant trade union philosophy of the time that 'Unity is Strength', organisations such as the Campaign Against Psychiatric Oppression and the British Network for Alternatives to Psychiatry were formed. The term 'survivor' is very particularly chosen by groups such as Survivors Speak Out, the UK Advocacy Network (UKAN) and the Hearing Voices Network to portray a positive image of people in distress, as those who had the strength to survive the mental health system. 'Survivor' also implies a notion of rejecting forms of professionally led and produced information.

Linked to this, the conceptualisation of users as 'providers' is reflected in the development of user-led services, which are found in the voluntary and statutory sector across the UK. User-led activities cover a spectrum of involvement, from patients being mutually supported in professionally led services to projects that are managed and staffed by users themselves. The latter include safe houses and drop-in day centres and often reflect the user movement priorities of voluntary relationships, alternatives to hospital admissions and personal support.

However, Pilgrim & Rogers (1999, p. 193) suggest that the main way in which users of mental health services have been portrayed is as 'patients' – as 'objects of the clinical gaze of mental health professionals'. With this representation, the danger is that users are seen in terms of their illness, perceived as irrational and therefore as incapable of having a valid view.

# Service users' perspectives on experiencing mental illness

Over the past 20 years, a growing body of work has explored how people who are experiencing something that might be called 'mental illness' (over which they may *or may not* agree with a professional) organise their thinking and action in order to 'make sense' of their own experiences. For health professionals, understanding and taking into account the ways in which individuals formulate their own problems are increasingly recognised as essential in collaboratively based treatment (Fowler *et al*, 1998). It is also important to remember that health professionals and service users can often be the same people.

## *Experiencing depression*

Khan *et al* (2007), who primarily looked at experiences in a UK setting, but across different ethnic groups, noted that external sources of stress or conflict were drawn upon most frequently to account for the presence of depression. These included conflict with work colleagues or family, chronic illness, events in childhood, material disadvantage and racism (Kadam *et al*, 2001; Rogers *et al*, 2001; Burr & Chapman, 2004; Grime & Pollock, 2004). Rather than emphasising symptoms or feelings of depression, respondents' personal experience was characterised by expressions of being unable to cope, and in particular disturbances to everyday functioning and social roles (with negative consequences for other family members) (Knudsen *et al*, 2002; Maxwell, 2005). Metaphors used by respondents to communicate the experience of depression included being 'on edge', 'churned-up inside', 'boxed in', 'a volcano bursting', 'broken in half', 'shut in my own little shell', 'a wall of pain' and 'prisoner in my own home'. Most importantly, service users' descriptions of the cause of their problems differed from the psychological model, which underlies cognitive–behavioural therapy, or the more biomedical notion underpinning the prescribing of antidepressants.

Traditional psychiatric transcultural wisdom about the experience and presentation of somatic symptoms of depression in South Asian communities was challenged by Burr & Chapman (2004). Their respondents freely described emotional experiences and reported how these also affected their overall physical well-being and their bodies, with effects including what psychiatrists would recognise as 'symptoms of depression' *in addition* to a range of physical experiences – nausea and vomiting, generalised aches and pains in the joints, headache, painful periods and asthma attacks, features that can be recognised across cultures (see also Chapter 21).

In-depth interviews with women with postnatal depression in Goa, India, revealed that, contrary to the assumption that sociocultural contexts associated with childbirth in non-Western societies protect mothers from depression, factors unique to culture, such as gender preference and the low involvement of husbands in child care, were perceived as major stressors by the women. Here, emotional distress was interpreted, just as found by Khan *et al* (2007), from the context of social adversity, poor marital relationships and cultural attitudes towards gender, rather than as a biomedical psychiatric category. Experiences of women with postnatal depression have also been explored in Chinese women in Hong Kong (Chan *et al*, 2002), some of whom described themselves as being trapped in a situation from which there was no way of escape except by violent means, such as homicide or suicide. Women's unhappiness was attributed to a non-caring husband, and controlling and powerful in-laws.

A Swedish study with a gender perspective (Danielsson & Johansson, 2005) noted how men seemed to talk more easily about physical distress, while women verbalised emotional distress more readily.

Age-related issues have been explored by Wisdom & Green (2004) and, at the other end of the age spectrum, Burroughs *et al* (2006). In Portland, Oregon, teenagers discussed their experiences of depression in a focus group and described experiences of an 'illness trajectory' similar to that found in adults: a slow growth of distress, a time of 'being in a funk', followed by a time of consideration of whether they were depressed. Elderly people with depression interviewed by Burroughs in Manchester, England, seemed to share the rather nihilistic views of their general practitioners (GPs) that depression in old age was 'understandable' and a product of social and contextual issues rather than an 'illness'.

## Experiencing psychosis

There is also a dearth of published literature examining the beliefs of people with a diagnosis of schizophrenia concerning the validity of their diagnosis and the cause of their illness. Indeed, the views of service users on diagnosis, causation and recovery are more likely to be found in the 'grey literature', particularly on user-led websites (see e-resources). While Lobban *et al* (2004) found that the majority of their participants ascribed their psychotic experiences to a mental health problem, Angermeyer & Klusmann (1988) showed that recent psychosocial factors, such as stressful live events, were the most often cited causal factors. Phillips *et al* (2006) interviewed individuals with schizophrenia and found that nearly 60% felt their main difficulty was something other than a psychiatric or psychological problem; instead they described physical, social or practical difficulties. They did not possess 'insight' in the strict medical model definition, but did recognise they had a problem. Indeed, individuals described on average five different causal factors as important in their illness, including 'out of the ordinary factors', 'nerves', life events, childhood experiences and relationship difficulties.

Bentall (2003) has suggested that psychosis in particular should be seen as just part of human variation, rather than as an illness. He cites studies showing that up to 11–13% of people have experienced hallucinations at some point in their lives (Tien, 1991) and the work of Marius Romme and

Sandra Escher (1989) in the Netherlands, who have suggested that many people hear voices, but have little difficulty coping with them and, indeed, have never sought psychiatric treatment for them. Bentall argues that the boundaries of madness are fluid and that many experiences that might be attributed to a psychotic illness (e.g. according to DSM criteria) are not necessarily pathological. His position is that:

> we should abandon psychiatric diagnoses altogether and instead try to explain and understand the actual experiences and behaviours of psychotic people.... Once these complaints have been explained, there is no ghostly disease remaining that also requires an explanation. Complaints are all there is ... an advantage of this approach is that it does not require us to draw a clear dividing line between madness and sanity. (Bentall, 2003, pp. 141–142)

## Service users' experience of primary care mental health

There has also been relatively little work addressing the views on primary care services of people with mental health problems. What work has been done has tended to concentrate on the content of the consultation and highlighted a perceived lack of information and explanation about diagnosis and treatment (Bailey, 1997), overuse of medication and delay in obtaining a diagnosis (Rogers & Pilgrim, 1993), as well as barriers created by stigmatising attitudes (Kai & Crosland, 2001).

Khan et al (2007) concluded, from the UK studies that they reviewed on the experience of depression, that engaging with primary care was problematic. People used primary care because it represented the only place where help was seen to be on offer, rather than through a specific expectation that accessing services would be helpful. In a study of adults with a diagnosis of depression in Manchester, some also exhibited an unquestioning attitude to the quality of care for their problems (Gask et al, 2003). A recurring theme was the sense of 'wasting the doctor's time'; that is, people with depression may feel that they do not deserve to take up the doctor's time and there was a sense that it was not possible for doctors to listen to them and understand how they felt. A study of people with depression, their supporters and GPs in Southampton showed that frequently they did not share the same views on the causes of depression and goals for treatment. GPs described encouraging patients to view depression as separate from the self and 'normal' sadness. People with depression and their supporters often questioned such boundaries, rejecting the notion of a medical cure and emphasising self-management (Johnston et al, 2007). All three groups of participants identified the importance of GPs listening more to patients, but often felt that this did not happen.

In interviews with people with chronic depression managed in primary care, Campbell et al (2007) found five key themes were identified in relation to the individual patient experience set against a generic patient experience:

1   the healthcare system provides a generic, 'one size fits all' service, which is incompatible with an individual service user's experience and sense of being as an individual and that privileges medical over social care

2   people with mild to moderate mental health problems often have feelings of powerlessness and of being 'lost' in a system that is more responsive to severe and acute episodes of illness than to chronic morbidity

3   people often have unmet needs in relation to the distress of living with mild to moderate mental health problems

4   there are substantial quality deficits in primary care for people with mild to moderate chronic mental health problems

5   GPs are rated highly, and the interpersonal attributes of a good GP can be clearly identified.

Patients also valued continuity of care, as echoed elsewhere (Freeman *et al*, 2002) (Box 5.1).

Primary care has been described as the 'cornerstone' of care for people with serious mental illness, with health professionals at the centre, able to advocate through the sometimes maze-like mental health services (Lester *et al*, 2005). There are, however, still considerable differences of opinion, particularly for people with a diagnosis of schizophrenia, over the possibility of recovery, with primary care professionals more pessimistic than both service users and the evidence base (Harrison *et al*, 2001; see also Chapter 15 for further details).

## Measuring users' views of primary care

Formal measurement of service users' experiences is an important way for practitioners to evaluate their work, challenge traditional assumptions and highlight key priorities patients would like to see addressed. It is also a major determinant in altering service provision (Glasby & Lester, 2004). Measuring users' views is particularly important in primary care mental health, where patients and providers often have different perspectives on what constitutes good care (Shield *et al*, 2003) and where patients experience poorer health and healthcare than the general population (see Chapter 21). Previous work has suggested that availability and access, health professional 'humanity', patient involvement in decision-making, provision of information and sufficient time are important to patients when assessing the generic quality of primary care (Wensing *et al*, 1998). There are, however, few validated tools available to assess the quality of primary care mental health services. Many questionnaires are largely relevant either only to secondary care or if relevant to primary care, for example Clinical Outcomes in Routine Evaluation (CORE) or Psychological Outcomes Profile (PSYCHLOPS), follow the clinical course of individual patients through the treatment process (Evans *et al*, 2000; Ashworth *et al*, 2004).

---

**Box 5.1** Service users' views of the value of primary care

In Faulkner & Layzell's (2000) study, a user-administered semi-structured question-naire with 76 mental health service users in six geographical areas across the UK emphasised that satisfaction is increased by longer consultations, and by a GP perceived as caring and who demonstrates respect for the patient's viewpoint. Access and continuity of care were also centrally important to service users.

Kai & Crosland's study (2001), involving in-depth interviews with 34 service users with enduring mental illness, found that participants valued an empathetic and continuing therapeutic relationship with professionals in primary care.

Lester *et al*'s (2003) study with 45 users with serious mental illness in Birmingham found that longitudinal and interpersonal continuity of care, relative ease of access and option of a home visit were valued features of primary care. This was often contrasted with the difficulty of seeing a constant stream of new faces in secondary care mental health services, with painful life stories told and retold for staff rather than patient benefit.

Gask *et al*'s (2003) study of the quality of care for service users with depression found that the ability to offer structured care and proactive follow-up was important, since non-attendance may signal deterioration rather than recovery and the illness itself may preclude the assertiveness sometimes required to negotiate access.

Lester *et al*'s (2005) focus group study of 45 patients with serious mental illness, 39 general practitioners and eight practice nurses found that where health profession-als perceived serious mental illness as a lifelong condition, patients emphasised the importance of therapeutic optimism and hope for recovery in consultations.

Campbell *et al*'s (2007) interview study of 19 people with chronic depression in primary care found that there are perceived shortfalls in the quality of mental healthcare for people who have chronic but non-psychotic mental health prob-lems, who may feel 'lost' in the system.

---

Recently in the UK, a 20-item Patient Experience Questionnaire (PEQ) has been developed and validated for use in evaluating patient experience of primary care mental health at practice level (Mavaddat *et al*, 2009) (Box 5.2). The overall ratings on the PEQ can give practices an indication of the views of their patients and closer examination of individual question items will enable practices to tailor their improvements.

# Positive practice in user involvement in primary care mental health services

## Why is user involvement important?

There are a number of often interrelated reasons for believing that mental health service user involvement is more than a politically mandated 'good thing' but is a worthwhile activity with a range of practical and ethical benefits (Box 5.3).

**Box 5.2** The Patient Experience Questionnaire

Patients are asked to read the following statements about their experiences of going to the GP's surgery for a consultation regarding any mental health difficulties. They are asked to circle the response they most agree with, and are offered the options 'Strongly disagree', 'Disagree', 'Neither agree nor disagree', 'Agree' or 'Strongly agree'. They are told, when answering the questions, to think about their experiences in the past 3 months, and to consider the GP they see most often.

1   My GP does not take anything I tell them seriously.
2   My GP always has time to listen.
3   My GP makes me feel like I'm wasting their time.
4   My GP never encourages me to talk about my worries and concerns.
5   My GP is too quick to blame my physical problems on stress.
6   If I need extra time with my GP, it is never available.
7   My GP always gives me clear information about my mental health difficulties and what help is available.
8   My GP never explains things to me in a way that I can understand.
9   My GP is always willing to discuss different options for managing my mental health problems.
10  My GP always gives me up-to-date information about how I can get more help with my mental health problems.
11  My GP offers me treatment choices besides taking medication.
12  I always have to insist that my GP refers me for counselling or other therapies.
13  My GP works closely with other mental health workers such as nurses and counsellors in helping me with my mental health difficulties.
14  My GP never offers me treatments other than tablets.
15  My GP does not deal with my concerns about tablets and their side-effects.
16  My GP regularly reviews my mental health problems and treatment.
17  My GP treats me as an individual and not just as a person with mental health problems.
18  I can always get the help I need from practice nurses when it comes to my mental health difficulties.
19  The practice does not respect people with mental health problems.
20  I am satisfied with the mental healthcare I have received.

First, there is widespread recognition that service users are experts, with an in-depth knowledge of services and of living with a mental health problem. By definition, no one else, no matter how well trained or qualified, can possibly have had the same experience of the onset of mental illness, the same initial contact with services or the same journey through the mental health system. Borrill (2000), for example, emphasises the way in which users can predict when they are about to become unwell and formulate appropriate responses at an early stage. If primary care health professionals can tap into this expertise, they make their own jobs much easier and more productive, by focusing on users' considerable strengths.

In addition, service users and mental health professionals often have very different perspectives. Lindow (1999, p. 154), for example, highlights

---

**Box 5.3** The benefits of user involvement

- Users are experts about their own illness and need for care.
- Users may have different but equally important perspectives on their illness and care.
- User involvement may increase the existing limited understanding of mental distress.
- Users are able to develop alternative approaches to mental health and illness.
- User involvement may of itself be therapeutic.
- User involvement may encourage greater social inclusion.

---

the way in which users and service providers may have very different priorities:

> Our discussions are seldom about new styles of management, or changes in service organisations: I have heard little interest [among users] in the idea of a GP-led National Health Service. There is, rather, much discussion of poverty, employment, housing; about services that control and rob our experiences of meaning and about dangerous treatment.

Involving users can therefore provide insights that prompt practitioners to re-evaluate their work, challenge traditional assumptions and highlight key priorities that users would like to see addressed.

At the same time, users have been able to develop alternative approaches to mental health that can complement existing services. The Strategies for Living group, for example, have highlighted the importance of alternative and complementary therapies (Mental Health Foundation, 2003), while the Hearing Voices Network encourages positive working practices with people who hear voices and works to promote greater tolerance and understanding of voice-hearing (see e-resources). For some people, moreover, user involvement can be therapeutic. Helping to shape services, particularly when users work together collectively, can help users increase their confidence, raise self-esteem and develop new skills (Clark *et al*, 2004).

Finally, user involvement may encourage greater social inclusion (Sayce & Morris, 1999). On almost any indicator, people with mental health problems are among the most excluded within society, particularly in terms of employment opportunities. Some users are excluded geographically from their community by 'nimby' ('not in my back yard') attitudes to the siting of services, and from communities of identity through negative stereotypes of irrationality and violence. Wilkinson (1996) has suggested that it is relative rather than absolute poverty within societies that creates health inequalities, through mediating factors such as powerlessness and social stress. Encouraging greater user involvement, including paid activity, can be empowering and address issues of poverty and therefore may act as one mechanism to encourage greater social inclusion.

**65**

## Rhetoric–reality gaps

User involvement in mental health has been encouraged for over a decade in the UK (Department of Health, 1992, 1994, 1995) and continues to be an important theme in mental health policy (Department of Health 2001; Crisp, 2005). However, while user involvement in primary mental healthcare is often acknowledged as a 'good thing', it is relatively rarely acted upon in practice.

Peck *et al* (2002) have constructed a useful schema in the context of secondary mental healthcare, with three distinct conceptions of patient involvement, as recipients, subjects of consultation or agents in control. At the same time, they suggest patient involvement within mental health services operates at four levels:

1   in the interaction between patients and in the form of self-help
2   in the interaction between individual patients and professionals working with them
3   in the management of local services
4   in the planning of overall services.

Peck *et al* argue that if these two frameworks are combined, it is possible to construct a matrix for patient involvement (Table 5.1). They suggest that although the matrix illustrates the sheer diversity of mental health patient involvement activities in the UK, at the present time, many initiatives are clustered in the 'subject of consultation' category rather than the 'agent in control' box.

In the context of primary care, although there are a number of positive examples of 'interactions between patients', particularly in terms of support and advice in the voluntary sector, interactions with health professionals appear to be far less widespread than in secondary care mental health services, and are predominantly in terms of being recipients of care (Lester *et al*, 2006). The matrix (Table 5.1) usefully highlights practical ways in which service user involvement from a secondary care perspective could be used to improve user involvement in primary mental healthcare. However, it is important to recognise that, for people with common mental health problems such as anxiety and depression managed wholly in primary care, the perceived potential stigma of self-identification as a 'user of services' may be problematic. With recovery may also come the understandable desire to return to 'normality' and dissociate from any notion of being linked with 'mental illness'. Considerable work needs to be done to explore ways in which people can feel comfortable being both 'patients' of their GP, in receipt of care, and actively engaged in having their voice heard in shaping how services are provided.

## Positive practice

Perhaps the most challenging example of user involvement for people with mental illness relates to employing them as part of the paid mental

**Table 5.1** Examples of patient involvement in England

| Levels of interaction | Conceptions of patient involvement | | |
|---|---|---|---|
| | Recipient of communication | Subject of consultation | Agent in control |
| Interaction between patients | Newsletters Periodicals | Advocacy schemes | Hearing voices Newsletters Periodicals |
| Interaction between patient and professionals | Receiving care plans | Agreeing care plans | Direct payments |
| Management of local services | Receiving information services | Patient councils Patient surveys 'User-focused monitoring' | Patient-run crisis houses Social firms |
| Planning of overall services | Community care plans | Mental health taskforce membership Stakeholder conferences Patients on local implementation teams | |

From Peck *et al* (2002), with permission.

health workforce. In the UK, recent mental health workforce developments include the implementation of 'support, time and recovery' (STR) workers (Department of Health, 2003*a*). STR workers include volunteers and existing and former services users who have the ability to listen to people without judging them. They work as part of a team that provides mental health services and focus directly on the needs of service users, working across boundaries, providing support, giving time and promoting their recovery. The Department of Health's (2003*b*) best practice guide *Graduate Primary Care Mental Health Workers* also includes recommendations for employing people with lived experience of mental illness in the role.

There is evidence to suggest that involving service users as paid workers is seen as a very positive move, particularly by people with serious mental illness, and could help them both express their problems and navigate their way through the healthcare system.

> The things, the experiences, the emotions, the feelings that we as people suffering from mental distress go through simply aren't experienced by people in good health. Trying to get that across to someone who hasn't ever felt like the Sword of Damocles is hanging round your neck for no apparently good reason, you know, you can't do it. It's like trying to explain colours to a blind man. You are trying to explain an emotive language, a set of emotions, which you know you shouldn't have and normal people don't have, and trying to get these across is an almost impossible task.... I would have found it very useful to have spoken to somebody who'd been through the system who could say 'You know I've been through it and you're probably very confused'.

Now, I could accept that coming from another patient but I'm damned if I could accept that coming from a doctor or a nurse. (Lester *et al*, 2006, pp. 417–418)

Paid employment can also help address wider issues of poverty and social isolation. However, employing service users in this way requires organisations to think about their own cultural environment. Service cultures that encourage involvement share a number of characteristics, including a commitment to genuine partnerships between users and professionals and to the development of shared objectives. As the National Schizophrenia Fellowship (now Rethink) observed:

> Everyone involved in the delivery of care ... should be treated as equal partners. Occasionally, some professionals may initially feel threatened by the involvement of service users and carers and if this is the case, then it is important that this issue is addressed so that all of the parties involved can work well together. (National Schizophrenia Fellowship, 1997, p. 10)

The approach and value base of individual practitioners are also critical. Some professionals may find it difficult to view service users as experts. This may reflect resistance to the notion of sharing and transferring power to users, or a clash of professional 'scientific' and users' more 'social' ways of thinking and working (Summers, 2003).

Strategies for greater service user involvement also have significant implications for funding in primary care, in terms of both employing patients in new roles and addressing the consequences of potentially longer consultation times required for shared decision-making. Perhaps, above all, a meaningful change in patient involvement requires commitment and belief from primary care practitioners that the views and experiences of people with mental health problems are valid and valuable, and need to be listened to at both a consultation and a practice level.

---

### Key points

- There has also been relatively little work addressing the views of people with mental health problems on primary care services.
- Health professionals need to understand and take into account the ways in which individuals formulate their own problems if they want to provide appropriate and collaborative care.
- Formal measurement of service users' experiences is an important way for practitioners to evaluate their work, challenge traditional assumptions and highlight key priorities patients would like to see addressed.
- A meaningful change in patient involvement requires commitment and belief from primary care practitioners that the views and experiences of people with mental health problems are valid and valuable, and need to be listened to at both a consultation and a practice level.

# Further reading and e-resources

Leudar, I. & Thomas, P. (2000) *Voices of Reason, Voices of Sanity: Studies of Verbal Hallucinations*. Brunner Routledge.

Solomon, A. (2001) *The Noonday Demon: An Anatomy of Depression*. Chatto and Windus.

Styron, W. (2001) *Darkness Visible*. Vintage.

http://www.hearing-voices.org

# References

Angermeyer, M. C. & Klusmann, D. (1988) The causes of functional psychoses as seen by patients and their relatives. 1 The patient's point of view. *European Archives of Psychiatry and Neurological Sciences*, **238**, 47–54.

Ashworth, M., Shepherd, M., Christey, J., *et al* (2004) A client-generated psychometric instrument: the development of 'PSYCHLOPS'. *Counselling and Psychotherapy Research*, **4**(2), 27–31.

Bailey, D. (1997) What is the way forward for a user-led approach to the delivery of mental health services in primary care? *Journal of Mental Health*, **6**, 101–105.

Bentall, R. (2003) *Madness Explained: Psychosis and Human Nature*. Allen Lane.

Borrill, J. (2000) *Developments in Treatment for People with Psychotic Experiences*. (Updates, volume 2, issue 9.) Mental Health Foundation.

Burr, J. & Chapman, T. (2004) Contextualising experiences of depression in women from South Asian communities: a discursive approach. *Sociology of Health and Illness*, **26**, 433–452.

Burroughs, H., Lovell, K., Morley, M., *et al* (2006) 'Justifiable depression': how primary care professionals and patients view late-life depression? A qualitative study. *Family Practice*, **23**, 369–377.

Campbell, S. M., Gately, C. & Gask, L. (2007) Identifying the patient perspective of the quality of mental healthcare for common chronic problems: a qualitative study. *Chronic Illness*, **3**, 46–65.

Chan, S. W., Levy, V., Chung, T. K., *et al* (2002) A qualitative study of the experiences of a group of Hong Kong Chinese women diagnosed with postnatal depression. *Journal of Advanced Nursing*, **39**, 571–9.

Clark, M., Glasby, J., Lester, H. E., *et al* (2004) Cases for change: user involvement in mental health services and research. *Research Policy and Planning*, **22**(2), 31–38.

Crisp, N. (2005) *Chief Executive's Report to the NHS*. Department of Health.

Danielsson, U. & Johansson, E. E. (2005) Beyond weeping and crying: a gender analysis of expression of depression. *Scandinavian Journal of Primary Health Care*, **23**, 171–177.

Department of Health (1992) *The Health of the Nation*. TSO (The Stationery Office).

Department of Health (1994) *Working in Partnership: A Collaborative Approach to Care – Report of the Mental Health Nursing Review*. HMSO.

Department of Health (1995) *Building Bridges: A Guide to the Arrangements for Interagency Working for the Care and Protection of Severely Disabled People*. Department of Health.

Department of Health (2001) *The Journey to Recovery: The Government's Vision for Mental Health Care*. Department of Health.

Department of Health (2003a) *Mental Health Policy Implementation Guide. Support, Time and Recovery Workers*. Department of Health.

Department of Health (2003b) *Mental Health Policy Implementation Guide. Fast Forwarding Primary Care Mental Health: Graduate Primary Care Mental Health Workers*. Department of Health.

Evans, C., Mellor-Clark, J., Margison, F., *et al* (2000) Clinical Outcomes in Routine Evaluation: the CORE-OM. *Journal of Mental Health*, **9**, 247–255.

Faulkner, A. & Layzell, S. (2000) *Strategies for Living: A Report of User-Led Research into People's Strategies for Living with Mental Distress*. Mental Health Foundation.

Fowler, D., Garety, P. & Kuipers, E. (1988) Understanding the inexplicable: an individually formulated cognitive approach to delusional beliefs. In *Cognitive Psychotherapy of Psychotic and Personality Disorders: Handbook of Theory and Practice* (eds C. Perris & P. D. McGorry), pp. 129–146. Wiley.

Freeman, G., Weaver, T., Low, J., *et al* (2002) *Promoting Continuity of Care for People with Severe Mental Illness whose Needs Span Primary, Secondary and Social Care*. National Coordinating Centre for Service Delivery and Organisation.

Gask, L., Rogers, A., Oliver, D., *et al* (2003) Qualitative study of patients' perceptions of the quality of care for depression in general practice. *British Journal of General Practice*, **53**, 278–283.

Glasby, J. & Lester, H. E. (2004) Cases for change in mental health: partnership working in mental health services. *Journal of Interprofessional Care*, **18**, 7–16.

Grime, J. & Pollock, K. (2004) Information versus experience: a comparison of an information leaflet on antidepressants with lay experience of treatment. *Patient Education and Counseling*, **54**, 361–368.

Harrison, G., Hopper, K., Craig, T., *et al* (2001) Recovery from psychotic illness: a 15 and 25 year international follow up study. *British Journal of Psychiatry*, **178**, 506–517.

Johnston, O., Kumar, S., Kendall, K., *et al* (2007) Qualitative study of depression management in primary care: GP and patient goals, and the value of listening. *British Journal of General Practice*, **57**, 872–879.

Kadam, U. T., Croft, P., McLeod, J., *et al* (2001) A qualitative study of patients' views on anxiety and depression. *British Journal of General Practice*, **51**, 375–380.

Kai, J. & Crosland, A. (2001) Perspectives of people with enduring mental ill health from a community-based qualitative study. *British Journal of General Practice*, **51**, 730–736.

Khan, N., Bower, P. & Rogers, A. (2007) Guided self-help in primary care mental health: meta-synthesis of qualitative studies of patient experience. *British Journal of Psychiatry*, **191**, 206–211.

Knudsen, P., Hansen, E., Traulsen, J., *et al* (2002) Changes in self-concept while using SSRI antidepressants. *Qualitative Health Research*, **12**, 932–944.

Lester, H. E., Tritter, J. & England, E. (2003) Satisfaction with primary care: the perspectives of people with schizophrenia. *Family Practice*, **20**, 508–513.

Lester, H. E, Tritter, J. Q. & Sorohan, H. (2004) Managing crisis: the role of primary care for people with serious mental illness. *Family Medicine*, **36**(1), 28–34.

Lester, H. E., Tritter, J. Q. & Sorohan, H. (2005) Patients' and health professionals' views on primary care for people with serious mental illness: focus group study. *BMJ*, **330**, 1122–1128.

Lester, H. E., Tait, L., England, E., *et al* (2006) Patient involvement in primary care mental health: a focus group study. *British Journal of General Practice*, **56**, 415–422.

Lindow, V. (1999) Power, lies and injustice: the exclusion of service users' voices. In *Ethics and Community in the Health Care Professions* (ed. M. Parker), pp. 154–177. Routledge.

Lobban, F., Barrowclough, C. & Jones, S. (2004) The impact of beliefs about mental health problems and coping on outcome in schizophrenia. *Psychological Medicine*, **34**, 1165–1176.

Mavaddat, N., Lester, H. E. & Tait, L. (2009) Development and validation of the PEQ. *Quality and Safety in Health Care*, **18**, 147–152.

Maxwell, M. (2005) Women's and doctors' accounts of their experiences of depression in primary care: the influence of social and moral reasoning on patients' and doctors' decisions. *Chronic Illness*, **1**, 61–71.

Mental Health Foundation (2003) *Surviving User-Led Research: Reflections on Supporting User-Led Research Projects*. Mental Health Foundation.

National Schizophrenia Fellowship (1997) *How to Involve Users and Carers in Planning, Running and Monitoring Care Services and Curriculum Development*. National Schizophrenia Fellowship.

Peck, E., Gulliver, P. & Towell, D. (2002) Information, consultation or control: user involvement in mental health services in England at the turn of the century. *Journal of Mental Health*, **11**, 441–451.

Phillips, C., Cooke, M. & Cooke, A. (2006) Identity and cause of problems: the perceptions of patients with a diagnosis of schizophrenia. *Behavioural and Cognitive Psychotherapy*, **35**, 237–240.

Pilgrim, D. & Rogers, A. (1999) *A Sociology of Mental Health and Illness* (2nd edition). Open University Press.

Rogers, A. & Pilgrim, D. (1993) *Experiencing Psychiatry: Users' Views of Services*. London: Macmillan.

Rogers, A. & Pilgrim, D. (2001) *Mental Health Policy in Britain* (2nd edition). Palgrave.

Rogers, A., May, C. & Oliver, D. (2001) Experiencing depression, experiencing the depressed: the separate worlds of patients and doctors. *Journal of Mental Health*, **10**, 317–333.

Romme, M. & Escher, A. (1989) Hearing voices. *Schizophrenia Bulletin*, **15**, 209–216.

Sayce, L. & Morris, D. (1999) *Outsiders Coming In? Achieving Social Inclusion for People with Mental Health Problems*. Mind Publications.

Shield, T., Campbell, S., Rogers, A., *et al* (2003) Quality indicators for primary care mental health services. *Quality and Safety in Health Care*, **12**, 100–106.

Summers, A. (2003) Involving users in the development of mental health services: a study of psychiatrists' views. *Journal of Mental Health*, **12**, 161–174.

Szasz, T. (2003) The psychiatric protection order for the 'battered mental patient'. *BMJ*, **327**, 1449–1451.

Tien, A. Y. (1991) The distribution of hallucinations in the population. *Social Psychiatry and Psychiatric Epidemiology*, **26**, 287–292.

Wensing, M., Jung, H., Mainz, J., *et al* (1998) A systematic review of the literature on patient priorities for general practice care. Part 1: Description of the research domain. *Social Science and Medicine*, **47**, 1573–1588.

Wilkinson, R. G. (1996) *Unhealthy Societies: The Afflictions of Inequality*. Routledge.

Wisdom, J. P. & Green, C. A. (2004) 'Being in a funk': teens' efforts to understand their depressive experience. *Qualitative Health Research*, **14**, 1227–1238.

# CHAPTER 6

# Low- and middle-income countries

Mohan Isaac and Oye Gureje

Summary

This chapter reviews the current status of integration of mental health into primary care services in low- and middle-income countries. More than 80% of the world's population of over 6 billion live in 128 countries which have widely varying overall status of development, health policies and health delivery systems. The focus of health policies in these countries has changed over the past three decades. Health delivery systems in most of them function suboptimally owing to a variety of chronic problems and need strengthening. Demonstration projects in many countries indicate that it is possible to train doctors and primary care workers and integrate mental health into primary care. However, there is a need to sustain, expand and evaluate programmes of primary care mental health.

In the early 1970s, comprehensive and authoritative reviews of psychiatric disorders in low- and middle-income (LAMI) countries in Latin America, sub-Saharan Africa and South-East Asia showed that all types of mental disorders were widely prevalent. The reviews highlighted the gross neglect of mental disorders in these countries for a variety of reasons, which included pervasive stigma, widespread misconceptions, grossly inadequate budgets and acute shortages of trained personnel. It was pointed out that, in these countries, basic mental healthcare should be decentralised and integrated with the existing system of general health services (German, 1972; Leon, 1972; Carstairs, 1973; Neki, 1973). The strategy of integrating mental health into primary care services was endorsed by a Mental Health Expert Committee of the World Health Organization (WHO) in 1974 (WHO, 1975). More than 25 years later, in 2001, the WHO devoted its *World Health Report* to mental health, focusing on the importance of integrating mental health into primary care (WHO, 2001a). Several other influential international reports have recommended the strengthening of existing systems of primary care services in LAMI countries to provide services for persons with mental disorders (Institute of Medicine, 2001;

Hyman *et al*, 2006). More recently, the *Lancet* series 'Global Mental Health' unequivocally recommended that mental health be recognised as an integral component of primary and secondary general healthcare, particularly in LAMI countries (Chisholm *et al*, 2007*a*; Gureje *et al*, 2007).

Better recognition of the societal burden of mental disorders, availability of effective interventions and high-profile recommendations often do not result in improved provision of mental healthcare in LAMI countries. This chapter reviews the widely varying nature of LAMI countries, their health policies, health systems, health personnel and barriers to better healthcare delivery in the context of the integration of mental health into primary healthcare.

# 'Developing countries'

More than 80% of the world's population of over 6 billion live in countries that are referred to as 'developing', a euphemism for poor countries. These countries are situated mostly in Africa, Latin America, Asia and some parts of eastern Europe. The typology of countries has changed over time. Terms such as 'Third World' have given way to newer operational ones, such as 'developing countries', 'less economically developed countries' (LEDC), 'emerging economies' and 'non-industrialised nations'. The World Bank (2006) classifies economies according to their gross national income per capita (Table. 6.1). Of the 208 nations in the world, the 54 that belong to the low-income group and the 58 in the lower-middle-income group constitute the 'developing countries' and are also referred to as 'low- and middle-income countries'.

## Are all 'developing countries' similar?

The LAMI countries are often described in ways that would suggest that they constitute a homogeneous group with similar colonial histories, an underdeveloped industrial base, an agriculture-based economy, low standards of living and similar problems of inadequate resources and capacities. However, there is considerable heterogeneity within these countries and there is no such thing as a 'typical' LAMI country. There are striking differences between various LAMI countries and between different regions

**Table 6.1** World Bank's classification of countries

| Country groupings | Gross national income, per capita (US$, 2006) |
| --- | --- |
| Low income | 905 or less |
| Lower middle income | 906–3595 |
| Upper middle income | 3596–11115 |
| High income | 11116 and above |

Source: World Bank (2006).

73

within countries. They have widely varying profiles of development. While some, notably in Asia (called the 'Asian tigers'), are growing very rapidly, countries in sub-Saharan Africa show indicators of declining growth and stagnation. In some countries with rapid growth in Asia, income inequalities as well as health inequalities have steadily increased (Asian Development Bank, 2007). Health inequalities across the globe are also on the rise (Vagero, 2007). Development in critical areas such as education and health has declined in many countries with histories of civil war, ethnic conflict, chronic large-scale breakdown of the rule of law and dictatorial regimes with scant regard for human rights and democratic governance. Such countries are sometimes referred to as 'failed states'. There is a strong association between low income and high fertility rates. Consequently, many low-income countries are experiencing rapid population growth. The steady growth in the populations of many LAMI countries in Africa and Asia is accompanied by rapid urbanisation. By the end of 2007, it was estimated that more than half of the world's population, about 3.3 billion, were living in urban areas, most of them in the developing world (United Nations Population Fund, 2007). In many LAMI countries, such urban cities are often characterised by high unemployment, insecurity and squalor.

The LAMI countries have varying abilities to translate their gross national income into tangible assets. Therefore, gross national income may not always provide a complete picture of a country's overall development. The United Nations Development Programme (2006) has developed a composite index called the Human Development Index (HDI) to better capture the complex relationship between a country's income and human progress (Box 6.1).

The United Nations Development Programme's annual *Human Development Reports* have stimulated global, regional and national discussions on issues that are relevant to health and human development. While the HDI of some countries such as China and Indonesia have shown an impressive rise over

---

**Box 6.1** The Human Development Index (HDI)

- The HDI is an alternative summary measure of development that indicates the average progress of a country in human development.
- It serves as a frame of reference for both social and economic development.
- It is a composite index of three dimensions of human development: life expectancy, educational attainment and standard of living.
- Educational attainment is measured by adult literacy and school enrolment at primary, secondary and tertiary levels.
- Standard of living is measured by income in purchasing power parity (PPP) US$.
- The United Nations Development Programme (UNDP) releases an annual *Human Development Report* (HDR), which ranks all countries according to their HDI.

the past two decades, some 21 countries had a lower HDI in 2003 than in 1990. Over the period, many countries in Africa had become poorer and life expectancy had fallen, largely owing to the HIV/AIDS epidemic. Other sensitive indices of the overall quality of healthcare of a population, such as infant mortality rate, the under-5 mortality rate and the maternal mortality rate, also show wide variations across and within LAMI countries.

# Changing focus of health policies

Until the mid-1970s, most LAMI countries in Africa and Asia, many of them newly decolonised, focused their health policies on the control of infectious diseases and reduction of mortality. A substantial proportion of their health budgets was spent on tertiary care hospitals, often located in state capitals and other large cities. The emergence of the concept of primary healthcare (PHC) in the 1970s provided a radically new way of formulating healthcare policy in these countries. A major international conference on primary healthcare organised in 1978 by the WHO and the United Nations Children's Fund, in Alma-Ata in the then Soviet Union (now Almaty, the capital of Kazakhstan), urged all governments, health and development agencies, and the world community to 'protect and promote the health of all the people of the world'. The famous 'Health for all by 2000' slogan was born and primary healthcare was declared the bedrock of healthcare provision globally, in the Alma-Ata Declaration (WHO, 1978; see also Chapter 2). The definition and essential components of primary healthcare as well as the place of mental health in primary healthcare, as formulated at Alma-Ata, have been critically reviewed by Sartorius in Chapter 2. 'Primary healthcare' was essentially an approach to the provision of basic health services, particularly in LAMI countries. However, it was soon realised that the primary healthcare strategy as envisaged in the Alma-Ata Declaration was too broad, utopian and unrealistic, and 'Health for all by 2000' was not feasible (Cueto, 2004; Magnussen et al, 2004). The available financial and human resources were considered to be grossly insufficient to achieve the goal.

## From 'comprehensive to 'selective' primary care

An interim alternative strategy, 'selective primary healthcare', with measurable and attainable goals and cost-effective planning was soon developed, aimed at the least developed countries. The focus of this programme was on four well-defined interventions, best known as 'GOBI', which stood for Growth monitoring, Oral rehydration techniques, Breastfeeding and Immunisation against diphtheria–pertussis–tetanus and measles (Walsh & Warren, 1979; Cueto, 2004). Over the years, universal provision of primary healthcare as well as efforts to achieve 'Health for all by 2000' were abandoned in most LAMI countries (Godley, 2007). Although the strategy of selective primary care was pursued with varying intensity in many countries, the emergence of HIV/AIDS in epidemic proportions, particularly in Africa, contributed to the revival of the earlier policy of strengthening disease-specific, vertical health programmes.

## Investing in health

The World Bank's *World Development Report* of 1993, *Investing in Health*, which reflected overall changes in economic philosophy, influenced health policy formulation in LAMI countries towards healthcare reform, primarily focusing on changes in financing and organisational structure (Whitehead *et al*, 2001). The role of the private sector in the delivery of healthcare was recognised. Policies and recommendations were influenced by new concepts such as user fees, cost recovery, private health insurance and public–private partnerships (Hall & Taylor, 2003; see also Chapter 2). Nevertheless, mortality rates due to maternal and perinatal conditions, vaccine-preventable diseases, diarrhoea, malnutrition (protein, energy and micronutrient), malaria, tuberculosis and HIV/AIDS continued to be high in many LAMI countries (Jha *et al*, 2002). The WHO Commission on Macroeconomics and Health led by economist Jeffrey Sachs concluded that an adequate investment in health is necessary for economic development (WHO, 2001*b*).

## Millennium Development Goals

With the dawn of the new millennium, a major global programme called the Millennium Project was initiated by the United Nations (UN) to deal with extreme poverty, including related health consequences (Box 6.2). At a UN millennium summit attended by a large number of world leaders and heads of state, the Millennium Declaration for development and poverty eradication was signed. The Declaration is translated into eight quantifiable goals referred to as the Millennium Development Goals (MDGs), which are to be achieved by 2015. Three of them – reducing child mortality, improving maternal health and combating malaria, tuberculosis and HIV/AIDS – are directly related to health (Sachs & McArthur, 2005). The Millennium Declaration and the MDGs have, no doubt, given tremendous visibility and momentum to achieving urgent public health priorities in LAMI countries. Increasing international assistance has also become available in the form of high-profile initiatives such as the Global Fund to Fight AIDS, Tuberculosis and Malaria, and the Global Alliance for Vaccines and Immunization, with financial support from global health charities such as the Bill and Melinda Gates Foundation.

The halfway mark of the Millennium Programme's 15-year course was passed in September 2007. Progress towards the agreed health goals has remained slow (Travis *et al*, 2004). It is increasingly being recognised that there are various critical challenges to achieving the MDGs in LAMI countries, related to their health systems. It is widely accepted that unless these health systems are substantially strengthened, many of the health

---

**Box 6.2** From Alma-Ata to the Millennium Declaration – the changing focus of health policies

- Alma-Ata Declaration (1978) – 'Health for all by 2000' by universal provision of comprehensive primary healthcare.
- Selective primary healthcare – focus on four measurable and attainable goals, namely Growth monitoring, Oral rehydration techniques, Breastfeeding and Immunisation (GOBI).
- World Bank's *World Development Report, Investing in Health* (1993) – emphasis on health sector reform, role of private sector, public–private partnerships, user fees, cost recovery, private health insurance, etc.
- WHO Commission on Macroeconomics and Health (2001) – highlighting the need for substantial financial investment in the health sector in developing countries, to promote economic development.
- UN Millennium Declaration (2000), for development and poverty eradication – eight quantifiable Millennium Development Goals (MDGs) to be achieved by 2015, including health-related goals such as reducing child mortality, improving maternal health and combating malaria, tuberculosis and HIV/AIDS.

---

targets are unlikely to be achieved (Mills *et al*, 2006). It has been argued that some of the time-limited health goals are either unmeasurable or cannot be adequately measured (Attaran, 2005). Some experts believe that the disease- or condition-specific programmes with a vertical nature will fragment the fragile health systems of LAMI countries, as these vertical programmes require separate planning, staffing and management from other health programmes (Travis *et al*, 2004; Brown, 2007). A wide variety of stakeholders all over the world continue to have an abiding interest and faith in primary healthcare. To mark the 30th anniversary of the Alma-Ata Declaration, the World Health Organization launched its World Health Report *Primary Health Care: Now More Than Ever* in October 2008 at Almaty, Kazakhstan (WHO, 2008). The report, which focuses on the role of primary healthcare in strengthening health systems, calls for a return to the primary healthcare approach.

## Mental health and the Millennium Development Goals

The United Nations' 'framework for development' does not include chronic non-communicable physical diseases, although many LAMI countries such as China and India are fast catching up with high-income countries in mortality and morbidity due to heart disease, cancer and diabetes. Mental health is also absent from the MDGs, although there is conclusive evidence that mental disorders constitute a significant health burden in LAMI countries (Prince *et al*, 2007). Poor mental health is linked to poverty, disadvantage, HIV/AIDS and poor maternal and child health (Miranda & Patel 2005; Gureje & Jenkins, 2007) and it is now clear that several of the MDGs are not achievable without a consideration of mental health issues.

# Health systems in LAMI countries

The exact nature of health systems varies widely across LAMI countries depending on a variety of socio-economic, cultural and political factors. In many LAMI countries, the health system is organised in such a way that, in rural and peripheral areas, healthcare is provided through a network of district hospitals and community health centres, primary health centres and health posts, which provide simple curative, preventive and outreach services. The population covered by a district hospital may range from about 100 000 to 1 000 000. The typical health post or health centre is run by health workers or nurses, commonly supervised by general physicians. Other tiers of the health service commonly comprise general and specialist hospitals, manned by various cadres of physicians and other health professionals. The population per doctor may range from 15 000 to 70 000.

Besides government-run public health services, there are private hospitals and general practitioners (GPs) who work independently. Most LAMI countries also have a vibrant traditional health sector, with a variety of complementary and alternative treatment practices. In addition, a large number of international agencies, and national and international non-governmental organisations contribute substantially to different aspects of health services, particularly in the poorest countries. Various disease-control programmes and programmes that promote maternal and child health are primarily the responsibility of government health services.

The coverage and effectiveness of health services are suboptimal in most LAMI countries. Health systems are constrained by a chronic shortage of motivated and adequately trained staff, low budgets, the high cost and irregular supply of drugs, lack of transportation, non-functioning equipment, and poor organisation and management. Health is a relatively low-priority area for many of these countries, as evidenced by low spending on health, commonly within the range of 2–4% of gross domestic product (GDP) (Table 6.2).

Urban-based hospitals and tertiary care services still consume a large share of health sector budgets. Health systems are known to be consistently

**Table 6.2** Health expenditure in high-income and LAMI countries

| Country | Share of gross domestic product (2005) | Per capita (2005) (US$, purchasing power parity) |
|---|---|---|
| USA | 15.3 | 6401 |
| Switzerland | 11.6 | 4177 |
| Canada | 9.5 | 3326 |
| UK | 8.3 | 2724 |
| Japan | 8.0 | 2358 |
| Low- and middle-income countries | 2–4 | No reliable data |

Source: Organisation for Economic Co-operation and Development (2007).

inequitable, often failing to reach disadvantaged sections of the population effectively (Gwatkin *et al*, 2004). Prescriptions for improving health system capacity and performance include contracting out service provision, especially to non-governmental organisations or private providers, encouraging staff retention and motivation through improved remuneration and non-monetary rewards (e.g. opportunities for training and career progression) and ensuring that the users of services have a voice in the local health system, to influence priorities (Mills *et al*, 2006). Tensions between vertical and horizontal strategies in programme implementation have not been resolved (Mills, 2005). The exact role of the private sector and the optimal public–private mix in health systems is unclear (Hanson & Berman, 1998). While the urgent need to strengthen health systems in LAMI countries is widely accepted, evidence-based strategies to achieve this aim are yet to emerge (Haines *et al*, 2004).

## Primary care mental health

The consequences of various efforts to integrate mental health into primary care in LAMI countries should be understood in the context of the changing focus of overall health policies and poorly functioning health systems, described above. The high prevalence of all forms of mental disorder in all parts of the developing world has been well documented by a large number of epidemiological studies carried out in different sections of the population of LAMI countries. The presence of mental disorders in about 25% of the attendees of primary care settings in LAMI countries has also been repeatedly shown (Harding *et al*, 1980; Üstün & Sartorius, 1995). The lack of uniform information about the nature and extent of available resources for mental healthcare delivery in different LAMI countries was filled to a great extent by the WHO's Mental Health Atlas project. The country profiles provided by the Atlas confirmed that mental health services are grossly inadequate when compared with the needs. The profiles also indicate that countries show wide variations in the availability of different components of mental health services (WHO, 2005). A recent review of the availability of resources for mental health in LAMI countries, which covered policy and infrastructure, human resources and funding, showed that resources were not only very scarce but were inequitably and inefficiently used (Saxena *et al*, 2007). As a consequence, the treatment gap for all mental disorders is big. Although effective treatment methods exist, most persons with mental disorders remain untreated (Kohn *et al*, 2004; Gureje & Lasebikan, 2006). The proportion of persons with mental disorders receiving services corresponds to a country's percentage spend of GDP on healthcare (Wang *et al*, 2007).

Widespread misconceptions about the causation and management of mental disorders continue to be rampant in most LAMI countries. Stigma towards mental disorders is rife (Gureje *et al*, 2005) and may contribute to the under-use of mental health services where they are provided (Gureje & Lasebikan, 2006). Utilisation of the public health service is often low

(Chisholm *et al*, 2000). The proportion of people on any kind of health insurance is also commonly low and services for mental health problems, even in primary care settings, may not be free. Consequently, out-of-pocket expenditure is the primary method of paying for mental health services in many countries (Saxena *et al*, 2003). This is considered neither efficient nor equitable (Dixon *et al*, 2006).

## Demonstration projects

Doctors and other primary healthcare workers in LAMI countries generally have little or no training or experience in the recognition and management of mental disorders. As a result, poor detection of mental disorders and inadequate treatment of those identified are common. During the past two-and-a-half decades, numerous mental health programmes in primary care settings have sprung up in different LAMI countries. One of the earliest initiatives was a collaborative programme, 'Strategies for Extending Mental Healthcare', initiated by the WHO in seven LAMI countries: Brazil, Colombia, Egypt, India, the Philippines, Senegal and Sudan (Sartorius & Harding, 1983). Since the early 1980s, training programmes and manuals in mental health for primary care workers have been developed, piloted and used in different LAMI countries (Isaac *et al*, 1982; WHO, 1990; Cohen, 2001). The WHO has produced a simple classification of mental disorders for use in primary care settings, with user-friendly diagnostic and management guidelines (WHO, 1998; see also Chapter 3). A comprehensive review of the effectiveness of primary care mental health services in LAMI countries as varied as Botswana, Guinea Bissau, India, Iran, Nicaragua, Nepal and Tanzania noted that adequate data on long-term effects were not available from any of these countries to make meaningful interpretations (Cohen, 2001).

While mental health training programmes for primary care personnel may bring about improvements in mental health knowledge and attitudes, there is rather little evidence of changes in the actual practice of health workers. Although the diagnostic sensitivity of trained workers increases, there is no evidence that such improvements result in better outcomes for patients. Many reports of demonstration projects in LAMI countries mention the numbers of patients with various mental disorders identified and treated in primary care but do not provide any information on long-term clinical outcomes, as the projects lacked rigorous evaluation (Cohen, 2001). Most training programmes consist of short courses focused on diagnosis and pharmacological management, without much emphasis on skill acquisition and application in clinical settings (Hodges *et al*, 2001).

Numerous other factors, such as erratic drug supplies, high rates of attrition of trained staff, lack of continued on-the-job training and inadequate support and supervision also influence the effectiveness and long-term sustainability of primary care mental health programmes. Even adequately funded programmes sometimes fail owing to factors such as a top-down approach to planning divorced from the realities on the ground, poor governance, managerial incompetence, and unrealistic expectations on the part of low-paid and poorly motivated primary care staff (Goel *et al*, 2004). Abas *et al* (2003), in a review of practice in delivering care to adults with common mental disorders in primary care settings of low-income countries, pointee out that 'much remains unknown, undocumented and unshared'. Whether primary care staff can improve outcomes for these disorders is yet to be established widely. While there is evidence that epilepsy can be treated effectively by primary care staff, evidence for effective management of severe mental disorders is largely inadequate (Cohen, 2001).

Even though the majority of persons with common mental disorders who receive treatment in LAMI countries, just as in high-income ones, do so in general or primary care settings (Gureje & Lasebikan, 2006; Wang *et al*, 2007), only a very small proportion receive even minimally adequate treatment. This inadequacy of service seems to reflect both the lack of adequate training for primary healthcare providers and the pattern of health service delivery in those settings. A large cross-national WHO collaborative study suggested that primary healthcare services in LAMI countries are often characterised by lack of continuity of care and poor record-keeping (Simon *et al*, 1999; Gureje, 2004).

## Traditional health in primary mental healthcare

Traditional healers continue to play a major role, particularly in rural areas of LAMI countries in Asia and Africa, and especially for severe (psychotic) mental disorders. They are easily accessible and affordable for most people. They also provide care that is consistent with the belief systems of patients and their families (Odejide & Morakinyo, 2003). In many countries, patients and families consult both traditional healers and modern doctors and are able to simultaneously follow the instructions of both quite comfortably (Thara *et al*, 2004). Religious institutions and places of worship are also important settings for the treatment of people who are mentally ill (Thara *et al*, 1998). A report on temple healing from South India showed that a brief stay at a healing temple improved objective measures of clinical psychopathology (Raguram *et al*, 2002). The authors suggested that the improvement was due to the supportive and non-threatening environment of a culturally valid refuge for people with severe mental illnesses.

Many psychiatrists, particularly from Africa, have argued for collaboration with traditional healers and for their involvement in the planning and delivery of mental health services (Ngoma *et al*, 2003; Ovuga *et al*, 2007; Patel *et al*, 2007). However, past attempts have shown that if such collaborations are to succeed, sound and workable programmes of integrating traditional healers with mental health service delivery will have to be carefully developed by all stakeholders. Since in many cases traditional treatments are characterised by unhealthy and injurious methods, the efficacy and safety of specific traditional interventions will have to be assessed. Minimum practice standards, a set of rules of practice, a code of ethics and lists of approved traditional practitioners will need to be developed (Gureje & Alem, 2000). Also, there is very little evidence to support the notion that patients with common mental disorders such as depression and anxiety in LAMI countries seek care from these healers for such problems rather than from orthodox health providers (Gureje & Lasebikan, 2006; Wang *et al*, 2007). The integration of traditional healing methods into the healthcare system is constrained by a lack of knowledge about the scientific bases of traditional practices and a poor evidence base documenting the efficacy and any untoward effects of the interventions provided. Research suggests that the views of traditional healers on the nature and causation of mental illness may be discordant with scientific evidence (Makanjuola, 1987) and that their treatment methods may often be at variance with present-day views about human rights and humane treatment.

## What next?

How can the current situation of primary care mental health in LAMI countries be improved? Large-scale improvements in the integration of mental health with primary care services can occur only with changes in healthcare policies and greater efficiency of health systems. It must be understood that health, including mental health, is a social, economic, political and cultural issue, too. A variety of social determinants – such as poverty, income inequality, gender bias, injustice, exploitation, social exclusion, conflict and violence – play a role in determining the overall health status of individuals and populations (WHO, 2007). Studies have also shown associations between indicators of poverty, in particular low levels of education, and risk of common mental disorders (Patel & Kleinman, 2003). Marmot (2006, p. 2081) has argued that 'failing to meet the fundamental human needs of autonomy, empowerment and human freedom is a potent cause of ill health'. Recent emphasis on inequalities in the health status of populations and a greater understanding of the social determinants of health should pave the way for a shift in the focus of health policies and health delivery back to comprehensive primary healthcare and 'health for all' in LAMI countries (Marmot, 2006; Haines *et al*, 2007; WHO, 2007). Mental health issues should be considered and included in further planning and implementation of MDGs.

A holistic understanding of local mental health problems and needs in each country is essential to develop country- or region-specific priorities of conditions and models of intervention. Since health systems vary widely in their design, inputs, outputs, efficiency and quality across and within countries, the optimal mix of skills and types of health personnel required for effective integration of mental health with primary care in each country or region should be identified. The proportion of GDP that goes on health spending should be increased and sustained in every LAMI country, as evidence shows that higher proportions contribute to smaller treatment gaps in mental health (Wang *et al*, 2007).

All the actors of the health system must be fully informed of mental health issues. Mental health should be introduced into the basic training programmes of doctors and all categories of health personnel. Mental health training should focus on skill acquisition and practical applications rather than on just the theoretical inputs of diagnostic categories and pharmacological management (see also Chapter 25). Primary care personnel require support, supervision and continued on-the-job training. Documentation and longer-term follow-up and evaluation of some of the existing projects will contribute to greater understanding of barriers to better primary care mental health.

# Conclusion

The large unmet need for mental health services in many LAMI countries, despite the availability of effective and relatively affordable interventions (Gureje *et al*, 2007), calls for an urgent effort to scale up primary care service in those countries. Efforts to scale up services must include a comprehensive review of the training provided for primary care providers in the recognition and treatment of mental health problems and a reorganisation of the primary healthcare system. Assumptions made about the relative professional autonomy of the primary healthcare system have led to an unsupported and unmotivated health workforce. A reorganisation

---

Key points

- Health is a comparatively low priority for many LAMI countries.
- The coverage and effectiveness of health services are suboptimal in most developing countries.
- Health systems are consistently inequitable and constrained by a variety of factors, which include low budgets and chronic shortage of adequately motivated and trained staff.
- Resources for mental health in LAMI countries are grossly inadequate and are inequitably and inefficiently spent.
- Pilot projects have established the feasibility of integration of mental health with primary care services; however, rigorous evaluation of such projects is lacking.
- Doctors and healthcare personnel working in primary health centres can be trained to identify and manage mental health problems.
- Traditional healers continue to play a significant role in many LAMI countries. Collaboration with such healers in the delivery of mental health services will have to be carefully planned and developed.

of the primary health system in LAMI countries must recognise the need for an effective secondary care level, with a sufficient number of specialist mental health workers to provide training and support for primary care providers and back-up for difficult cases requiring specialist interventions. Adequate resources are also needed. However, it has been estimated that the investment needed to scale up mental healthcare is not large in absolute terms, when considered at the population level and in comparison with other health sector investments (Chisholm *et al*, 2007*b*). Efforts to integrate mental health effectively into primary care services are unlikely to work until public funded health systems are better resourced and made more effective.

## Further reading and e-resources

Cohen, A., Kleinman, A. & Saraceno, B. (2002) *World Mental Health Casebook: Social and Mental Health Programs in Low-Income Countries*. Kluwer Academic/Plenum Publishers. Provides seven descriptive narratives of mental health-related programmes that were implemented in various countries, including China, India and Nepal.

WHO (2001) *World Health Report 2001. Mental Health: New Understanding, New Hope*. WHO. Highlights the fact that mental health is crucial to the well-being of all individuals, societies and countries. It makes several useful recommendations for the improvement of mental health services all over the world.

Disease Control Priorities Project, http://www.dcp2.org/Home.html – gives valuable information about disease control priorities in LAMI countries including mental health.

Institute of Medicine of the National Academies (USA), http://www.iom.edu/CMS/3783/3957/5469.aspx – provides access to a seminal work entitled 'Neurological, psychiatric and developmental disorders: meeting the challenges in the developing world', which presents a comprehensive plan to help remedy this problem.

WHO's mental health programme, http://www.who.int/mental_health/en – has links to many useful WHO publications, documents and reports, including reports from the Atlas project, which maps mental health resources in the world.

## References

Abas, M., Baingana, F., Broadhead, J., *et al* (2003) Common mental disorders and primary health care: current practice in low-income countries. *Harvard Review of Psychiatry*, **11**, 166–173.

Asian Development Bank (2007) *Inequality in Asia: Key Indicators 2007. Special Chapter Highlights*. Downloadable from http://www.adb.org/Documents/Books/Key_Indicators/2007/pdf/Inequality-in-Asia-Highlights.pdf

Attaran, A. (2005) An immeasurable crisis? A criticism of the Millennium Development Goals and why they cannot be measured. *PLoS Medicine*, **2**(10), e318.

Brown, H. (2007) Great expectations. *BMJ*, **334**, 874–876.

Carstairs, G. M. (1973) Psychiatric problems in developing countries. *British Journal of Psychiatry*, **123**, 271–277.

Chisholm, D., James, S., Sekar, K., *et al* (2000) Integration of mental health care into primary care: demonstration cost-outcome study in India and Pakistan. *British Journal of Psychiatry*, **176**, 581–588.

Chisholm, D., Flisher, A., Lund, C., et al (2007a) Scale up services for mental health: a call for action. Lancet, 370, 1241–1252.

Chisholm, D., Lund, C. & Saxena, S. (2007b) Cost of scaling up mental health care in low and middle income countries. British Journal of Psychiatry, 191, 528–535.

Cohen, A. (2001) The Effectiveness of Mental Health Services in Primary Care: The View from the Developing World. WHO.

Cueto, M. (2004) The origins of primary health care and selective primary health care. American Journal of Public Health, 94, 1864–1874.

Dixon, A., McDaid, D., Knapp, M., et al (2006) Financing mental health services in low- and middle-income countries. Health Policy and Planning, 21, 171–182.

German, G. A. (1972) Aspects of clinical psychiatry in sub-Saharan Africa. British Journal of Psychiatry, 121, 461–479.

Godley, F. (2007) The fight for primary care. BMJ, 335, 532.

Goel, D. S., Agarwal, S. P., Ichhpujani, R. L., et al (2004) Mental health 2003: the Indian scene. In Mental Health: An Indian Perspective (1946–2003) (eds S. P. Agarwal, D. S. Goel, R. N. Salhan, et al), pp. 3–24. Elsevier.

Gureje, O. (2004) What can we learn from a cross-national study of somatic distress? Journal of Psychosomatic Research, 56, 409–412.

Gureje, O. & Alem, A. (2000) Mental health policy in Africa. Bulletin of the World Health Organization, 78, 475–482.

Gureje, O. & Jenkins, R. (2007) Mental health in development: re-emphasising the link. Lancet, 369, 447–449.

Gureje, O. & Lasebikan, V. O. (2006) Use of mental health services in a developing country: results from Nigerian survey of mental health and well-being. Social Psychiatry Psychiatric Epidemiology, 41, 44–49.

Gureje, O., Lasebikan, V. O., Ephraim-Oluwanuga, O., et al (2005) A community study of knowledge of and attitude to mental illness in Nigeria. British Journal of Psychiatry, 186, 436–441.

Gureje, O., Chisholm, D., Kola, L., et al (2007) Cost effectiveness of an essential mental health intervention package in Nigeria. World Psychiatry, 6, 42–48.

Gwatkin, D. R., Bhuiya, A. & Victoria, C. G. (2004) Making health systems more equitable. Lancet, 364, 1273–1280.

Haines, A., Kuruvilla, S. & Borchert, M. (2004) Bridging the implementation gap between knowledge and action for health. Bulletin of the World Health Organization, 82, 724–732.

Haines, A., Horton, R. & Bhutta, Z. (2007) Primary health care comes of age: looking forward to the anniversary of Alma Ata: call for papers. Lancet, 370, 911–913.

Hall, J. J. & Taylor, R. (2003) Health for all beyond 2000: the demise of the Alma-Ata declaration and primary health care in developing countries. Medical Journal of Australia, 178, 17–20.

Hanson, K. & Berman, P. (1998) Private health provision in developing countries: a preliminary analysis of levels of composition. Health Policy and Planning, 13, 195–211.

Harding, T. W., De Arango, M. V., Baltazar, J., et al (1980) Mental disorders in primary health care: a study of their frequency in four developing countries. Psychological Medicine, 10, 231–241.

Hodges, B., Inch, C. & Silver, I. (2001) Improving the psychiatric knowledge, skills and attitudes of primary care physicians, 1950–2000: a review. American Journal of Psychiatry, 150, 1579–1586.

Hyman, S., Chisholm, D., Kessler, R., et al (2006) Mental disorders. In Disease Control in Developing Countries (eds D. T. Jamison, J. G. Breman, A. R. Measham, et al), pp. 605–621. Oxford University Press.

Institute of Medicine (2001) Neurological, Psychiatric and Developmental Disorders: Meeting the Challenges in the Developing World. National Academy Press.

Isaac, M. K., Kapur, R. L., Chjandrashekar, C. R., et al (1982) Mental health delivery through rural primary care: development and evaluation of a pilot training programme. Indian Journal of Psychiatry, 24, 131–138.

Jha, P., Mills, A., Hanson, K., *et al* (2002) Improving the health of the global poor. *Science*, **295**, 2036–2039.

Kohn, R., Saxena, S., Levav, I., *et al* (2004) The treatment gap in mental health care. *Bulletin of the World Health Organization*, **82**, 856–866.

Leon, C. A. (1972) Psychiatry in Latin America. *British Journal of Psychiatry*, **121**, 121–136.

Magnussen, L., Ehiri, J. & Jolly, P. (2004) Comprehensive versus selective primary health care: lessons from global health policy. *Health Affairs*, **23**, 167–176.

Makanjuola, R. O. A. (1987) Yoruba traditional healers in psychiatry. 1. Healers' concepts of the nature and aetiology of mental disorders. *African Journal of Medicine and Medical Sciences*, **16**, 53–59.

Marmot, M. (2006) Health in unequal world. *Lancet*, **368**, 2081–2094.

Mills, A. (2005) Mass campaigns versus general health services: what have we learnt in 40 years about vertical versus horizontal approaches? *Bulletin of the World Health Organization*, **83**, 315–322.

Mills, A., Rasheed, F. & Tollman, S. (2006) Strengthening health systems. In *Disease Control Priorities in Developing Countries* (2nd edition) (eds D. T. Jamison, J. G. Breman, A. R. Measham, *et al*), pp. 87–102. Oxford University Press.

Miranda, J. J. & Patel, V. (2005) Achieving the millennium development goals: does mental health play a role? *PLoS Medicine*, **2**, 962–965.

Neki, J. S. (1973) Psychiatry in South-East Asia. *British Journal of Psychiatry*, **123**, 257–269.

Ngoma, M. C., Prince, M. & Mann, A. (2003) Common mental disorders among those attending primary health clinics and traditional healers in urban Tanzania. *British Journal of Psychiatry*, **183**, 349–355.

Odejide, O. & Morakinyo, J. (2003) Mental health and primary care in Nigeria. *World Psychiatry*, **2**, 164–165.

Organisation for Economic Co-operation and Development (2007) *OECD Health Data 2007*. Downloadable from http://www.oecd.org/dataoecd/46/4/38980557.pdf

Ovuga, E., Boardman, J. & Wasserman, W. (2007) Integrating mental health into primary health care: local initiatives from Uganda. *World Psychiatry*, **6**, 60–61.

Patel, V. & Kleinman, A. (2003) Poverty and common mental disorders in developing countries. *Bulletin of the World Health Organization*, **81**, 609–615.

Patel, V., Saribine, A. P. F. & Soares, I. C. (2007) Prevalence of severe mental and neurological disorders in Mozambique: a population based survey. *Lancet*, **370**, 1055–1060.

Prince, M., Patel, V., Saxena, S., *et al* (2007) No health without mental health. *Lancet*, **370**, 859–877.

Raguram, R., Venkateswaran, A., Ramakrishna J., *et al* (2002) Traditional community resources for mental health: a report of temple healing from India. *BMJ*, **325**, 38–40.

Sachs, J. D. & McArthur, J. W. (2005) The Millennium Project: a plan for meeting the millennium development goals. *Lancet*, **365**, 347–353.

Sartorius, N. & Harding, T. W. (1983) The WHO collaborative study on strategies for extending mental health care, I: the genesis of the study. *American Journal of Psychiatry*, **140**, 1470–1473.

Saxena, S., Sharan, P. & Saraceno, B. (2003) Budget and financing of mental health services: baseline information on 89 countries from AHO's project Atlas. *Journal of Mental Health Policy and Economics*, **6**, 135–143.

Saxena, S., Thornicroft, G. & Knapp, M. (2007) Resources for mental health: scarcity, inequity and inefficiency. *Lancet*, **370**, 878–889.

Simon, G. E., Von Korff, M., Piccinelli, M., *et al* (1999) An international study of the relation between somatic symptoms and depression. *New England Journal of Medicine*, **341**, 1329–1335.

Thara, R., Islam, A. & Padmavati, R. (1998) Beliefs about mental illness: a study of a rural South Indian community. *International Journal of Mental Health*, **27**, 70–85.

Thara, R., Padmavathi, R. & Srinivasan, N. (2004) Focus on psychiatry in India. *British Journal of Psychiatry*, **184**, 366–373.

Travis, P., Bennett, S., Haines, A., *et al* (2004) Overcoming health-systems constraints to achieve the millennium development goals. *Lancet*, **364**, 900–906.

United Nations Development Programme (2006) *Human Development Report 2006*. Downloadable from http://hdr.undp.org/hdr2006/statistics/

United Nations Population Fund (2007) State of the World's Population 2007. Downloadable from http://www.unfpa.org/swp/2007/presskit/pdf/sowp/2007_eng.pdf

Üstün, T. B. & Sartorius, N. (1995) *Mental Illness in General Health Care: An International Study*. Wiley.

Vagero, D. (2007) Health equities across the globe demand new global policies. *Scandinavian Journal of Public Health*, **35**, 113–115.

Walsh, J. A. & Warren, K. S. (1979) Selective primary health care: an interim strategy for disease control in developing countries. *New England Journal of Medicine*, **301**, 967–974.

Wang, P. S., Aguilar-Gaxiola, A., Alomo, J., *et al* (2007) Use of mental health services for anxiety, mood and substance disorders in 17 countries in the WHO world mental health surveys. *Lancet*, **370**, 841 850.

Whitehead, M., Dahlgren, G. & Evans, T. (2001) Equity and health sector reforms: can low-income countries escape the medical poverty trap? *Lancet*, **358**, 833–836.

WHO (1975) *Organization of Mental Health Services in Developing Countries*. Technical Report Series 564. WHO.

WHO (1978) *Declaration of Alma-Ata*. WHO. Downloadable from http://www.who.int/hpr/NPH/docs/declaration_almaata.pdf

WHO (1990) *The Introduction of a Primary Care Component into Primary Health Care*. WHO.

WHO (1998) *Mental Disorders in Primary Care: A WHO Education Package*. WHO.

WHO (2001a) *The World Health Report 2001. Mental Health: New Understanding, New Hope*. WHO.

WHO (2001b) *Commission on Macroeconomics and Health: Investing in Health for Economic Development*. WHO.

WHO (2005) *Mental Health Atlas*. WHO.

WHO (2007) *Achieving Health Equity: From Root Causes to Fair Outcomes*. Commission on Social Determinants of Health, Interim Statement. WHO.

WHO (2008) *The World Health Report 2008. Primary Health Care: Now More Than Ever*. WHO.

World Bank (1993) *World Development Report 1993: Investing in Health*. Oxford University Press.

World Bank (2006) *Classification of World Bank Member Countries*. Downloadable at www.worldbank.org/data/countryclass/classgroups.htm.

# CHAPTER 7

# Diagnosis and classification of mental illness: a view from primary care

Linda Gask, Christopher Dowrick, Michael Klinkman and Oye Gureje

Summary

This chapter considers the nature of 'mental illness' before it moves on to review the problems with existing concepts of classification of mental illness when they are applied to the primary care setting. It considers the shortcomings in some detail before conclusions are drawn concerning what a diagnostic system should provide to have both validity and utility in primary care settings.

Differences between mental health and illness, and what is considered normal and abnormal in psychological terms, are perhaps not so easily determined in mental healthcare as in physical medicine. The term 'mental illness' is generally used in psychiatry when a clear syndrome can be identified *and* there has been a definite change from how the person used to be (which is important in differentiating illness from 'personality disorder', which is not viewed as 'illness') *and* there is a deterioration in the person's ability to function effectively. Dependence on alcohol or drugs is similarly not viewed as being mental illness but, again, mental health services are involved in treatment in order to attempt to relieve suffering, as experienced by either the persons themselves or those around them. Various different models of mental illness and health exist (Table 7.1). The biological perspective is often that to which a medically trained individual can particularly contribute. However, the psychological, social and spiritual perspectives are equally important in fully understanding the causes of a person's problems, what investigations to carry out and what treatment is required.

Diagnosis was, in the past, considered within psychiatry to be useful only if it conferred some utility, such as being able to predict what treatment would be indicated or predict response to treatment or prognosis (Kendell, 1975). In practice, categorical diagnoses continue to have practical utility in making simple treatment decisions, but they also have their limitations. In

**Table 7.1** Models of mental illness and mental healthcare

| | Biological | Psychological | | Social | | | Spiritual |
|---|---|---|---|---|---|---|---|
| | | Psychodynamic | Cognitive–behavioural | Stress models | Family models | Conspiratorial | |
| Influences | Strongly supported by doctors/nurses; some support from carers | Remains a powerful model in lay terms though 'out of fashion' in healthcare provision | Powerful model in psychology and current mental health policy | Influential in thinking of social workers and in primary care | Influences social work, child and family work and primary care | Survivor groups, radical professionals and anti-psychiatrists | Religious belief |
| Causal models | Physical changes in brain | Early experiences | Inappropriate learning, poor coping skills | Social and cultural stress | Whole family is 'sick' and person acts in response to family pressures | Myth of mental illness – result of the way a person is expected to behave by others | Variety of spiritual theories, reflecting culture/religion |
| Treatment models | Drugs, electro-convulsive therapy | Psychodynamic psychotherapy – one-to-one and group | Cognitive–behavioural therapy, behavioural therapy, social skills training | Social change and interventions | Family therapy | None – empower and advocate for person who is labelled as mentally ill | Faith-based therapies, retreat and meditation |
| Rights and duties of client/ patient | Right to sick role but must cooperate | Responsible – but spared moral judgement | Responsible – with contract to cooperate | Right to help but must cooperate | Whole family duty to participate | Right to privacy and same rights as others | Obligation depends on personal faith |

Adapted from Colombo *et al* (2003).

recent years, the need for more standardised approaches to diagnosis, driven by both research and billing requirements in some healthcare systems, has resulted in classification systems encompassing an ever-increasing variety of human experiences; for example, 'tobacco use disorder' and 'pre-menstrual dysphoric disorder' (PMDD) both appear in the US classification DSM–IV (the fourth edition of the *Diagnostic and Statistical Manual* of the American Psychiatric Association, 1995). Outside the USA, the World Health Organization's *International Classification of Diseases* (in its 10 revision, ICD–10, World Health Organization, 1992) is more generally used, and in some countries (notably the Netherlands, Belgium and Denmark) its *International Classification of Primary Care* (ICPC) is used in the primary healthcare setting (in its second revision, ICPC–2, World Health Organization, 2003). While the ICD and DSM have some notable differences, their criteria for specific diagnoses such as major depressive disorder (MDD) are quite similar. The criteria listed for diagnosis of 'depressive disorder' in the ICPC reflects a broader, primary care view of depression, with fewer specific criteria (Table 7.2).

# Mad or bad? The problem of personality disorder

People with lifelong personality difficulties are not viewed as suffering from mental illness. However, this does not mean that mental health services should not be involved in trying to help them. Abnormal personality traits are common in the community and some confer considerable advantages on those who demonstrate them. Many people will have both abnormal personality traits and mental illness, and the former may result in both their being more impaired by their symptoms and slower recovery, as they may

**Table 7.2** Comparison of the diagnostic criteria for depression across three classifications: DSM–IV (major depressive disorder), ICD–10 (major depressive disorder) and ICPC–2 (depressive disorder)

| Symptoms of depression | DSM–IV | ICD–10 | ICPC–2 |
| --- | --- | --- | --- |
| 1 Depressed mood | + | + | + |
| 2 Markedly diminished interest or pleasure in activities | + | + | + |
| 3 Loss of energy or fatigue | + | + | + |
| 4 Loss of confidence or self-esteem | – | + | + |
| 5 Unreasonable self-reproach or guilt | + | + | – |
| 6 Recurrent thoughts of death or suicide, or any suicidal behaviour | + | + | – |
| 7 Diminished ability to think or concentrate, or indecisiveness | + | + | + |
| 8 Psychomotor agitation or retardation | + | + | – |
| 9 Insomnia or hypersomnia | + | + | + |
| 10 Change in appetite | + | + | + |

lack the necessary social support required. Problems come with those with very severe personality disorders, who in lay terms may appear to be 'mad', as what they do is beyond the realms of normal human understanding, but they do not have symptoms of a specific mental illness that is treatable. In an increasingly risk-averse society, mental health professionals are under pressure to be involved in detaining such people under mental law *before* they commit a crime. This poses considerable threats to civil liberty and problems for already overcrowded hospital services, and is unlikely to be particularly cost-effective in terms of the number of people who would need to be detained to prevent a single crime.

# Diagnosis and classification of mental health problems in primary care

Patients in primary care settings are much less likely to present with clearly identifiable diagnostic syndromes. People present with a wide variety of symptoms, concerns, worries and problems. These are not only undifferentiated, as originally described by Balint (1964), but also, crucially, at least at first presentation, unrehearsed by prior discussion with doctors versed in the agenda and language of diagnosis. Primary care clinicians will often encounter unfiltered and unrecognised symptoms that may or may not be identifiable as mental health syndromes, while specialist mental health clinicians will encounter filtered symptoms that are recognised and understood as representative of a mental health problem.

Thus, diagnosis is a less precise (and less frequent) activity in primary care than it is in specialist care. Family doctors are more likely to think in terms of problems than diagnoses. They are more likely to make a diagnosis of depression if they believe they can manage and treat it; that is, diagnosis tends to follow management decisions, not precede them (Dowrick *et al*, 2000). In particular, family doctors and patients may see making and accepting a mental health diagnosis as a social and moral decision. Women with depression, for example, may seek and accept help (e.g. medication) for the sake of others, when they feel they are not adequately fulfilling their social roles. Doctors may offer diagnosis and treatment in order to demonstrate that they are taking their patient's suffering seriously, despite considering that their problems are primarily social in origin (Maxwell, 2005).

Current classification systems are generally based upon research and experience in psychiatric settings. There is mounting evidence that there are indeed important differences between patients seen in primary care and specialty mental health settings. Patients who present with emotional symptoms in primary care are generally less distressed, are less likely to have a discernible mental disorder and are less impaired than are psychiatric cohorts within secondary care (Zinsbarg *et al*, 1994; Coyne *et al*, 1997).

**91**

## Distress versus disorder

Emotional distress can be present in patients for many reasons other than the presence of a mental health disorder, and patients with threshold disorders may not display any distress. Many primary care patients are clearly distressed, but do not exhibit other symptoms of mental illness (Katerndahl et al, 2005) – yet primary care physicians often recognise this distress and manage these patients differently from those without distress. They do so without guidance from most existing classification systems, which (with one or two exceptions – see below) do not account for 'distress'.

## The relationship between physical, mental and social problems

Primary care patients frequently present a mixture of psychological, physical and social problems. Mental health problems occur more frequently in those with common chronic physical illness, such as diabetes, chronic obstructive pulmonary disease and heart disease, and their comorbid mental health problems may not be recognised, as attention is focused on their physical illness. One of the most important aspects of a classification of mental disorders for primary care is that it should enable primary care workers accurately to record core elements of the context of care, such as life events, undifferentiated symptoms, and patient perceptions, goals and preferences for care; this will in turn allow clinicians more effectively to help patients with 'mixed' physical, mental and social suffering. The traditional biomedical model, which still dominates the training pattern of health professionals, makes it difficult for them to deal with these patients, as there is often not a specific problem that can be solved.

## Transient, recurrent or chronic symptoms

When primary care patients meet diagnostic criteria for specific disorders, their symptoms often fluctuate over time and their 'caseness' may be transient. Nosological diagnoses (nosology is the term in medicine that refers to classification of disease) have been demonstrated to last less than 4 weeks 30% of the time and less than 6 months 65% of the time (Lamberts & Hofmans-Okkes, 1993). There is an absence of good research on the long-term validity and prognosis of 'threshold' mental health diagnoses in primary care patient samples. Community-based epidemiological studies have confirmed that many patients have recurrent or chronic depression (Judd et al, 1998; Gask, 2005; Kessler et al, 2005), but the relative risk of recurrence or of developing chronic depression, and the level of disability associated with these potential outcomes are not clear (Van Weel-Baumgarten et al, 1999; Vuorilehto et al, 2005).

The fluctuating nature of symptoms has made it difficult to assess the performance of primary care workers in recognising and treating mental health problems. Recognition of their potential long-term impact on health and function has led to aggressive case-finding and treatment efforts in primary care settings to prevent disability. Although primary care workers have frequently been criticised for their lack of skill in recognising threshold mental disorders, recognition in primary care is itself a complex phenomenon, related in part to the transience of symptoms. Higher rates of detection (and treatment) have been found for patients with more severe symptoms and higher levels of disability (Dowrick & Buchan, 1995; Thompson *et al*, 2001; MaGPIe Research Group, 2003) and there is some evidence that short-term outcomes for 'detected' and 'undetected' depression in primary care do not differ (Coyne *et al*, 1997).

# How valid are existing diagnostic systems for application in primary care?

There are a number of ways in which existing diagnostic systems may have limited validity when applied in primary care settings.

## *The problem of comorbidity*

Overlapping psychopathology may exist along a spectrum of anxiety (Fig. 7.1), depression, somatisation and substance misuse in primary care. This coexistence may be cross-sectional, in that all these symptoms appear together at the same time, or it may be longitudinal, in the sense that one set of symptoms is followed closely in time by another (Katerndahl, 2005). Much of the evidence regarding comorbidity was assembled during

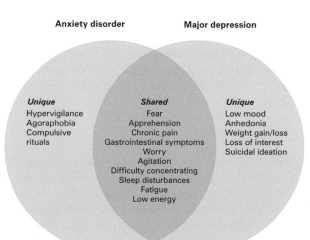

**Fig. 7.1** Symptom overlap between anxiety and depression. Derived from Baldwin *et al* (2002).

the 1990s in the WHO Collaborative Study of Psychological Problems in General Healthcare (Üstün & Sartorius, 1995), conducted in 15 centres in Asia, Africa, Europe and the Americas (see Chapter 2). Consecutive primary care attendees between the age of majority (typically 18 years) and 65 years were screened (n = 25 916) and stratified random samples interviewed (n = 5438). The study found that 'well-defined' psychological problems (according to ICD–10) are frequent in general healthcare settings (median 24% of attendees) and among the most common were depression, anxiety, alcohol misuse, somatoform disorders and neurasthenia. The most common co-occurrence was depression and anxiety (Sartorius et al, 1996).

Medically unexplained symptoms pose a particular problem. There is now considerable empirical evidence suggesting that persistent medically unexplained symptoms frequently coexist with mood or anxiety disorders in primary care settings (Kirmayer & Robbins, 1991; Kessler et al, 1996; Garcia-Campayo et al, 1998; Toft et al, 2005). In Toft et al's study in Denmark, comorbidity was highest for anxiety disorders – 89% of these patients had another diagnosis – but lowest for somatoform disorders (39%). The concept of somatisation is difficult because of the finding by Simon & Gureje (1999) that the majority of these symptoms (61%) will not be recalled as a problem a year later.

Substance misuse may also commonly coexist with anxiety and depression. A study by the MaGPIe Research Group (2003) in New Zealand revealed that more than one-third of people attending their general practitioner (GP) had had a diagnosable mental disorder during the previous 12 months. The most common disorders identified by accepted and well-validated psychological instruments were anxiety disorders, depression, and substance-use disorders, and there was high comorbidity of these three groups, with the experience of mixed pictures as common as disorders occurring alone.

Do all these findings constitute evidence of true comorbidity (i.e. coexistence of two or more discrete disorders), or rather an overlap between – and therefore confusion of – diagnostic categories? We consider the latter far more likely.

## Subthreshold disorders

Subthreshold conditions (i.e. conditions meeting some but not all diagnostic criteria for a specific disorder in DSM–IV or ICD–10) are prevalent and associated with significant costs and disability. Pincus et al (1999) have shown how varying conceptualisations have been applied to define these conditions. Considerable attention was paid to the presence of sub-threshold disorders in the WHO study, where it was noted that roughly 9% of patients suffered from a 'subthreshold condition' that did not meet diagnostic criteria but led to clinically significant symptoms and functional impairment (Üstün & Sartorius 1995).

## Cross-cultural application of systems

The complete DSM–IV and ICD–10 classifications in current use are the direct descendants of clinical and research diagnostic classifications developed in the USA and Western Europe. As such, they are based upon a Western conceptual framework of mental health and mental illness, and it is highly likely that some of their diagnostic categories will have limited validity in other parts of the world. It is also highly likely that some conditions important in other, non-Western cultures will have limited or inaccurate representation in DSM or ICD (Mezzich *et al*, 1999). This issue may be of particular relevance in cross-cultural primary care settings.

# Classification systems developed or modified for use in primary care

Three classifications are in current use for mental health diagnosis in primary care: DSM–IV–PC, ICD–10–PHC and ICPC. Both DSM–IV–PC and ICD–10–PHC are simplified versions of the 'full' classification intended to be more accessible to primary care clinicians. However, the extent to which these systems have been adopted in *routine* data collection within primary care and monitoring across the world is unclear, although ICD–10–PHC has been widely disseminated. In contrast, ICPC was developed specifically for use in the primary healthcare setting. Translation between the three systems is possible but complex, and clinical comparability of the same diagnosis in different systems is limited by the characteristics of the different systems (Lamberts *et al*, 1998).

## ICD–10–PHC

The primary care version of ICD–10's Chapter 5 (mental and behavioural disorders) was published first in 1995 (Üstün *et al*, 1995) and was finalised after a series of field trials in different countries (Jenkins *et al*, 2002). It is now the most widely used system for the diagnosis of mental health problems in primary care, although it has a range of uses and can be used as much for education and training as for data collection and coding. The classification bears a rough correspondence to ICD–10 categories, is user friendly, is based upon the different types of management that the various conditions require and includes detailed advice about the sort of psychological help that has been shown to be effective; it also provides the information about each disorder that should be given to the patient and family. Advice is given about drug treatments, where these are indicated, as well as features that require specialist referral. The system consists of 25 conditions (Box 7.1) that are common in primary care settings, but each country is encouraged to adapt the system to its own needs.

This classification was field tested in 30 different centres in 19 countries and published evidence is available from two large studies (Goldberg *et*

**Box 7.1** The 25 ICD–10–PHC disorders

The 25 included disorders, along with their full ICD–10 codes, are as follows:

**Addictive disorders**
1 Alcohol use disorder (F 10)
2 Drug use disorder (F 11)
3 Tobacco use disorder (F 17.1)

**Common mental disorders**
4 Depression (F 32)
5 Phobic disorders (F 40)
6 Panic disorders (F 41.0)
7 Generalised anxiety (F 41.1)
8 Mixed anxiety depression (F 41.2)
9 Adjustment disorder (F 43)
10 Dissociative disorder (conversion hysteria) (F 44)
11 Unexplained somatic complaints (F 45)
12 Neurasthenia (F 48.0)
13 Eating disorders (F 50)
14 Sleep problems (F 51)
15 Sexual disorders (F 52)
16 Bereavement (Z 63)

**Organic disorders**
17 Dementia (F 00)
18 Delirium (F 05)

**Psychotic disorders**
19 Chronic psychotic disorders (F 20)
20 Acute psychotic disorders (F 23)
21 Bipolar disorders (F 3)

**Disorders of childhood**
22 Mental retardation (F 70)
23 Hyperkinetic (attention deficit) disorder (F 90)
24 Conduct disorder (F 91)
25 Enuresis (F 98.0)

For multi-purpose health workers, an even simpler version is available, which consists of the following six categories:

26 Cognitive disorders
27 Alcohol and drug use disorder
28 Psychotic disorders
29 Depression
30 Anxiety disorders
31 Unexplained somatic complaints

*al*, 1995; D'A Busnello *et al*, 1999). In the UK study, a total of 478 GPs completed all stages of the study. Nearly all the participating GPs found the classification 'very useful' or 'useful'. Each category was also rated and most received high ratings; those that were criticised were amended by the group at a later meeting.

In the UK, the classification has been modified since the original publication, and the whole system has been re-issued twice, with a number of additional features, including information leaflets for the patient and information about voluntary agencies (see e-resources at the end of the chapter). ICD–10–PHC is simple and easy to use, and links diagnosis to treatment. However, it does not address issues of measurement of severity, associated disability or chronicity, or the accompanying social problems manifest in primary care settings. It is also important to note that simply disseminating guidelines developed from ICD–10–PHC did not improve outcomes in a British primary care study (Upton *et al*, 1999).

## DSM–IV–PC

The primary care adaptation of DSM–IV was introduced in 1995 and contains a number of symptom-based clinical algorithms designed to guide the primary care physician through the diagnostic process (American Psychiatric Association, 1995).

A number of limitations are evident (Pingitore & Sansone, 1998). It is a large and complex volume that requires some level of familiarity before it can be used. The complexity of the diagnostic schemes, and the amount of time needed to reach a diagnosis, have been cited as conspicuous limitations.

## ICPC

The *International Classification of Primary Care* (ICPC), first published in 1987 under the auspices of Wonca (the World Organization of Family Doctors) and now in its second edition (International Classification Committee of Wonca, 1998), represents a departure from the two classifications described above. ICPC was designed to capture and code three essential elements of each clinical encounter: the patient's *reason for encounter*, the clinician's *diagnosis*, and the (diagnostic and therapeutic) *interventions*, all organised in an *episode of care* data structure that links initial to all subsequent encounters for the same clinical problem. This approach permits coding of 95% or more of primary care visits and enables the calculation of prior and posterior probabilities for important diseases (Okkes *et al*, 2002).

Although the limited diagnostic specificity available in ICPC is problematic, ICPC offers a major advantage in its more complete capture of the context of mental health problems (Box 7.2). The episode structure of ICPC automatically accommodates mental health and biomedical comorbidity by simply noting all active problems at a point in time or over a specified time interval. The inclusion of symptoms as reasons for encounter at the beginning of a longitudinal data stream enables investigation of the relationship between somatic symptoms and mental health disorders at a level of resolution not possible when using other classifications. The routine coding of social problems provides detail about the social context in which mental heath problems occur that is not available anywhere else. Pilot studies to embed codes for additional context elements, such as

**Box 7.2** ICPC–2 diagnostic terms in Chapter P (Psychosocial)

Note: P01 to P29 can be recorded as symptoms or diagnoses. P70 to P99 are diagnostic terms. Each term has a definition as well as inclusion and exclusion criteria.

P01 feeling anxious/nervous/tense
P02 acute stress reaction
P03 feeling depressed
P04 feeling/behaving irritable/angry
P05 senility, feeling/behaving old
P06 sleep disturbance
P07 sexual desire reduced
P08 sexual fulfilment reduced
P09 sexual preference concern
P10 stammering, stuttering, tics
P11 eating problems in children
P12 bed-wetting, enuresis
P13 encopresis/bowel training problem
P15 chronic alcohol abuse
P16 acute alcohol abuse
P17 tobacco abuse
P18 medication abuse
P19 drug abuse
P20 memory disturbance
P22 child behaviour symptom/complaint
P23 adolescent behaviour symptom/complaint
P24 specific learning problem
P25 phase of life problems in adults
P27 fear of mental disorder
P28 limited function/disability psychosocial
P29 psychological symptom/complaint, other

P70 dementia
P71 organic psychosis, other
P72 schizophrenia
P73 affective psychosis
P74 anxiety disorder/anxiety state
P75 somatisation disorder
P76 depressive disorder
P77 suicide/suicide attempt
P78 neurasthenia, surmenage
P79 phobia, compulsive disorder
P80 personality disorder
P81 hyperkinetic disorder
P82 post-traumatic stress disorder
P85 mental retardation
P86 anorexia nervosa, bulimia
P98 psychosis not otherwise specified/other
P99 psychological disorder, other

severity of illness and disability, into ICPC have been completed (Parkerson *et al*, 1996).

# Tools developed for primary care

Four types of tools used as *aids to diagnosis* in primary care are briefly reviewed here: interview schedules designed for use in primary care; screening tools; and tools for the measurement of severity and of disability.

## *Interview schedules*

Interview schedules have primarily been used for research purposes. The exception is the PRIME–MD, which has been widely used across the world and generates DSM–IV diagnoses (Spitzer *et al*, 1994). However, it remains unclear to what extent such a formal schedule might be adopted into routine primary care consultations, particularly in low- and middle-income countries, given the very brief time available in the primary care consultation (see Chapter 6).

## *Screening tools*

Screening instruments have also been widely used in research. The best-known is the General Health Questionnaire (GHQ; Goldberg & Williams, 1988), available in four versions (comprising 12, 28, 30 or 60 items) and translated into numerous languages. The GHQ is non-specific and does not provide specific diagnoses, unlike the Hospital Anxiety and Depression Scale (HAD; Zigmond & Snaith 1983) or the self-completion measures derived from PRIME–MD, the original comprehensive Patient Health Questionnaire (PHQ; Spitzer *et al*, 1999) and the depression-specific PHQ-9 (Kroenke *et al*, 2001), the Generalised Anxiety Disorder Scale (GAD-7; Spitzer *et al*, 2006) and the PHQ-15 for severity of somatic symptoms (Kroenke *et al*, 2002).

However, although a variety of other tools have been developed for screening, there is considerable disagreement in the literature about whether screening is of benefit in improving the psychosocial outcomes of those with psychiatric disorder managed in non-psychiatric settings (Gilbody *et al*, 2001). A brief screening tool consisting of only two written screening questions, plus the addition of a question enquiring whether help is needed, which can be completed in the waiting room and handed directly to the primary care worker (or the questions can be asked directly), has recently shown promising results in terms of diagnostic validity (Arroll *et al*, 2005). But, as some studies in Brazil have demonstrated, self-answered questionnaires in low-income countries usually have to be read by an interviewer, even for research purposes, as a significant proportion of the patients attending primary care units are only semi-literate (Mari & Williams, 1985)

## Measuring severity

Screening questionnaires can also be used to measure the severity of symptoms. The PHQ has been widely used for this purpose in depression. Other tools include the Inventory to Diagnose Depression (Zimmerman et al, 1986), the Primary Care Screener for Affective Disorder (PC-SAD) (Rogers et al, 2002), and the 21-item major depressive disorder (MDD) subscale of the Psychiatric Diagnostic Screening Questionnaire (PDSQ; Zimmerman & Mattia, 2001). All perform as well as the Beck Depression Inventory (Rogers et al, 2005), although most of these have not been validated for use in countries other than the USA or in languages other than English. Measurement of severity has been introduced in the UK through the Quality Outcomes Framework (QOF) in primary care, which has enabled assessment of severity to be directly linked to treatment guidelines for depression recommended by the National Institute for Health and Clinical Excellence (NICE).

## Measuring impairment and disability

A 'clinical significance' criterion is a part of many DSM diagnoses, generally expressed in terms of functional impairment. In contrast, an explicit attempt has been made to separate functional impairment from diagnostic criteria in ICD. There has been a working assumption that increasing severity of disorders is directly associated with increasing disability and hence with worse outcomes.[1] However, there are two problems with this assumption. The first, as noted above, is that it tends to play down the considerable levels of impairment experienced by people with subthreshold disorders. The second is that severity and impairment may not after all be directly associated, but may rather form separate but overlapping domains. Research by Foley et al (2003) on the Virginia twin register found that, while the risk factors for major depression and associated functional impairment were substantially correlated, they were not identical. The most parsimonious model suggests that over a quarter of the variance in associated functional impairment was due to factors unrelated to risk of major depression.

This is potentially important in primary care. Family doctors are probably better at assessing impairment than at making formal psychiatric diagnoses. If impairment is indeed a separate problem from diagnosis, then awareness of and emphasis on this difference may well play to the strengths of primary care.

Disability in relation to depression has commonly been measured using the Sheehan Disability Scale (Sheehan, 1983), a three-item self-

---

1 Note that disability differs from impairment: disability is the functional consequence of impairment and the relationship between them is open to debate in the mental health arena (Mulvany, 2000).

report scale measuring the severity of disability in the domains of work, family life/home responsibilities and social/leisure activities. The Social Functioning Questionnaire (SFQ), an eight-item self-report scale (score range 0–24), was developed from the Social Functioning Schedule (SFS), a semi-structured interview that has been used primarily with non-psychotic patients and that has good test–retest and inter-rater reliability as well as construct validity (Tyrer *et al*, 2005).

The World Health Organization Disability Assessment Schedule (WHO–DAS II) is a brief instrument which comes in a variety of versions for rating by observer, self or caregiver (see e-resources). The WHO–DAS has been largely supplanted by the new International Classification of Functioning, Disability, and Health (ICF) (see e-resources), now available for use worldwide.

# Conclusion

Existing classification systems are unsatisfactory for primary care. Most have been *adapted for*, rather than *developed in*, primary care settings; the exception is ICPC. In general, they do not capture the complexity of psychological disorder as it manifests in primary care settings, with associated physical illness and social problems. Revision of both ICD and DSM is currently underway, and there is a strong desire for a simpler classification for use in primary care than in specialist settings, one that will prove to be clinically useful.

A classification system for primary care should: be characterised by simplicity; address *not only* categorical diagnosis, but also severity and chronicity; be linked to disability assessment; be linked to routine data-gathering, including gathering information on outcomes; be linked to training; and be useful in facilitating communication between primary and specialist care.

---

Key points

- There are a number of different 'models of mental illness'.
- Primary care patients frequently present a mixture of psychological, physical and social problems.
- Patients in primary care settings are much less likely to present with clearly identifiable diagnostic syndromes.
- There are a number of ways in which existing diagnostic systems may have limited validity when applied in primary care settings. Specifically, they do not address in a satisfactory way the problems of comorbidity; subthreshold disorders; cross-cultural applications; or the differences between severity and impairment/disability. A satisfactory diagnostic system for primary care needs to address all these factors.

# Further reading and e-resources

ICPC (2nd edn) http://www.who.int/classifications/icd/adaptations/icpc2/en/index. html

International Classification of Functioning, Disability, and Health (ICF), http://www. who.int/classifications/icf/site/icftemplate.cfm

UK version of ICD–10PC, http://www.mentalneurologicalprimarycare.org

World Health Organization Disability Assessment Schedule (WHO–DAS II), http://www. who.int/icidh/whodas/index.html

# References

American Psychiatric Association (1995) *Diagnostic and Statistical Manual of Mental Disorders (4th edition), Primary Care Version*. APA.

Arroll, B., Goodyear-Smith, F., Kerse N., *et al* (2005) Effect of the addition of a 'help' question to two screening questions on specificity for diagnosis of depression in general practice: diagnostic validity study. *BMJ*, **331**, 884–886.

Baldwin, D. S., Evans, D. L., Hirschfeld, R. M., *et al* (2002) Can we distinguish anxiety from depression? *Psychopharmacology Bulletin*, **36** (suppl. 2), 158–165.

Balint, M. (1964) *The Doctor, His Patient and the Illness*. Pitman.

Colombo, A., Bendelow, G., Fulford, B., *et al* (2003) Evaluating the influence of implicit models of mental disorder on processes of shared decision making within community-based multi-disciplinary teams. *Social Science and Medicine*, **56**, 1557–1570.

Coyne, J. C., Klinkman, M. S., Gallo, S. M., *et al* (1997) Short-term outcomes of detected and undetected depressed primary care patients and depressed psychiatric patients. *General Hospital Psychiatry*, **19**, 333–343.

D'A Busnello, E., Tannous, L., Gigante, L., *et al* (1999) Diagnostic reliability of mental disorders of the International Classification of Diseases – primary care. *Rev Saúde Pública*, **33**, 487–494.

Dowrick, C. & Buchan, I. (1995) Twelve month outcome of depression in general practice: does detection or disclosure make a difference? *BMJ*, **311**, 1274–1276.

Dowrick, C., Gask, L., Perry, R., *et al* (2000) Do general practitioners' attitudes towards the management of depression predict their clinical behaviour? *Psychological Medicine*, **30**, 413–419.

Foley, D., Neale, M. C., Gardner, C. O., *et al* (2003) Major depression and associated impairment: same or different genetic and environmental risk factors? *American Journal of Psychiatry*, **160**, 2128–2133.

Garcia-Campayo, J., Lobo, A., Perez-Echeverria, M. J., *et al* (1998) Three forms of somatisation presenting in primary care settings in Spain. *Journal of Nervous and Mental Disease*, **186**, 554–560.

Gask, L. (2005) Is depression a chronic illness? *Chronic Illness*, **1**, 101–106.

Gilbody, S. M., House, A. O. & Sheldon, T. A. (2001) Routinely administered questionnaires for depression and anxiety: systematic review. *BMJ*, **322**, 406–409.

Goldberg, D. & Williams, P. (1988) *A User's Guide to the General Health Questionnaire*. NFER-Nelson.

Goldberg, D., Sharp, D. & Nanayakkara, K. (1995) The field trial of the mental disorders section of ICD–10 designed for primary care (ICD10–PHC) in England. *Family Practice*, **12**, 466–473.

International Classification Committee of Wonca (1998) *ICPC–2: International Classification of Primary Care* (2nd edn). Oxford University Press.

Jenkins, R., Goldberg, D., Kiima, D., *et al* (2002) Classification in primary care: experience with current diagnostic systems. *Psychopathology*, **35**, 127–131.

Judd, L. L., Akiskal, H. S., Maser, J. D., *et al* (1998) A prospective 12-year study of subsyndromal and syndromal depressive symptoms in unipolar major depressive disorders. *Archives of General Psychiatry*, **55**, 694–700.

Katerndahl, D. (2005) Variations on a theme: the spectrum of anxiety disorders and problems with DSM classification in primary care settings. In New Research on the Psychology of Fear (ed. P. Gower), pp. 181–221. NovaScience Publishers.

Katerndahl, D., Larne, A. C., Palmer, R. F., et al (2005) Reflections on DSM classification and its utility in primary care: case studies in 'mental disorders'. Primary Care Companion Journal of Clinical Psychiatry, 7, 91–99.

Kendell, R. (1975) The Role of Diagnosis in Psychiatry. Blackwell.

Kessler, R. C., Nelson, C. B., McGonagle, K. A., et al (1996) Comorbidity of DSM–III–R major depressive disorder in the general population: results from the US National Comorbidity Survey. British Journal of Psychiatry, 168 (suppl. 30), 17–30.

Kessler, R. C., Berglund, P., Demler, O., et al (2005) Lifetime prevalence and age-of-onset distributions of DSM–IV disorders in the National Comorbidity Survey replication. Archives of General Psychiatry, 62, 593–602.

Kirmayer, L. J. & Robbins, J. M. (1991) Three forms of somatization in primary care: prevalence, co-occurrence and socio-demographic characteristics. Journal of Nervous and Mental Disease, 179, 647–655.

Kroenke, K., Spitzer, M. & Williams, J. B. (2001) The PHQ-9: validity of a brief depression severity measure. Journal of General Internal Medicine, 16, 606–613.

Kroenke, K., Spitzer, M. & Williams, J. B. (2002) The PHQ-15: validity of a new measure for evaluating the severity of somatic symptoms. Psychosomatic Medicine, 64, 258–266.

Lamberts, H. & Hofmans-Okkes, I. M. (1993) Classification of psychological and social problems in general practice. Huisarts Wet, 36, 5–13.

Lamberts, H., Magruder, K., Katholm R. G., et al (1998) International classification of mental disorders in primary care: a guide through a difficult terrain. International Journal of Psychiatry and Medicine, 28, 159–76.

MaGPIe Research Group (2003) The nature and prevalence of psychological problems in New Zealand primary healthcare: a report on Mental Health and General Practice Investigation (MaGPIe). Journal of the New Zealand Medical Association, 116, u379. Downloadable from http://www.nzma.org.nz/journal/116-1171/379/

Mari, J. J. & Williams, P. (1985) A comparison of the validity of two psychiatric screening questionnaires (GHQ-12 and SRQ-20) in Brazil using relative operating characteristic (ROC) analysis. Psychological Medicine, 15, 651–659.

Maxwell, M. (2005) Women's and doctors' accounts of their experiences of depression in primary care: the influence of social and moral reasoning on patients' and doctors' decisions. Chronic Illness, 1, 61–71.

Mezzich, J. E., Kirmayer, L. J., Kleinman, A., et al (1999) The place of culture in DSM–IV. Journal of Nervous and Mental Diseases, 187, 457–464.

Mulvany, J. (2000) Disability, impairment or illness? The relevance of the social model of disability to the study of mental disorder. Sociology of Health and Illness, 22, 582–681.

Okkes, I., Oskam, S. K. & Lamberts, H. (2002) The probability of specific diagnoses for patients presenting with common symptoms to Dutch family physicians. Journal of Family Practice, 51, 31–36.

Parkerson, G. R., Bridges-Webb, C., Gervas, J., et al (1996) Classification of severity of health problems in family/general practice: an international field trial. Family Practice, 13, 303–309.

Pincus, H. A., Davis, W. W. & McQueen, L. E. (1999) 'Subthreshold' mental disorders. A review and synthesis of studies on minor depression and other 'brand names'. British Journal of Psychiatry, 174, 288–296.

Pingitore, D. A. & Sansone, R. A. (1998) Using DSM–IV Primary Care Version: a guide to psychiatric diagnosis in primary care. American Family Physician, 58, 1447–1452.

Rogers, W. H., Wilson, I. B., Bungay, K. M., et al (2002) Assessing the performance of a new depression screener for primary care (PC-SAD©). Journal of Clinical Epidemiology, 55, 164–175.

Rogers, W. H., Adler, D. A., Bungay, K. M., *et al* (2005) Depression screening instruments made good severity measures in a cross-sectional analysis. *Journal of Clinical Epidemiology*, **58**, 370–377.

Sartorius, N., Üstün, T. B. & Lecrubier, Y., *et al* (1996) Depression comorbid with anxiety: results from the WHO study on psychological disorders in primary health care. *British Journal of Psychiatry*, suppl. 30, 38–43.

Sheehan, D. V. (1983) *The Anxiety Disease*. Scribner.

Simon, G. & Gureje, O. (1999) Stability of somatization disorder and somatization symptoms among primary care patients. *Archives of General Psychiatry*, **56**, 90–95.

Spitzer, R. L., Kroenke, K. & Williams, J. B. (1999) Validation and utility of a self-report version of PRIME-MD: the PHQ primary care study. *JAMA*, **282**, 1737–1744.

Spitzer, R. L., Kroenke, K., Williams, J. B., *et al* (2006) A brief measure for assessing generalized anxiety disorder: the GAD-7. *Annals of Internal Medicine*, **166**, 1092–1097.

Thompson, C., Ostler, K., Peveler, R. C., *et al* (2001) Dimensional perspective on the recognition of depressive symptoms in primary care. *British Journal of Psychiatry*, **179**, 317–323.

Toft, T., Fink, P., Oernboel, E., *et al* (2005) Mental disorders in primary care: prevalence and co-morbidity among disorders: results from the functional illness in primary care (FIP) study. *Psychological Medicine*, **35**, 1175–1184.

Tyrer, P., Nur, U., Crawford, M., *et al* (2005) The Social Functioning Questionnaire: a rapid and robust measure of perceived functioning. *International Journal of Social Psychiatry*, **51**, 265–275.

Upton, M. W., Evans, M., Goldberg, D. P., *et al* (1999) Evaluation of ICD–10 PHC mental health guidelines in detecting and managing depression within primary care. *British Journal of Psychiatry*, **175**, 476–482.

Üstün, T. B. & Sartorius, N. (1995) *Mental Illness in General Health Care*. Wiley.

Üstün, T. B., Goldberg, D., Cooper, J., *et al* (1995) New classification for mental disorders with management guidelines for use in primary care: ICD–10 PHC chapter five. *British Journal of General Practice*, **45**, 211–215.

Van Weel-Baumgarten, E., van den Bosch W., van den Hoogen, H., *et al* (1999) Ten year follow-up of depression after diagnosis in general practice. *British Journal of General Practice*, **48**, 1643–1646.

Vuorilehto, M., Melartin, T. & Isometsa, E. (2005) Depressive disorders in primary care: recurrent, chronic and co-morbid. *Psychological Medicine*, **35**, 673–682.

World Health Organization (1992) *The ICD–10 Classification of Mental and Behavioural Disorders. Clinical Descriptions and Diagnostic Guidelines*. WHO.

World Health Organization (2003) *International Classification of Primary Care* (2nd revision) (ICPC–2). WHO.

Zigmond, A. S. & Snaith, R. P. (1983) The Hospital Anxiety and Depression Scale. *Acta Psychiatrica Scandinavica*, **67**, 361–370.

Zimmerman, M. & Mattia J. I. (2001) A self-report scale to help make psychiatric diagnoses: the Psychiatric Diagnostic Screening Questionnaire. *Archives of General Psychiatry*, **58**, 787–794.

Zimmerman, M., Coryell, W. & Wilson, S., *et al* (1986) Evaluation of symptoms of major depressive disorder: self-report vs clinician ratings. *Journal of Nervous and Mental Disease*, **174**, 150–153.

Zinsbarg, R., Barlow, D., Liebowitz, M., *et al* (1994) DSM–IV field trial for mixed anxiety-depression. *American Journal of Psychiatry*, **151**, 1153–1162.

# Part II: Clinical issues

This section outlines the clinical features of the main mental health problems that general practitioners are likely to encounter in their daily work. We have tried to keep the content of this part focused on the needs of the busy practitioner, providing practical advice and guidance, as well as pointing to supporting resources such as relevant websites. In addition we have asked authors to provide links to further reading for those who wish to delve more deeply into the subject matter of each chapter.

As far as possible, management advice is supported by evidence, but of course in many cases the evidence base that supports treatment recommendations comes from settings other than primary care. We have tried to make this clear as far as possible, and so these chapters are also a useful guide to where gaps in the evidence exist and where further research is needed. Because all the editors of this book work in the UK, current management guidance leans heavily on UK recommendations, but we have tried as far as possible to broaden this to include guidance from other sources where it is available.

# CHAPTER 8

# Depression

Tony Kendrick and Andre Tylee

Summary

This chapter covers the diagnosis and classification of depression, including major depressive disorder, mild depression and dysthymia. A stepped-care approach to depression, including screening and detection, guided self-help, drug treatment, psychological therapies and referral, is described, based on guidelines from the UK National Institute for Health and Clinical Excellence. Measures of the severity of depression are discussed in relation to the challenging issue of deciding when to intervene in primary care.

## Defining depression

Depressive symptoms range along a continuum from everyday sadness to suicidal depression, and any cut-off between a 'normal' and a 'depressed' person is to an extent arbitrary, but categorical diagnoses are necessary in clinical practice to make decisions about intervening. Psychiatric classification systems identify a category of 'major depression' which predicts the need for active treatment, irrespective of environmental factors, except for bereavement (American Psychiatric Association, 2000).

Around three times as many depressed patients have symptom levels below the cut-off for major depression, which, though relatively mild, are still associated with significant distress and impairment of social functioning (Rapaport *et al*, 2002). Depression very commonly occurs with anxiety (see Chapter 10).

## Epidemiology

The multi-country survey of 2000–2001 undertaken by the World Health Organization (WHO) found that major depression affected around 5% of women and 3% of men per year. Depression was the fourth leading cause of disease burden among all diseases, responsible for, on average, 4.4% of total disability-adjusted life-years lost (ranging from 1.2% in Africa to 8.0% in the Americas), which had increased from 3.7% in 1990. Depression caused the largest amount of non-fatal burden among all diseases: 12.1% of total years lived with disability on average, which had increased from 10.7% in 1990 (Üstün *et al*, 2004).

Cross-sectional surveys have shown an increasing prevalence of depression, prompting talk of an epidemic of depression. The prevalence of major depression doubled among US adults between 1992 and 2002 (Compton *et al*, 2006). Depression is now the second (for women) or third (for men) biggest cause of long-term sickness benefits in the UK (Moncrieff & Pomerleau, 2000) and all high-income countries have seen year-on-year increases in antidepressant prescribing in primary care since the selective serotonin reuptake inhibitors (SSRIs) were introduced in 1990 (Middleton *et al*, 2001). Depression is predicted to be second after ischaemic heart disease in global health burden by 2020 (Murray & Lopez, 1997).

## Recognition of depression

Depression is much more likely to be recognised when patients present with psychosocial symptoms as opposed to somatic symptoms (Kirmayer *et al*, 1993; Tylee *et al*, 1995). However, the old notion that general practitioners (GPs) tend to miss 50% or more of cases of depression among their patients can now be discounted, as GPs have been found to be very good at recognising moderate to severe depression (Thompson *et al*, 2001), where the evidence of treatment benefit is stronger. In a large WHO naturalistic study in 15 cities around the world (and in 11 languages), patients whose depression went unrecognised had milder depression at baseline and were not found to be at a disadvantage in terms of outcome (Goldberg *et al*, 1998).

## Risk factors

Higher rates of attendance and treatment for depression are associated with socially disadvantaged populations: people living in deprived areas, especially the inner city but also deprived rural areas; people who are unemployed and living on benefits; and victims of violence, including domestic violence, and those living in violent areas. Depression is also associated with a lack of social support: it is more common among: people who are divorced or separated; single parents (usually women); widowed elderly people; non-religious communities; and communities with fewer extended families, where people are more likely to be living alone. Other risk factors are listed in Box 8.1.

Bereavement is often followed by 3–6 months of symptoms, which may reach the level of major depression. Most bereaved people do not need active

---

**Box 8.1** Risk factors for depression

- A history of depression.
- A family history of depression.
- Recent unemployment, bereavement or divorce.
- Financial or housing problems.
- Recent childbirth, demanding child care.
- Menopausal symptoms.
- Caring for a disabled relative.
- Living in residential accommodation.
- Chronic physical illness.

---

treatment beyond a listening ear, but if symptoms persist beyond 6 months, or are severe enough to affect daily functioning, particularly in a person who has a history of depression, then active treatment is warranted.

## Classification and diagnosis

In the DSM–IV classification, the diagnosis of major depression rests on the identification of at least five out of nine symptoms (Box 8.2), one of which must be depressed mood or loss of interest and pleasure in usual activities (American Psychiatric Association, 2000).

'Trigger' symptoms with a high predictive value for depression include sleep problems, fatigue and irritability, and should prompt enquiry about all nine symptoms. Symptoms must have been present most of every day for a minimum of 2 weeks, and ideally for much longer, to be sure of the diagnosis. Patients who fulfil criteria for major depression of recent onset can improve spontaneously and best practice is to ask patients to come back for a review of symptoms in a week or two, as a proportion will respond to support alone

---

**Box 8.2** The DSM–IV criteria for major depression

Low mood *or* loss of interest and pleasure for at least 2 weeks, plus four out of the seven following symptoms:

- change in sleep pattern
- change in appetite or weight
- poor energy, tiredness
- poor concentration, forgetfulness
- guilt, worthlessness
- agitation/retardation
- suicidal ideas.

---

within a few weeks. As well as being persistent, the depressive symptoms must cause clinically significant distress or impairment in functioning for the diagnosis of major depression to be made.

## Mild depression

Mild depression is diagnosed if low mood or loss of pleasure is accompanied by up to three other symptoms of depression, and the patient's day-to-day functioning is not significantly impaired. The distinction between mild or minor depression and major depression is important, as the treatment is different (see below). However, patients with less severe depression of recent onset should be monitored, under a policy of 'watchful waiting', in case they go on to develop major depression.

## Dysthymia

Dysthymia is mild depression which has persisted for 2 years or more. A systematic review of 15 randomised controlled trials (RCTs) of a variety of antidepressants for the treatment of dysthymia found that they improved outcomes, but these were mostly small studies, of variable quality, and all in secondary care populations (de Lima *et al*, 1999). This suggests that duration is an important factor as well as severity in determining whether to prescribe for depression.

# Detection and management of depression: a stepped-care model

A guideline produced by the UK National Institute of Health and Clinical Excellence (NICE) (National Collaborating Centre for Mental Health, 2004) recommend a stepped-care model:

Step 1   recognition of depression
Step 2   mild depression in primary care
Step 3   moderate to severe depression in primary care
Step 4   refractory, recurrent, atypical and psychotic depression in specialist mental health services
Step 5   depression requiring in-patient care.

NICE recommendations are graded according to the level of supporting evidence (Box 8.3). At the time of writing, the NICE guidelines are being updated, but they are unlikely to change significantly.

## Step 1. Recognition of depression

### Detection/screening

The NICE guidance recommends that screening for depression should be undertaken in high-risk groups (grade C evidence), including:

> **Box 8.3** Levels of recommendations in NICE guidelines
>
> A    Based on level I evidence (meta-analysis of randomised controlled trials, or at least one randomised controlled trial)
>
> B    Based on level II or III evidence (well-conducted clinical studies but no randomised controlled trials) or extrapolated from level I evidence
>
> C    Based on level IV evidence (expert opinion)
>
> GPP  Good practice point (panel experience)
>
> N    Evidence from NICE technology appraisal

- patients with significant physical illnesses
- patients with other mental health problems, such as dementia
- patients who have faced significant life events –
  - unemployment and financial difficulties
  - childbirth, and the care of young children
  - bereavement, or loss of significant relationships
  - past physical or sexual abuse.

Two questions concerning mood and interest are recommended (grade B evidence), specifically:

1 'During the last month, have you often been bothered by feeling down, depressed or hopeless?'
2 'During the last month, have you often been bothered by having little interest or pleasure in doing things?'

These two questions are highly sensitive for depression (Arroll *et al*, 2003). However, this policy has been questioned since the guidance was issued, in part because the available screening tests may not fulfil the required criteria of precision and acceptability (Gilbody *et al*, 2006). The *relatively* low prevalence of major depression in primary care (less than 10%) means that the positive predictive value (PPV, which is a measure of the accuracy of a test in identifying a true positive result) of even very sensitive and specific instruments will be low when used in the general population of primary care patients (false positives are more of an issue when the prevalence of true positives is low in the population being screened).

However, the specificity of screening has been shown to be improved by the addition of a third 'help' question asked of patients answering 'yes' to either of the first two questions (Arroll *et al*, 2005):

3 'Is this something with which you would like help?'

This third question has three possible responses: 'no', 'yes, but not today', and 'yes'. A 'no' response to this third question makes major depression highly unlikely (negative predictive value, NPV, 94%). It is important to stress, therefore, that a negative result to this two- or three-item screen can usually be taken to indicate that the patient does not have depression (Mitchell & Coyne, 2007). It is also important to stress that those screening positive need further clinical assessment to determine whether they are true cases or false positives.

A further objection to population screening is that it has not been shown to lead to better outcomes, often because effective treatment has not been in place to deal with identified cases (Gilbody et al, 2003). Therefore case-finding should be undertaken only for groups of patients for whom there is good evidence that available treatments actually improve outcomes.

## Quality indicators for depression in the UK general practice contract

In the UK, GPs are rewarded financially for performance against two quality indicators for the detection and management of depression, through a points system, called the Quality and Outcomes Framework (QOF). First, points are awarded for case-finding for depression among patients with diabetes or coronary heart disease (CHD), among whom the prevalence of depression is two to three times that of the general population. Second, points are awarded in the QOF for the use of validated questionnaire measures for the diagnosis and severity of depression, at the outset of treatment. In 2009, a third indicator was introduced into the contract, awarding more points for a follow-up measure of severity 1–3 months after diagnosis.

Among patients with heart disease or diabetes there is grade A evidence that treatment improves outcomes for depression (and may also improve outcomes for their physical health problems, although that is less certain). The presence of depression in people with CHD is associated with reduced compliance with treatment, increased use of health resources, increased social isolation and poorer outcomes. A meta-analysis of 20 trials found that depression was an independent risk factor for mortality in people with CHD (Barth et al, 2004). There is also grade A evidence that treatment with selective serotonin reuptake inhibitors (SSRIs) for people with CHD is safe and effective in reducing depression, at least among those with a prior history of depression and more severe symptoms (Glassman et al, 2002; Taylor et al, 2005). Patients treated with an SSRI were also found to have a 42% reduction in death or recurrent myocardial infarction in a subgroup analysis of outcomes in a trial of cognitive–behavioural therapy (CBT), although this was a post hoc observation, and assignment to antidepressants was not randomised (Lesperance et al, 2007). The CBT given in that trial was effective in reducing depressive symptoms, but had no effect on death or recurrent infarction.

People with both diabetes and depression are less physically and socially active and less likely to comply with diet and treatment than people with diabetes alone, leading to worse long-term complications and higher mortality. It may also be that practitioners provide poorer care to patients with comorbid depression and diabetes because depression impairs communication with patients. There is grade A evidence that effective treatment with either antidepressants or CBT improves the outcome of depression in patients with diabetes. While treatment has not been shown consistently to improve glycaemic control (Williams *et al*, 2004), psychological well-being has been identified by the St Vincent Declaration (International Diabetes Federation, 1989) as an important goal of diabetes management in its own right.

## Depression and other comorbid physical illnesses

One in three stroke survivors experiences depression, which impedes rehabilitation, through poorer physical and cognitive function, and is associated with an increased risk of death, including suicide. However, a Cochrane review concluded that there was insufficient evidence to support the routine use of antidepressants for the prevention of depression or to improve recovery from stroke, and recommended further research be carried out (Hackett *et al*, 2005). Depressive and anxious symptoms are common in chronic obstructive pulmonary disease (COPD), and case-finding should be considered for all COPD patients, although trials of psychological treatments and antidepressants have had varying findings. Clinically significant depression is also common in heart failure, where it is related to increased rates of death and secondary events. However, only a small number of intervention studies have been carried out and the results are inconclusive.

## Measuring depression severity at the outset of treatment

Three alternative questionnaires are suggested for use in the UK GP contract QOF: the Patient Health Questionnaire (PHQ-9; Kroenke *et al*, 2001), the Hospital Anxiety and Depression Scale (HAD; Zigmond & Snaith, 1983) and the Beck Depression Inventory (BDI; Arnau *et al*, 2001). The aim of using these measures is to help the practitioner to distinguish mild from moderate to severe depression, as NICE recommends different treatments for the different levels of severity. The HAD includes depressive (HAD-D) and anxiety (HAD-A) symptoms and relies less on somatic symptoms, being specifically designed for physically ill populations.

Table 8.1 shows the approximate thresholds for considering active treatment of depression according to the scores on the three suggested measures. It has recently been shown that a score of 12 or more on the PHQ-9 has greater specificity, and the same sensitivity, as a score of 10 for major depression in a UK population (Gilbody *et al*, 2007). Furthermore, when used concurrently in the same group of patients, the PHQ-9 at a cut-off of 10 was shown to classify significantly more patients as depressed and in need of treatment than the HAD-D (Cameron *et al*, 2008). So a PHQ-9 score of 12 rather than 10 may be a better cut-off to use when deciding whether or not to offer active treatment.

It is important to use *clinical judgement* in interpreting severity scores on questionnaires, in particular taking into account the degree of interference

**Table 8.1** Approximate thresholds on questionnaire measures of depression for considering active treatment

| Measure | PHQ-9 score | HAD-D score | BDI-II score |
| --- | --- | --- | --- |
| Minimal or no depression, no need for action | 1–4 | 0–7 | 0–13 |
| Mild depression, monitor for any deterioration | 5–9 | 8–10 | 14–19 |
| Moderate to severe depression, consider active treatment | 10 or greater* (max. 27) | 11 or greater (max. 21) | 20 or greater (max. 63) |

*Recent evidence suggests a PHQ-9 score of 12 may be a more specific cut-off (see text).

with daily activities caused by the patient's symptoms. Some patients have a greater likelihood of reporting symptoms than others, and so diagnoses should not be based on symptom counts alone. The available measures have not been validated for use with all ethnic groups and so the results should be interpreted with caution, and the meaning of symptoms should be explored with individual patients. Also, a previous history and previous treatment for depression are important predictors of future problems and so even low levels of symptoms in patients with previous depression should be taken seriously.

## Step 2. Mild depression in primary care: guided self-help

The NICE guideline states that antidepressants should not normally be prescribed for mild depression. However, mild depression should not be ignored, but should be monitored for at least 2 weeks, with 'watchful waiting' in case the patient goes on to develop more severe symptoms (grade C evidence). During this period, a variety of self-help measures are recommended, including advice on sleep hygiene and anxiety management, and regular exercise at least three times per week for 45–60 minutes, which has been shown to improve symptoms (grade C evidence).

A range of resources are now available to provide guided self-help based on the principles of CBT. These encourage patients to identify and tackle their depressive thoughts, and to develop more positive thoughts and behaviours, which in turn can reduce their depressive symptoms.

Informal support from a GP, practice nurse, health visitor or primary care mental health worker is crucial, as simply providing a listening ear can be therapeutic in itself. Patients need to feel accepted and to be reassured they are not going mad; as well as providing this 'normalising' function, primary care practitioners can, even if all else fails, bear witness to patients' sadness, acknowledge their resilience in the face of adversity and provide encouragement that they will get through their difficulties (Johnston *et al*, 2007).

## Bibliotherapy

Written material for self-help, or 'bibliotherapy', involves more than just giving the patient a book; the material needs to be introduced by a practitioner (doctor, nurse or primary care mental health worker) and progress monitored at intervals over 6–8 weeks while the patient works through the material. One example of bibliotherapy is the *Overcoming Depression* programme (see 'Resources for patients' at the end of this chapter).

## Computerised CBT

Self-help based on CBT is now available through computer programs which patients can work through either at home or on computers at the practice. *Beating the Blues* (Proudfoot *et al*, 2004) was recommended for mild to moderate depression following a NICE (2006) technology appraisal (see 'Resources for patients'). The *Overcoming Depression* programme has been computerised, although NICE found insufficient evidence to recommend that particular programme. 'Mood gym' and 'Living life to the full' are also available free online. More extended CBT is also becoming available through the internet.

## Brief psychological treatments

Chapter 26 on covers psychological therapies in primary care more generally. In relation to depression, counselling has been shown, through a systematic review and meta-analysis of seven trials, to improve short-term outcomes over 4 months, although the benefits of counselling over usual care were found not to persist by 12 months (Bower *et al*, 2002). More research is needed to establish whether counselling is cost-effective in the medium to longer term. The trials showed that a minimum severity of depression was required for counselling to be likely to benefit patients, specifically a score of 14 on the BDI (equivalent to 5 on the PHQ-9 or 8 on the HAD-D).

Problem-solving therapy (PST) is a brief CBT-based therapy which lasts for 6–8 sessions rather than 15–20 for full CBT. PST has been shown to be as effective as antidepressants for moderate depression (Dowrick *et al*, 2000; Mynors-Wallis *et al*, 2000). As with counselling, PST should be offered only to patients with a minimum severity of symptoms, equating to moderate depression, as PST was found to be no more effective than usual GP care for mild depression and anxiety disorders (Kendrick *et al*, 2006*b*).

The NICE depression guideline (National Collaborating Centre for Mental Health, 2004) also covers interpersonal therapy, in which the person's relationships with others are looked at, which has a similar efficacy to CBT but is more widely available in the USA than in the UK. The guideline also includes marital therapy, in which both members of a relationship are involved, and the efficacy for this is lower than for the other types of therapy described.

### Antidepressant treatment

Antidepressants are not recommended by NICE for the initial treatment of mild depression, as the cost–benefit ratio is thought to be less favourable than for moderate depression. An early trial of amitriptyline found no advantage over placebo for minor depression (Paykel *et al*, 1988), although a later study using paroxetine found some advantage for dysthymia and for minor depression in patients aged over 60 with more functional impairment (Barrett *et al*, 2001; Williams *et al*, 2000). A trial of fluoxetine found a small advantage over placebo (Judd *et al*, 2004), but a significant proportion of patients recovered on placebo alone, and it is questionable whether such a small difference in outcome is clinically significant. A recent *post hoc* analysis of two trials of duloxetine against placebo also found evidence of benefit for mild depression (Perahia *et al*, 2006). The THREAD study of SSRIs for mild to moderate depression in primary care has shown that their use is probably cost-effective at the levels of cost per quality adjusted life year (QALY) recommended by NICE, when compared with support from the GP without medication (Kendrick *et al*, 2009).

However, even if antidepressants are cost-effective in mild depression, they are clearly not acceptable to many patients, and more psychological treatments should be made available as an alternative for those who do not wish to take drugs.

Antidepressants are recommended by NICE only for patients with mild depression whose symptoms persist after other interventions have been tried, for patients with a history of more severe depression, and for those with mild depression associated with psychosocial problems (grade C recommendation). However, in practice, antidepressants may be all there is to offer in primary care, particularly for persistent mild depression, as psychological treatments are often in short supply, even in the richest countries.

## Step 3. Moderate to severe depression in primary care

### Antidepressant treatment

The SSRIs are recommended by NICE as first-line treatment for moderate to severe depression, as they are as effective as the older tricyclics but better tolerated, and fluoxetine and citalopram are now just as cost-effective since coming off patent in the UK (Kendrick *et al*, 2006*a*).

Patient preference is an important consideration, and patients who have responded well to tricyclics in the past may prefer to have them again for recurrent depression. The tricyclics have some advantage over the SSRIs in terms of sedation if this is required, but the SSRIs are less cardiotoxic and therefore preferable for patients who are at greater risk of overdose. Tricyclics should not be used for patients with cardiovascular problems or epilepsy, as they can lower the seizure threshold. Lofepramine is a reasonable alternative if sedation is required.

Another advantage of the SSRIs is that they can be started at a therapeutic dose, unlike the tricyclics, which need titrating upwards, adjusting the dose frequently in the first few weeks of treatment. However, the SSRIs are not without side-effects, including weight loss, insomnia and agitation among some patients in the early stages of treatment, and occasional severe restlessness and agitation (akathisia).

Patients should be advised about the benefits and side-effects of treatment, in particular that it may take some weeks to take effect, although recent evidence suggests SSRIs may start to work within days rather than weeks (Taylor *et al*, 2006*b*). Patients should be reviewed every 1–2 weeks until they have improved, then monthly. At each visit, the doctor should evaluate the patient's response to treatment, adherence, side-effects and suicide risk. If suicide seems to be a possibility, the doctor should limit the amount of drug prescribed.

The initial dose should be continued for at least 4 weeks before the dose is reviewed (6 weeks for elderly patients). After 6 weeks (9 weeks for elderly patients), the patient may be switched to another SSRI if there has been no response (research is currently addressing whether an antidepressant from a different class, such as a tricyclic, should be used instead of another SSRI). If the patient fails to respond to a 6-week (or 9-week) course of two different first-line antidepressants, then a second-line drug should be considered. Advice is available on safe switching between antidepressants in the Maudsley Prescribing Guidelines (Taylor *et al*, 2006*a*).

## Second-line antidepressants

Mirtazapine is a pre-synaptic alpha-2 antagonist and the most sedative of the newer antidepressants, but it frequently causes weight gain, so it is a better choice if the patient has suffered weight loss and agitation. Reboxetine is a noradrenaline reuptake inhibitor which is more energising, so it is more useful if the patient is suffering from retarded depression. Venlafaxine has a dual action on the reuptake of both serotonin and noradrenaline and may be more effective for more severe or resistant depression, but it can cause arrhythmias and hypertension at higher doses, so the patient's heart rhythm and blood pressure should be monitored during the first few weeks of treatment. Duloxetine is a newer, dual-action antidepressant, which has been shown to be effective for mild to moderate depression (Perahia *et al*, 2006).

If successful, antidepressant drug treatment should be continued for at least 4 months after remission (usually at least 6 months in all), as studies have shown that earlier cessation is associated with a greater risk of relapse. Continuing treatment for at least 2 years is recommended by NICE for patients who have suffered two episodes of major depression.

## Stopping treatment

A significant proportion of patients established on SSRIs experience withdrawal symptoms on trying to stop them, including anxiety, dizziness, headaches, and odd sensations like electric shocks, so in general they should not be stopped suddenly but withdrawn gradually. Paroxetine in particular must be gradually withdrawn, as it has a shorter half-life. In theory, fluoxetine may be stopped suddenly, as it has a longer half-life, although in practice many patients suffer withdrawal effects even with the longer-acting drugs.

### Targeting treatments to the patients who really need them

Longitudinal studies of antidepressant prescribing have shown that many patients stop taking them within 1–2 months (Dunn *et al*, 1999; Olfson *et al*, 2006). This is perhaps not surprising, because studies using validated measures of severity show that GPs often prescribe for patients with very mild depression, who are likely to recover quickly in the majority of cases without antidepressants (Kendrick *et al*, 2001, 2005). It is important therefore that patients are assessed carefully before they are begun on drug treatment. Patients with very mild symptoms should not be prescribed antidepressants immediately on presentation, but should be brought back for review in case of progression to major depression.

The use of validated severity measures should help doctors discriminate between mild and moderate depression, and in addition a careful assessment of the patient's attitudes towards taking treatment is recommended before a prescription is made, as the majority of people think antidepressants are addictive (Kendrick *et al*, 2005). Qualitative research has shown that patients often reject the notion of depression as a disease, along with the notion of a medical 'cure' for life's ills (Johnston *et al*, 2007).

The year-on-year rise in antidepressant prescribing (Prescription Pricing Authority, 2007) is due to a small but increasing proportion of patients remaining on SSRIs for years, often without a justifiable indication for long-term use. Such patients may experience worrying symptoms of anxiety on trying to stop medication and so continue them long after they could be stopped (Leydon *et al*, 2007). Long-term users of SSRIs need careful review at regular intervals and counselling about the withdrawal effects and support to taper off medication slowly when it is appropriate to do so. Patients often confuse discontinuation symptoms with a relapse of depressive symptoms, so it is advisable to explain that relapse symptoms are generally more likely to emerge after 2–3 weeks.

## Step 4. Referral to mental health services

Patients with refractory, recurrent, atypical and psychotic depression, suicidal intention or severe self-neglect should be referred to specialist mental health services, but in countries with well-developed primary care services this should be required for fewer than 20% of patients with depression. Box 8.4 lists the indications for referral to secondary care.

### Psychological treatments

Cognitive–behavioural therapy is as effective as antidepressant drug treatment for major depression, and may be preferred to drugs by the

---

**Box 8.4** Indications for referral of patients with depression to specialist mental health services

- Poor response to three courses of antidepressants
- Recurrent episode within 1 year of last episode
- Patient or relatives request referral
- Self-neglect
- Postnatal depression
- Suicidal ideas and plans (urgent referral)
- Psychotic symptoms (urgent referral)

---

majority of patients. Unfortunately, however, CBT is not readily available in most countries, although access is being increased in the UK, USA, Australia and New Zealand.

A full course of CBT involves 15–20 one-hour sessions with a trained therapist, and so is expensive in relation to drug treatment. However, it may be more effective than drugs at preventing relapse (Evans *et al*, 1992) and so it may be more cost-effective in the long run. CBT involves the patient in homework between sessions, working on identifying and tackling self-defeating automatic negative thoughts, and practising more positive and self-affirming behaviours. It is not suitable therefore for patients who have difficulty engaging in a dialogue with the therapist, or whose functioning is so impaired that they are unable to undertake the required exercises. Combined CBT and drug treatment is indicated for resistant or severe depression.

In the UK, a policy of massively expanding the availability of CBT is being followed, in combination with employment counselling, with the aim of getting patients with long-standing depression back to work. It is thought that CBT could pay for itself through reductions in sickness benefits and increases in tax contributions from patients returning to employment (Layard & Centre for Economic Performance's Mental Health Policy Group, 2006).

### Collaborative care management

In relation to depression, the treatment of major depression has been shown to be much improved through collaborative care management (detailed in Chapter 27), which includes active follow-up of patients by a dedicated care manager, specific counselling about the need to continue treatment, and increased access to psychiatric and psychological treatment through primary–secondary care collaboration (Katon *et al*, 1995; Wells *et al*, 2000; Dietrich *et al*, 2006). However, such care is expensive and has not been rolled out to everyday practice, even in the USA, where most of the research showing its effectiveness has been carried out.

## Improving access to primary care treatment

An important prospective study of primary care service provision for depression in six countries showed that its availability varied enormously. Receipt of antidepressant treatment in primary care varied from 38% of patients in the USA to 0% in Russia, and receipt of specialist care from 29% of patients in Australia to 3% in Russia. Cost was the most important barrier to treatment (Simon *et al*, 2004).

Mental and behavioural disorders cause 12% of the global burden of disease, yet mental health budgets are less than 1% of total health expenditures, and health insurance programmes do not cover mental health at the same level as other illnesses. More than 30% of countries have no mental health programme and over 90% have no mental health policy for children and adolescents (World Health Organization, 2001) (see Chapter 6 on low- and middle-income countries). The World Health Organization (2001) has developed a ten-point plan to tackle depression globally, which emphasises the need for primary care treatments to be made more available, and for social agencies to work together to effect social change (Box 8.5).

## Primary care research priorities for depression

Depression is so common that even higher-income countries cannot afford to provide specialist mental healthcare and extensive psychological treatments for the large majority of sufferers. More innovative non-drug treatment strategies need to be developed and evaluated, based on self-help, and administered by non-specialists.

Prevention is clearly better than cure, and more work needs to go into mental health promotion (see Chapter 24), including micro-finance to allow people to climb out of poverty, a reduction of domestic and other violence, befriending, increasing social networks and improving parenting

---

**Box 8.5** The World Health Organization's ten-point plan to tackle depression globally

1  Provide treatment in primary care
2  Make psychotropic drugs available
3  Give care in the community
4  Educate the public
5  Involve communities, families and consumers
6  Establish national policies, programmes and legislation
7  Develop human resources
8  Link with education, labour, welfare and law
9  Monitor community mental health
10 Support more research

skills (Lancet Global Mental Health Group, 2007). The idea that depression can be tackled by pills, diets or other quick fixes is a seductive but false hope. In the longer term, the 'depression epidemic' will be reversed only through difficult but essential social changes to increase people's support for each other and reverse some of the trends towards the fragmentation of society in the 21st century.

---

Key points

- Depression may be difficult to detect in primary care settings, where patients commonly present with physical symptoms.
- Screening of the whole population is not justified but case-finding in high-risk groups is important.
- Depressive symptoms range along a continuum from normal sadness, and categorisation is, to an extent, arbitrary.
- The diagnosis of major depressive disorder requires five or more symptoms most of the day for at least 2 weeks, preferably several, accompanied by impaired functioning.
- Structured questionnaires are helpful in assessing severity.
- Mild depression should be treated with guided self-help and watchful waiting.
- Antidepressants are the first-line treatment for depression of at least moderate severity, but patients often prefer psychological treatments.
- Access to psychological therapies such as problem-solving treatment and cognitive–behavioural therapy needs to be improved, even in the richest countries.

---

# Further reading and e-resources

Mild depression in general practice: time for a rethink? *Drug and Therapeutics Bulletin* (2003), **41**, 60–64.
NICE Depression Guideline (2004), at http://www.nice.org.uk
Patient Health Questionnaire (© Pfizer Inc.), at http://www.depression-primarycare.org

## Resources for patients

Depression Alliance, http://www.depressionalliance.org
Royal College of Psychiatrists, patient information sheets, http://www.rcpsych.ac.uk
Williams, C. (2006) *Overcoming Depression and Low Mood: A Five Areas Approach*. Arnold.

## Computerised CBT

Beating the Blues, http://www.media-innovations.ltd.uk
Internet-based CBT, http://www.psychologyonline.co.uk
Living life to the full, http://www.livinglifetothefull.com
Mood gym, http://www.moodgym.anu.edu.au
More extended CBT is also becoming available through the internet at http://www.psychologyonline.co.uk
Overcoming Depression, http://www.calipso.co.uk

# References

American Psychiatric Association (2000) *Diagnostic and Statistical Manual of Mental Disorders* (4th edn, text revision) (DSM–IV–TR). APA.

Arnau, R., Meagher, M. W., Norris, M. P., *et al* (2001) Psychometric evaluation of the Beck Depression Inventory–II with primary care medical patients. *Health Psychology*, **20**, 112–119.

Arroll, B., Khin, N. & Kerse, N. (2003) Screening for depression in primary care with two verbally asked questions: cross sectional study. *BMJ*, **327**, 1144–1146.

Arroll, B., Goodyear-Smith, F., Kerse, N., *et al* (2005) Effect of the addition of a 'help' question to two screening questions on specificity for diagnosis of depression in general practice: diagnostic validity study. *BMJ*, **331**, 884.

Barrett, J. E., Williams, J. W., Oxman, T. E., *et al* (2001) Treatment of dysthymia and minor depression in primary care: a randomized trial in patients aged 18 to 59 years. *Journal of Family Practice*, **50**, 405–412.

Barth, J., Schumacher, M. & Herrmann-Lingen, C. (2004) Depression as a risk factor for mortality in patients with coronary heart disease: a meta analysis. *Psychosomatic Medicine*, **66**, 802–813.

Bower, P., Rowland, N., Mellor Clark, J., *et al* (2002) Effectiveness and cost effectiveness of counselling in primary care. *Cochrane Database of Systematic Reviews*, **(1)**, CD001025.

Cameron, I. M., Crawford, J. R., Lawton, K., *et al* (2008) Psychometric comparison of PHQ-9 and HADS for measuring depression severity in primary care. *British Journal of General Practice*, **58**, 32–36.

Compton, W. M., Conway, K. P., Stinson, F. S., *et al* (2006) Changes in the prevalence of major depression and comorbid substance use disorders in the United States between 1991–1992 and 2001–2002. *American Journal of Psychiatry*, **163**, 2141–2147.

de Lima, M. S., Hotopf, M. & Wessely, S. (1999) The efficacy of drug treatments for dysthymia: a systematic review and meta-analysis. *Psychological Medicine*, **29**, 1273–1289.

Dietrich, A., Oxman, T. E., Williams, J. W., *et al* (2006) Re-engineering systems for the treatment of depression in primary care: cluster randomised controlled trial. *BMJ*, **329**, 602.

Dowrick, C., Dunn, G., Ayuso-Mateos, J. L., *et al* (2000) Problem solving treatment and group psychoeducation for depression: multicentre randomised controlled trial. *BMJ*, **321**, 1450–1454.

Dunn, R. L., Donoghue, J. M., Ozminski, R. J., *et al* (1999) Longitudinal patterns of antidepressant prescribing in primary care in the UK: comparison with treatment guidelines. *Journal of Psychopharmacology*, **13**, 136–143.

Evans, M. D., Hollon, S. D., DeRubeis, R. J., *et al* (1992) Differential relapse following cognitive therapy and pharmacotherapy for depression. *Archives of General Psychiatry*, **49**, 802–808.

Gilbody, S., Whitty, P., Grimshaw, J., *et al* (2003) Educational and organizational interventions to improve the management of depression in primary care. A systematic review. *JAMA*, **289**, 3145–3151.

Gilbody, S., Sheldon, T. & Wessely, S. (2006) Should we screen for depression? *BMJ*, **332**, 1027–1030.

Gilbody, S. M., Richards, D. & Barkham, M. (2007) Diagnosing depression in primary care using self-completed instruments: UK validation of PHQ-9 and CORE-OM. *British Journal of General Practice*, **57**, 650–652.

Glassman, A. H., O'Connor, C. M., Cailff, R. M., *et al* (2002) Sertraline treatment of major depression in patients with acute MI or unstable angina. *JAMA*, **288**, 701–709.

Goldberg, D., Privett, M., Ustun, B., *et al* (1998) The effects of detection and treatment on the outcome of major depression in primary care: a naturalistic study in 15 cities. *British Journal of General Practice*, **48**, 1840–1844.

Hackett, M. L., Anderson, C. S. & House, A. O. (2005) Management of depression after stroke. A systematic review of pharmacological therapies. *Stroke*, **36**, 1092–1097.

International Diabetes Federation (1989) *The St Vincent Declaration 1989*. International Diabetes Federation (http://www.idf.org/st-vincents-declaration-svd).

Johnston, O., Kumar, S., Kendall, K., *et al* (2007) Qualitative study of depression management in primary care: GP and patient goals, and the value of listening. *British Journal of General Practice*, **57**, 872–879.

Judd, L. J., Rapaport, M. H., Yonkers, K. A., *et al* (2004) Randomized, placebo-controlled trial of fluoxetine for acute treatment of minor depressive disorder. *American Journal of Psychiatry*, **161**, 1864–1871.

Katon, W., von Korff, M., Lin, E., *et al* (1995) Collaborative management to achieve treatment guidelines. Impact on depression in primary care. *JAMA*, **273**, 1026–1031.

Kendrick, T., Stevens, L., Bryant, A., *et al* (2001) Hampshire Depression Project: changes in the process of care and cost consequences. *British Journal of General Practice*, **51**, 911–913.

Kendrick, T., King, F., Albertella, L., *et al* (2005) GP treatment decisions for depression: an observational study. *British Journal of General Practice*, **55**, 280–286.

Kendrick, T., Peveler, R., Longworth, L., *et al* (2006a) Cost-effectiveness and cost-utility of tricyclic antidepressants, selective serotonin reuptake inhibitors, and lofepramine. Randomised controlled trial. *British Journal of Psychiatry*, **188**, 337–345.

Kendrick, T., Simons, L., Mynors-Wallis, L., *et al* (2006b) Cost-effectiveness of referral for generic care or problem-solving treatment from community mental health nurses, compared with usual general practitioner care for common mental disorders. *Randomised controlled trial. British Journal of Psychiatry*, **189**, 50–59.

Kendrick, T., Chatwin, J., Dowrick, C., *et al* (2009) Randomised controlled trial to determine the clinical effectiveness and cost-effectiveness of selective serotonin reuptake inhibitors plus supportive care, versus supportive care alone, for mild to moderate depression with somatic symptoms in primary care: the THREAD (THREshold for AntiDepressant response) study. *Health Technology Assessment*, **13**, 22.

Kirmayer, L. J., Robbins, J. M., Dworkind, M., *et al* (1993) Somatization and the recognition of depression and anxiety in primary care. *American Journal of Psychiatry*, **150**, 734–741.

Kroenke, K., Spitzer, R. L. & Williams, J. (2001) The PHQ-9: validity of a brief depression severity measure. *Journal of General Internal Medicine*, **16**, 606–613.

Lancet Global Mental Health Group (2007) Scale up services for mental disorders: a call for action. *Lancet*, **370**, 1241–1252.

Layard, R. & Centre for Economic Performance's Mental Health Policy Group (2006) *The Depression Report: A New Deal for Depression and Anxiety Disorders*. London School of Economics.

Lesperance, F., Frasure-Smith, N., Koszycki, D., *et al* (2007) Effects of citalopram and interpersonal psychotherapy on depression in patients with coronary artery disease: the Canadian Cardiac Randomized Evaluation of Antidepressant and Psychotherapy Efficacy (CREATE) Trial. *JAMA*, **297**, 367–379.

Leydon, G. M., Rodgers, L. & Kendrick, T. (2007) A qualitative study of patient views on discontinuing long-term selective serotonin reuptake inhibitors. *Family Practice*, **24**, 570–575.

Middleton, N., Gunnell, D., Whitley, E., *et al* (2001) Secular trends in antidepressant prescribing in the UK, 1975–1998. *Journal of Public Health Medicine*, **23**, 262–267.

Mitchell, A. J. & Coyne, J. C. (2007) Do ultra-short screening instruments accurately detect depression in primary care? *British Journal of General Practice*, **57**, 144–151.

Moncrieff, J. & Pomerleau, J. (2000) Trends in sickness benefits in Great Britain and the contribution of mental disorders. *Journal of Public Health Medicine*, **2**, 59–67.

Murray, C. & Lopez, A. D. (1997) Alternative projections of mortality and disability by cause 1990–2020: Global Burden of Disease Study. *Lancet*, **349**, 1498–1504.

Mynors-Wallis, L. M., Gath, D. H., Day, A., *et al* (2000) Randomised controlled trial of problem solving treatment, antidepressant medication, and combined treatment for major depression in primary care. *BMJ*, **320**, 26–30.

National Collaborating Centre for Mental Health (2004) *Depression: Management of Depression in Primary and Secondary Care*. Clinical Guideline 23. National Institute for Health and Clinical Excellence.

NICE (2006) *Computerised Cognitive Behaviour Therapy for Depression and Anxiety. Review of Technology Appraisal 51*. NICE.

Olfson, M., Marcus, S. C., Tedeschi, M., *et al* (2006) Continuity of antidepressant treatment for adults with depression in the United States. *American Journal of Psychiatry*, **163**, 101–108.

Paykel, E. S., Hollyman, J. A., Freeling, P., *et al* (1988) Predictors of therapeutic benefit from amitriptyline in mild depression: a general practice placebo-controlled trial. *Journal of Affective Disorders*, **14**, 83–95.

Perahia, D., Kajdasz, D. K., Walker, D. J., *et al* (2006) Duloxetine 60 mg once daily in the treatment of milder major depressive disorder. *International Journal of Clinical Practice*, **60**, 613–620.

Prescription Pricing Authority (2007) Prescribing Analysis and Cost (PACT) data, at http://www.nhsbsa.nhs.uk/Documents/Oct_-_Dec_2007_Drugs_used_in_Mental_Health.pdf .

Proudfoot, J., Ryden, C., Everitt, B., *et al* (2004) Clinical efficacy of computerised cognitive–behavioural therapy for anxiety and depression in primary care: randomised controlled trial. *British Journal of Psychiatry*, **185**, 46–54.

Rapaport, M. H., Judd, L. J., Schettler, P. J., *et al* (2002) A descriptive analysis of minor depression. *American Journal of Psychiatry*, **159**, 637–643.

Simon, G., Fleck, M., Lucas, R., *et al* (2004) Prevalence and predictors of depression treatment in an international primary care study. *American Journal of Psychiatry*, **161**, 1626–1634.

Taylor, C. B., Youngblood, M. E., Catellier, D., *et al* (2005) Effects of antidepressant medication on morbidity and mortality in depressed patients after myocardial infarction. *Archives of General Psychiatry*, **62**, 792–798.

Taylor, D., Kerwin, R. & Paton, C. (2006*a*) The Maudsley Prescribing Guidelines 2005–2006 (8th edn). Taylor and Francis.

Taylor, M. J., Freemantle, N., Geddes, J. R., *et al* (2006*b*) Early onset of selective serotonin reuptake inhibitor antidepressant action: systematic review and meta analysis. *Archives of General Psychiatry*, **63**, 1217–1223.

Thompson, C., Ostler, K., Peveler, R. C., *et al* (2001) Dimensional perspective on the recognition of depressive symptoms in primary care. *British Journal of Psychiatry*, **179**, 317–323.

Tylee, A., Freeling, P., Kerry, S., *et al* (1995) How does the content of consultations affect the recognition by general practitioners of major depression in women? *British Journal of General Practice*, **45**, 575–578.

Üstün, T. B., Ayuso-Mateos, J. L., Chatterji, S., *et al* (2004) Global burden of depressive disorders in the year 2000. *British Journal of Psychiatry*, **184**, 386–392.

Wells, K. B., Sherbourne, C., Schoenbaum, M., *et al* (2000) Impact of disseminating quality improvement programs for depression in managed primary care. *JAMA*, **283**, 212–220.

Williams, J. W., Barrett, J., Oxman, T. E., *et al* (2000) Treatment of dysthymia and minor depression in primary care: a randomized controlled trial in older adults. *JAMA*, **284**, 1519–1526.

Williams, J. W., Katon, W., Lin, E., *et al* (2004) The effectiveness of depression care management on diabetes-related outcomes in older people. *Annals of Internal Medicine*, **140**, 1015–1024.

World Health Organization (2001) *The World Health Report 2001. Mental Health: New Understanding, New Hope*. WHO.

Zigmond, A. S. & Snaith, R. P. (1983) The Hospital Anxiety and Depression Rating Scale. *Acta Psychiatrica Scandinavica*, **67**, 361–370.

# CHAPTER 9

# Suicide and self-harm

Sandra Dietrich, Lisa Wittenburg, Ella Arensman, Airi Värnik
and Ulrich Hegerl

Summary

There are many underlying causes of suicidal acts and complex, multiple risk factors are involved. An awareness of these risk factors can alert primary care professionals to particular areas of patients' lives. With a large number of suicide completers suffering from a diagnosable psychiatric disorder and an increased risk of suicide in virtually all psychiatric disorders, a key prevention strategy is improved care of patients with depression and other psychiatric disorders. This chapter outlines the epidemiology of suicide and self-harm, goes on to describe the clinical management of individual cases, and reviews the literature on wider strategies for suicide reduction. (Management of suicide risk is also discussed in Chapter 16.)

## Terminology and definitions

There has been much discussion about the most suitable terminology for suicidal acts and researchers have tried to find a common terminology and classification as well as operational definitions for the range of suicidal behaviours (O'Carroll et al, 1996; Maris, 2002; De Leo et al, 2004). In this chapter, we use the outcome-based term 'fatal suicidal acts' for suicidal behaviour that results in death and 'non-fatal suicidal acts' for suicidal actions that do not result in death.

There is no consensus on the definition of fatal suicidal acts, making it difficult, for instance, to collect accurate, comparable total rates of suicide. Numerous definitions are used, the most widely accepted being the definition produced by the World Health Organization (WHO, 2007a): 'the act of deliberately killing oneself'. Apart from fatal suicidal acts, it is also of great importance to consider non-fatal suicidal acts, because they are one of the strongest predictors of suicide and have significant economic, medical and social costs. Non-fatal suicidal acts are also often called 'attempted suicide' (especially in the USA), 'parasuicide' and 'deliberate self-harm' (especially in Europe), but also 'non-fatal suicidal behaviour', 'non-fatal self-inflicted harm', 'self-injury' and 'self-directed violence'. The usage of these terms varies considerably between countries.

# Epidemiology

Approximately one million people died from fatal suicidal acts in the year 2000, reflecting a 'global' mortality rate of 16 per 100000, or one death every 30 seconds. Suicide is now among the three leading causes of death among those aged 15–45 years (both sexes) and in a growing number of countries the first cause of mortality among men aged 15–34. These figures do not include non-fatal suicidal acts, which are up to 20 times more frequent than fatal suicidal acts (WHO, 2007b). According to WHO estimates, approximately 1.53 million people will die from fatal suicidal acts in 2020, and 10–20 times more people will attempt suicide worldwide. This represents on average one death every 20 seconds and one attempt every 1–2 seconds (WHO, 1999).

# Risk factors for suicidal behaviour

There are many underlying causes of suicidal acts and complex, multiple factors are involved. These factors interact with one another and they are likely to be operating simultaneously. Among the multitude of factors that are closely associated with a heightened risk of suicidal acts, mental disorders are positioned in the first rank. Estimates of up to over 90% are reported for the proportion of suicide completers who have a diagnosable psychiatric illness, and an increased risk of suicide is present in virtually all psychiatric disorders, but particularly in major depression, other affective disorders, schizophrenia, alcohol dependence and other addictions (Robins et al, 1959; Rich et al, 1988; Brent et al, 1994; Wasserman & Värnik, 1998; Lonnqvist, 2000; Zhang et al, 2004). Other contributing factors are choice of methods (which may be more or less lethal), access to lethal means, age and gender, cultural and social factors (including attitudes towards suicide and imitation effects) and personality-associated factors, such as impulsivity and (auto-)aggression. In addition, suicidal acts are more likely to occur during periods of rapid socio-economic and political change (Värnik et al, 1998a; Mäkinen, 2000) and also during family and individual crises, such as loss of a loved one or unemployment (WHO, 2007b).

Non-fatal suicidal acts are one of the strongest predictors of completed suicide, especially in males (Hawton et al, 1998). Table 9.1 gives an overview of factors which have been proposed to be associated with non-fatal suicidal acts/self-harm and fatal suicidal acts. It must be noted, however, that this list represents a selection of risk factors studied in large populations. When assessing suicide risk, each patient must be regarded individually, as a

**Table 9.1** Selected risk factors associated with self-harm and suicide

| | Demographic characteristics (age, gender, race/ethnicity, marital status, occupation, place of living, sexual orientation, immigration status, etc.) | Health status (physical and mental health) | Social factors (family characteristics, childhood experiences, social isolation, lack of social support, cultural stress, mass media culture, etc.) | Economic factors (employment status, level of education, income, etc.) | Interpersonal/ psychological characteristics | Situational factors (stressful events, media influence, availability of means of self-harm or suicide, etc.) | Other factors (forensic history, seasonal variation, deliberate self-harm, etc.) |
|---|---|---|---|---|---|---|---|
| Self-harm/non-fatal suicidal acts | Youth (women, age 15–24, men age 25–34), female gender; white population and young Asian women, separated or divorced, homosexual or bisexual orientation | Presence of mental disorder: major depression, substance misuse, anxiety disorders, personality disorder, schizophrenia, comorbidity. Presence of physical disorder: epilepsy, HIV infection, past head injury | Dysfunctional family, separated or divorced parents, marital discord, emotional, physical and sexual abuse during childhood, abandonment, neglect, traumatic events, poor social support/ relationships, mass-media culture | Unemployment, low socio-economic status, low level of education, low income, poverty | Impulsivity, rage towards others or self; feelings of abandonment, guilt or desperation; poor problem-solving skills | Adverse life event, death of celebrity, awareness of peers who have self-harmed, media influence, availability of means of self-harm | Religious aspects |
| Fatal suicidal acts | Old age, adult men up to 45, male, white population and young Asian women. Divorced, single, widowed. Living in urban areas (except China and men). Certain professions (e.g. farming, medicine, dentistry, police, anaesthesiology). Homosexual or bisexual orientation. Immigrants | Presence of mental disorder: current episode of mental illness, major depression, other mood (affective) disorders, schizophrenia, anxiety, and disorders of conduct and personality, alcohol dependence and substance misuse, recent discharge from in-patient care, major history of hospitalisation for psychiatric disorder. Physical disorder: chronic medical illness, HIV/AIDS, visual impairment | Single, cohabiting, loss of a child. Poor social support/ social relationships. History of abuse in childhood, breakdown of traditional or primary family group structures, domestic violence, greater inter-generational pressure, mass-media culture | Unemployment, low income, financial problems, receipt of disability pension, low wealth status, socio-economic disadvantage (e.g. poverty, homelessness) | Impulsive behavioural style, poor problem-solving ability, negative or hopeless outlook, acquired capability to enact lethal self-injury | Recent loss/bereavement (job, partner or health, recent diagnosis of chronic or terminal illness such as HIV, cancer). Sense of being trapped. Insufficient capacity to solve problems. Absence of protective factors, deficient prospective cognitive processes, feelings of hopelessness. Availability of means of suicide | Previous or current history of self-harm, previous suicide attempt, history of violent crime. Season – spring (for prisoners, autumn) |

Sources: Department of Human Services (1997); Maris (2002); Phillips *et al* (2002); McAllister (2003); Buck (2004); Gunnell *et al* (2004); Packman *et al* (2004); Zhang *et al* (2004); Bouch & Marshall (2005); Qin *et al* (2005); Skegg (2005); Steele & Doey (2007).

unique person. An awareness of these risk factors, however, can alert health professionals in primary care to look at particular areas of people's lives.

# Changing patterns within the population

Suicide rates are not distributed equally throughout the general population of single countries. Social and economic changes as well as the availability of methods of suicide have influenced national trends in suicide. Taking a closer look at changing patterns within the population, the suicide rates of men and women, for instance, are consistently different in most places, as are rates in different age groups, and regions within countries.

## Gender

Rates of suicide are generally higher among men. There are about three male suicides for every female one (with the exception of rural China and parts of India, discussed below). However, women have higher rates of non-fatal suicidal acts. An explanation might be that women have higher levels of healthcare utilisation and exhibit more favourable intentions to seek help from mental health professionals (Bertakis *et al*, 2000; Ladwig *et al*, 2000; Adamson *et al*, 2003; Mackenzie *et al*, 2006); thus, for instance, they are more likely to receive treatment for depression, and to receive it earlier than men.

## Age

Suicide rates tend to increase with age (Värnik *et al*, 1998*b*). However, although, traditionally, suicide rates have been highest among elderly men, 'rates among young people have been increasing to such an extent that they are now the group at highest risk in a third of countries, in both lower-income and higher-income countries' (WHO, 2007*b*).

One of the reasons why suicide rates have been higher among elderly people might be that their determination to die is greater than that of other age groups and that they tend to choose more violent methods – such as shooting, hanging or jumping from a height (De Leo & Ormsker, 1991). Furthermore, ageing-related biological and/or psychological processes may contribute to increased risk for suicide in elderly people, as do living alone and losses, and physical frailty (Conwell & Duberstein, 2005).

## Ethnicity, cultural background and immigration

Sharing a common ancestry seems to be associated with similar suicide rates; for instance, both Finland and Hungary (whose common ancestors were Uralic-speaking herdsmen, known as the Magyars) have very high rates, even though Hungary is geographically quite distant from Finland (Krug *et al*, 2002; Gunnell, 2005). Kliewer (1991) compared immigrant suicide in Australia, Canada, England and Wales, and the USA during the period 1959–73 and found significant correlations between the suicide rates of the immigrants and those of the origin populations, indicating that the suicide rates for individual immigrant groups were to some extent influenced by their experiences in the origin countries. This study and another, by Kliewer & Ward (1988), found that factors in the destination country also influenced immigrant suicide rates, as the rates of the majority of the immigrant groups had a tendency to converge towards the rates of the native-born over time.

Finally, within countries, suicide rates are frequently higher among indigenous groups – notable examples include the Aboriginal and Torres Strait Islander populations in Australia and the Inuit in Canada's arctic north (WHO, 2002).

## Region

The incidence of suicide varies between urban and rural regions of the same country. Suicide rates are generally higher in urban areas than in rural areas. However, several studies have reported higher rates in rural areas, for example in Australia (Taylor et al, 2005), China (Qin & Mortensen, 2001), England and Wales (Middleton et al, 2003), India (Gajalakshmi & Peto, 2007), Iran (Abbasi-Shavazi, 2004) and the USA (Fiske et al, 2005). Reasons for higher rates in rural areas may include the limited access to healthcare, lower levels of education and social isolation. In addition, in contrast to urban areas, highly toxic herbicides and pesticides are more readily available in some countries, making poisoning a frequently used means of suicide.

# Assessment and management of patients at risk of suicide

As the rate of contact with clinicians in primary care in the year preceding suicide averages approximately 77% across all age groups and as persons with mental health problems are more likely to seek services in the primary care sector rather than from mental health professionals (Luoma et al, 2002), primary care professionals' ability to assess and manage suicide risk must be strengthened.

## What should clinicians do when faced with a suicidal patient?

At the primary care level, many patients at risk of suicide will not talk spontaneously about their despair, their suicide ideations or suicidal plans. Therefore, these have to be actively explored in every individual patient who is showing signs of despair or who belongs to a high-risk group (Table 9.1 and Box 9.1).

However, talking about suicide is often considered to be difficult for both the patient and the primary care provider. The emotional burden associated

---

**Box 9.1** Assessing the risk of suicide – risk groups

- Older single men (in some countries also younger men)
- Persons with mental disorders (depression; addictive disorders; psychoses)
- Persons in acute crisis (e.g. social isolation, unemployment, debt, divorce, traumatic experience)
- Access to potentially lethal means
- Chronic physical illness
- Family history of fatal suicidal acts and/or non-fatal suicidal acts/self-harm
- Previous non-fatal suicidal acts/self-harm
- Recent discharge from psychiatric hospital

---

with suicidal behaviour as well as fears that speaking about it might induce suicide are barriers to an active exploration of suicidal ideas, often with the result that the topic is addressed only briefly and the conversation rapidly switches to a less complex topic, or that trivialisation leads to an underestimation of the suicidal risk. In order to avoid this, primary care providers must be aware of these psychodynamic mechanisms and must be able to deal competently with suicidal behaviour. This begins with finding the right words for starting the exploration of suicide in a direct way. Every primary care worker should prepare a sentence or two or some questions to lead into the topic gradually, with due attention to the patient, in an empathic and non-judgemental but clear and focused manner. Examples would be:

- Do you feel unhappy and hopeless?
- Do you feel life is a burden?
- Do you feel unable to face each day?

If the answer to any of these questions indicates a possible suicide risk, active exploration should address the points listed in the Suicide Risk Screen (Harrison *et al*, 2004) (Box 9.2; see also Chapter 16).

When assessing a suicidal patient, it is particularly helpful to explore ideas of hopelessness, the feeling that not only is the current situation intolerable, but that it is unlikely to improve in future. This is particularly strongly associated with suicide risk. Active wishes to end one's life are more serious than passive wishes to be dead. Useful questions are listed in Box 9.3.

General practitioners may be called upon to assess someone following a suicidal act. The risk of suicide in such individuals is 100 times higher than the background rate in the general population. While some people may use self-harm as a coping strategy, and have no plans of suicide, or as a way of communicating intense distress, others may have continuing active plans to end their life. A suggested assessment framework is shown in Box 9.4.

**Box 9.2** Suicide Risk Screen

The presence of a larger number of the following suggests a greater level of risk:

- previous self-harm
- previous use of violent means
- suicidal plan/expressed intent
- current suicidal thoughts/ideation
- hopelessness/helplessness
- depression
- evidence of psychosis
- alcohol and/or drug misuse
- chronic physical illness/pain
- family history of suicide
- unemployed/retired
- male gender
- separated/widowed/divorced
- lack of social support
- family concerned about risk
- disengaged from services
- poor adherence to psychiatric treatment
- access to lethal means of harm.

Source: Harrison *et al* (2004)

**Box 9.3** Assessing suicide risk

1  General interview skills
    - Establish rapport
    - Open questioning style
    - Pick up verbal and non-verbal cues
    - Demonstrate acceptance of the patient
    - Clarify ambiguities
    - Summarise
2  Clarify current problems
3  Specific questioning about suicide intent
    - Explore hopelessness (e.g. 'How do you see the future?')
    - Does the patient have any wishes to be dead (fleeting or persistent)?
    - Specific plans for suicide (questions could include: 'Have you ever felt that you would prefer to get away from it all?', 'Have you ever felt that life isn't worth living?', 'Have you ever thought that you would do something to harm yourself?', 'What exactly would you do? Do you have plans?', 'What has stopped you from carrying that out so far?')
    - Measures to prevent detection
4  Background: past suicide attempts, coping mechanisms
5  Symptoms of mental disorder

Box 9.4 Assessment of a person who has recently self-harmed

The interviewer should ask about:

**Antecedents**
- Duration and degree of planning suicide attempt (greater risk of suicide if attempt was planned, especially if planning occurred over some time)
- Detailed account of events in preceding 48 hours
- Final acts (suicide note, will, etc.)

**The attempt**
- Lethality (hanging, shooting, drowning, carbon monoxide poisoning are all very high risk)
- Expectation of outcome (the expectation of the person engaging in self-harm is more important than the clinician's own expectation: professionals may be aware that a handful of aspirin is unlikely to be fatal – the person taking them may not)
- Precautions against discovery

**Mental state**
- Mood (especially hopelessness/worthlessness)
- Suicidal thoughts
- Current attitude (regret or guilt concerning the recent suicide attempt is less likely to be associated with completed suicide).

Further information can be obtained at www.medicine.manchester.ac.uk/storm.

Following initial assessment by the primary care worker, different types of aftercare may be appropriate, such as referral to psychological treatment, including cognitive–behavioural therapy and problem-solving therapy, or pharmacological treatment. It sometimes may be necessary to refer the patient for a detailed psychiatric assessment. Box 9.5 presents a list of possible steps. However, primary care workers should be aware that acute suicide risk can be an emergency, where even hospitalisation against the patient's will may be necessary. Psychotic depression, for example, is associated with an extremely high suicide risk and requires in-patient treatment in most cases.

# Evidence for the effectiveness of prevention strategies – an international perspective

Depending on the risk factors involved in suicidal acts, specific preventive interventions are used in individual countries, for instance restricting access to herbicides and pesticides in China or gun possession control in the USA. In addition, because a large number of suicide completers suffer from a diagnosable psychiatric disorder and because there is an increased

Box 9.5 Managing suicidal behaviour

- Arrange short-term follow-up
- Consult a specialist
- Involve family and relatives
- Draw up a suicide prevention contract
- Establish an emergency plan
- Ensure there is a safe home environment
- Administer appropriate medication
- If necessary, refer to in-patient treatment (also against the person's will)

risk of suicide in virtually all psychiatric disorders, a key prevention strategy is improved care of patients with depression and other psychiatric disorders.

For a categorisation of prevention strategies see Mann *et al* (2005) (Box 9.6).

## The Gotland study

In 1983–84, all 18 general practitioners (GPs) working on the Swedish island of Gotland (population 56 000) were invited to attend a 2-day education programme on the diagnosis and treatment of depression, given by the Swedish branch of the International Committee for the Prevention and Treatment of Depression (Swedish PTD Committee). The intervention was evaluated in relation to referrals to psychiatry, in-patient treatment, psychopharmacological prescription rates, sick leave from work and suicide rates (Rutz *et al*, 1989*b*). Two years after the intervention, referrals of patients with depression to psychiatry had increased, in particular for those

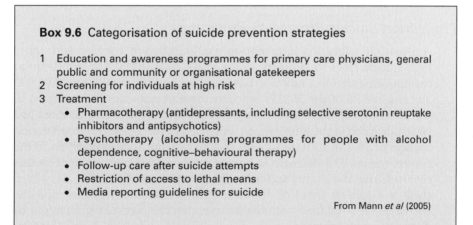

Box 9.6 Categorisation of suicide prevention strategies

1 Education and awareness programmes for primary care physicians, general public and community or organisational gatekeepers
2 Screening for individuals at high risk
3 Treatment
   - Pharmacotherapy (antidepressants, including selective serotonin reuptake inhibitors and antipsychotics)
   - Psychotherapy (alcoholism programmes for people with alcohol dependence, cognitive–behavioural therapy)
   - Follow-up care after suicide attempts
   - Restriction of access to lethal means
   - Media reporting guidelines for suicide

From Mann *et al* (2005)

suffering severe depression. The same was observed for the prescription of antidepressants. Sick leave and in-patient treatment decreased. The suicide rate on Gotland fell from 19.7 per 100000 at baseline ($n = 11$) in 1982 to 7.1 per 100000 in 1985 ($n = 4$) (Rutz et al, 1989a). However, the population observed and the number of suicides were too small and the random fluctuation in suicide numbers in the preceding years was too high to allow strong conclusions concerning the efficacy of the intervention in preventing suicide. Yet the Gotland study has drawn attention to the relevance of healthcare structure (such as the availability of trained GPs) for suicide prevention and has stimulated and inspired other research groups to follow this approach.

## The STORM Project

The suicide prevention training intervention STORM (Skills Training on Risk Management), which is based within the University of Manchester in the UK, is aimed at the improvement of clinical skills in primary care needed to assess and manage suicide risk. The target group of this intervention are front-line workers in health, social and criminal justice services (Green & Gask, 2005). Skills are developed through a short lecture, demonstration scenario of the skills to be learned, role rehearsal for practice, self-reflection and video-feedback on performance in four modules covering assessment, crisis management, problem-solving and crisis prevention.

To date, three evaluation projects of STORM have been carried out (Morriss et al, 1999; Appleby et al, 2000; Gask et al, 2006;) and these have shown positive changes in attitudes and confidence towards suicide. A before-and-after STORM training analysis showed no change in suicide rate (Morriss et al, 2005). A conclusion from this is that brief educational interventions to improve the assessment and management of patients at risk of suicide may not be sufficient to reduce the suicide rate and must be considered as a part of an overall, multifaceted suicide prevention strategy (Morriss et al, 2005).

## Hungarian Suicide Prevention Programme

A 5-year GP education intervention was launched in a region with quite high suicide rates in Hungary in the years 2001–2005. The intervention was implemented in a mixed urban/rural area with a population of 73000 and reached 28 of the 30 GPs working there. A non-contiguous region in the same county was chosen as a control. After 5 years, suicide rates had clearly dropped in the intervention region (from the 5-year pre-intervention average of 59.7 in 100000 to 49.9 in 100000) but they also did so in the control region. The decrease in suicide rates was larger than the decreases reported from the county and from Hungary (Szanto et al, 2007). However, there is a general trend of decreasing suicide rates in Hungary, and the decreases reported from both the intervention and control region might be due to this general trend.

## US Air Force Suicide Prevention Programme (AFSPP)

This programme, a population-based approach to reducing the risk of suicide, was first implemented with active-duty personnel in late 1996. Eleven initiatives were developed, aimed at strengthening social support, promoting development of effective social and coping skills, promoting awareness of the range of risk factors related to suicide, changing policies and norms to encourage effective help-seeking, and reducing the stigma related to help-seeking.

Personnel exposed to the programme experienced a 33% reduction of risk of fatal suicidal acts compared with personnel before the implementation ($P < 0.001$) (Registry of Evidence-Based Suicide Prevention Programs, 2005; Pflanz, 2007). When the project began, fatal suicidal acts were the second leading cause of death in the US Air Force. Thereafter, the suicide rate declined statistically significantly over three consecutive years. It must be noted that suicide rates in the USA also declined in the second half of the 1990s. This decline, however, was small compared with that measured in the Air Force (US Air Force Medical Service, 2002). As the Air Force community represents a select population, the generalisability of findings to other communities has been questioned (Knox *et al*, 2003).

## Multi-level approaches to suicide prevention – 'Choose Life' in Scotland

In 2002, the Scottish government launched 'Choose Life', a 10-year national strategy and long-term action plan to reduce suicide in Scotland by 20% by 2013 through improved early prevention and crisis response, engagement with the media, and adoption of an evidence-based approach (Mackenzie *et al*, 2007). The main aim of Choose Life is to set out a framework to achieve seven multifaceted objectives:

1    early prevention and intervention
2    responding to immediate crisis
3    longer-term work to provide hope and support recovery
4    coping with suicidal behaviour and completed suicide
5    promoting greater public awareness and encouraging people to seek help early
6    supporting the media
7    knowing 'what works' to prevent suicide.

MacKenzie *et al* argue that it is difficult to show that Choose Life has played a causal role in the reduction of suicide rates, because the massive reduction in male suicide and 'undetermined' deaths between 2002 ($n = 673$, rate $= 34.1/100\,000$) and 2003 ($n = 577$, rate $= 29.1/100\,000$) occurred when Choose Life had been only very partially implemented (Mackenzie *et al*, 2007). This reduction might also have been due to other factors, such as legislation restricting paracetamol sales. At the time of writing, the evaluation was still in progress.

## The Nuremberg Alliance Against Depression in Germany

In the years 2001 and 2002, an intervention for the improvement of care for patients with depression and the prevention of suicidality was implemented in the city of Nuremberg, Germany (population 500 000), with Würzburg (population 270 000) as a control region. The intervention took place on four levels (Fig. 9.1):

1 intervention with primary care physicians
2 initiation of a professional public media campaign
3 intervention with community facilitators
4 intervention with persons with depression, suicide attempters and their relatives.

The intervention was intense; for example, more than 2000 community facilitators were trained and more than 100 000 leaflets on depression were distributed. The evaluation was ambitious and included data from a 1-year baseline (year 2000) and a control region. The number of suicidal acts was defined as the primary outcome criterion. During the two intervention years, the number of suicidal acts (fatal plus non-fatal) decreased by 24% in the intervention region, significantly more than in the control region, where the rate remained stable (Hegerl *et al*, 2006). Interestingly, this was not a short-term effect, because a further decrease was observed in the follow-up year, 2003 (−32% compared with the baseline year). When taking into consideration fatal and non-fatal suicidal acts (secondary outcome criteria) independently, a significant effect was only observed for the latter. The base

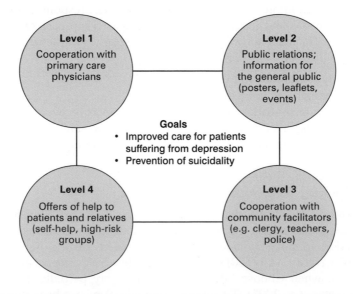

**Fig. 9.1** The four-level suicide prevention strategy of the Nuremberg Alliance Against Depression and the European Alliance Against Depression.

rate of fatal suicidal acts was too low to allow for the statistical detection of moderate, though clinically relevant, intervention effects.

The Nuremberg Alliance Against Depression has provided strong evidence that its four-level intervention concept and its materials are effective in the prevention of suicidality. The success of this multi-level intervention is most likely based not only on the effectiveness of the single intervention on all levels but also on synergistic effects between them. This view is clearly supported by WHO recommendations which advocate choosing a multifaceted approach in the prevention of mental disorders and suicidality (WHO, 2004). Meanwhile, the four-level intervention concept and materials of the Nuremberg Alliance Against Depression have been taken up by 50 regions in Germany, where similar alliances against depression are run, by the European Alliance Against Depression (http://www.eaad.net) and by the Seventh Framework Programme 'Optimised Suicide Prevention Programmes' (OSPI-Europe, http://www.ospi-europe.com/).

# International comparisons

Differences in the definition and the procedure for assessing suicide rates between countries pose challenges to the collection of accurate, comparable rates of suicide. Such differences represent a significant challenge for field work and reduce the validity of available official suicide statistics and influence the rates of 'hidden' suicides. Categories such as 'unknown reason of death' or 'ill-defined and unknown causes of mortality' (ICD–10, R96–R99) might be used more often in some regions than in others, for a variety of reasons, and changes in these rates of recording deaths may show an inverse relationship to those of suicide rates. For instance, there is considerable variation in undetermined deaths across countries and this appears to have an effect on the accuracy of national suicide statistics.

## International total suicide rates

Among countries reporting suicide rates to the WHO, the highest total rates (per 100 000 population) are found in eastern European countries – for instance, for Lithuania, 40.2 in 2004; for the Russian Federation, 34.3 in 2004; and for Hungary, 27.7 in 2003 (WHO, 2007c). Within Europe, however, there are considerable cross-national differences in published total suicide rates. Some of the lowest rates are found in Armenia (1.8 in 2003) and Greece (3.2 in 2004) (WHO, 2007c). Other European countries show total rates somewhere between these extremes.

High total rates of suicide have also been reported in Sri Lanka, at 21.6 in 1996, in Japan, at 24.0 in 2004, in selected rural areas in China, at 22.5 in 1999, and in Guyana, at 27.2 in 2003. In contrast, people in Latin America (e.g. Brazil, at 4.3 in 2002, and Paraguay, at 3.1 in 2003), a few Asian nations (e.g. the Philippines, at 2.1 in 1993, and Thailand, at 7.8 in 2002) and in Muslim countries (0.2 in Iran in 1991 and 2.0 in Kuwait in 2002) are least likely to end their own life. Countries in other parts of North America, parts of Asia and the Pacific fall in between these total rates (e.g. in the USA 11.0 in 2002, and in New Zealand 11.9 in 2000). Almost no data are available from the WHO African region. Information is also scarce from the WHO South-East Asia and Eastern Mediterranean regions.

The rate of non-fatal suicidal acts is estimated to be about 20 times higher than that of fatal suicidal acts. In Europe, the highest rates for non-fatal suicidal acts are found in younger women, whereas the highest rates for fatal suicidal acts are found in older men and in a growing number of European countries such as Lithuania, Estonia, Latvia, Finland and Ireland also among young men aged 15–34. The lowest rates are found mainly in Latin America and a few countries in Asia.

## Explaining the difference

It is difficult to explain the diverse geographical variation in international suicide rates in detail. From what we know today, it is likely that a combination of factors contribute to the variation, such as differences in historical, socio-cultural and societal factors, in the prevalence of psychiatric morbidity or access to means of suicide, and in the availability and effective delivery of primary and secondary healthcare services. For a thorough discussion see Gunnell (2005).

## Taking a closer look at gender and region

In almost all regions of the world, more men commit suicide than women – with the exception of rural China and parts of India. The highest suicide rate (of women) in the world has been reported among young women in South India, where the average suicide rate for women aged 15–19 years living around Vellore in Tamil Nadu was 148 per 100 000 (Bhattacharya, 2007). In comparison, the highest suicide rate for men has been reported for Lithuania, at 70.1 per 100 000 (WHO, 2007c).

There are numerous possible explanations for the high suicide rate among females in rural China and South India. A major factor appears to be that highly toxic pesticides are easily available in these regions (Bertolote et al, 2006). Since women prefer intoxication as method of suicide attempts, the lethality of this method is far higher than in countries where these pesticides have been banned. Other reasons may be that political and economic changes have partially eroded the social structures in rural areas and women, who have little opportunities to participate in economic and cultural transformation, are especially hit by the shock of modernisation. In addition, women in these countries still have a lower social status. Finally, there are fewer legal or religious sanctions against suicide, compared with other countries (Gunnell, 2005).

## Taking a closer look at religion

Several but not all studies have provided evidence that a higher level of religious affiliation is associated with lower suicide rates (Neeleman *et al*, 1997; Neeleman & Lewis, 1999; Clarke *et al*, 2003; Dervic *et al*, 2004; van Tuberger *et al*, 2005). However, again there are variations: official suicide rates in many Islamic countries are much lower than in countries of other religions; for example, the total suicide rate per 100 000 in Kuwait was 2.0 in 2002, whereas in largely Hindu India it was 10.5 in 2002, and in broadly Buddhist Japan it was 24.0 in 2004. This might be because Islam specifically forbids suicide.

# Conclusion

From a global perspective, the variation in suicide rates between countries – and also within countries – indicates that it is important for each country to watch epidemiological trends, to identify at-risk populations and to derive effective suicide prevention strategies. It is likely that the adoption of similar prevention strategies will be successful and effective in countries that share similar historical, social and economic characteristics and also show similar total suicide rates.

One example of a cross-European prevention strategy is the four-level community-based intervention programme based on the Nuremberg Alliance Against Depression, which has been implemented in 17 regions across Europe within the European Alliance Against Depression. The concept used in Nuremberg has been complemented with local materials and adapted for use in the different European partner countries (Hegerl *et al*, 2007, 2009).

---

Key points

- Approximately 1.53 million people will die from fatal suicidal acts in 2020, and 10–20 times more people will attempt suicide worldwide.
- Multiple and interacting risk factors are involved in suicidal acts.
- Up to over 90% of suicide completers suffer from a diagnosable psychiatric disorder.
- When assessing suicide risk, each patient must be regarded individually.
- Suicide risk must be actively explored by clinicians.
- There is geographical variation in international suicide rates and a combination of factors, such as differences in historical, socio-cultural and societal factors, in the prevalence of psychiatric morbidity and in access to means of suicide, contribute to the variation.
- Specific suicide prevention interventions have been evaluated in individual countries and regions.

# Acknowledgements

We would like to thank the following authors for their valuable contribution to this chapter: Esa Aromaa MSc, Lapuan psykiatrinen poliklinikaa, Finland; Chantal Van Audenhove PhD, LUCAS – Katholieke Universiteit Leuven, Belgium; Jean-Hervé Bouleau MD, Fédération de Psychiatrie, Hôpital René Dubos, France; Christina M. van der Feltz-Cornelis MD PhD, Trimbos instituut, Utrecht, and VU Medical Centre Institute of Extramural Research, Amsterdam, The Netherlands; Ricardo Gusmão MD PhD, Universidade Nova de Lisboa, Faculdade de Ciências Médicas, Lisbon, Portugal; Maria Kopp MD PhD, Semmelweis University Budapest, Hungary; Andrej Marusic MD PhD, Institute of Public Health of the Republic of Slovenia, Slovenia; Margaret Maxwell PhD, Department of Applied Social Science, University of Stirling, UK; Ullrich Meise MD PhD, Society for Mental Health – pro mente tirol, Austria; Högni Óskarsson MD, Directorate of Health, Icelandic Alliance Against Depression, Seltjarnarnes, Iceland; Roger Pycha MD, Autonome Provinz Südtirol, Assessorat für das Gesundheitswesen, Italy; Charles Pull MD PhD, Centre Hospitalier de Luxembourg, Luxembourg; Thomas Reisch MD, University Hospital of Psychiatry, University of Bern, Switzerland; Armin Schmidtke PhD, Klinik und Poliklinik für Psychiatrie und Psychotherapie der Universität Würzburg, Germany; Victor Pérez Sola MD, Hospital de la Santa Creu i Sant Pau Psychiatry Department, Barcelona, Spain.

# Further reading and e-resources

De Leo, D. & Evans, R. (2004) *International Suicide Rates and Prevention Strategies*. Hogrefe & Huber.

De Leo, D., Bille-Brahe, U., Kerkhof, A., *et al* (eds) (2004) *Suicidal Behaviour: Theories and Research Findings*. Hogrefe & Huber.

Hawton, K. (ed.) (2005) *Prevention and Treatment of Suicidal Behaviour: From Science to Practice*. Oxford University Press.

Hawton, K. & van Heeringen, K. (eds) (2000) *The International Handbook of Suicide and Attempted Suicide*. Wiley.

Jacobs, D. G. (1999) *The Harvard Medical School Guide to Suicide Assessment and Intervention*. Jossey-Bass.

Kutcher, S. & Chehil, S. (2007) *Suicide Risk Management: A Manual for Health Professionals*. Blackwell Publishing.

Maris, R. W., Berman, A. L. & Silverman, M. M. (2000) *Comprehensive Textbook of Suicidology*. Guilford Press.

Shea, S. C. (2002) *The Practical Art of Suicide Assessment: A Guide for Mental Health Professionals and Substance Abuse Counselors*. Wiley.

Shneidman, E. S. (1998) *The Suicidal Mind*. Oxford University Press.

Simon, R. I. (2004) *Assessing and Managing Suicide Risk. Guidelines for Clinically Based Risk Management*. American Psychiatric Publishing.

Simon, R. I. & Hales, R. E. (eds) (2006) *The American Psychiatric Publishing Textbook of Suicide Assessment and Management*. American Psychiatric Publishing.

http://www.awp.nhs.uk/FOI%20Documents/Support%20documents/Guidance%20Note%203.pdf – Integrated Care Pathway, Assessment of Suicide Risk in Primary Care Settings, Guidance Note 3

http://www.chooselife.net/ – more information about Choose Life

http://www.eaad.net/ – more information about the European Alliance Against Depression

http://www.eaad.net/enu/information-material.php – screening instruments, structured patient file for the detection and diagnosis of depression, treatment guidelines and informational films http://www.medicine.manchester.ac.uk/storm/ – more information about the STORM project

http://www.mentalneurologicalprimarycare.org/ – WHO guide to mental and neurological health in primary care

http://www.nrepp.samhsa.gov/programfulldetails.asp?PROGRAM_ID=68 – more information about the US Air Force Suicide Prevention Program

http://sdsuicideprevention.org/toolsforcommunities/index.php?id=31 – suicide prevention, clinician guidelines, links to guidelines and booklets of the Risk Management Foundation, American Psychiatric Association and Harvard Medical School Guide

http://www.who.int/mental_health/resources/suicide/en/ – WHO list of different suicide prevention publications, such as preventing suicide – a resource for general practitioners

# References

Abbasi-Shavazi, M. J. (2004) Preliminary notes on trends and emerging issues of mortality in Iran, http://www.unescap.org/esid/psis/meetings/health_mortality_sep_2004/H_M_Iran.pdf.

Adamson, J., Ben Shlomo, Y., Chaturvedi, N., *et al* (2003) Ethnicity, socio-economic position and gender – do they affect reported health-care seeking behaviour? *Social Science and Medicine*, **57**, 895–904.

Appleby, L., Morriss, L., Gask, L., *et al* (2000) An educational intervention for front-line health professionals in the assessment and management of suicidal patients (the STORM Project). *Psychological Medicine*, **30**, 805–812.

Bertakis, K. D., Azari, R., Helms, L. J., *et al* (2000) Gender differences in the utilization of health care services. *Journal of Family Practice*, **49**, 147–152.

Bertolote, J. M., Fleischmann, A., Eddleston, M., *et al* (2006) Deaths from pesticide poisoning: a global response. *British Journal of Psychiatry*, **189**, 201–203.

Bhattacharya, S. (2007) Indian teens have world's highest suicide rate. *Lancet*, **363**, 1117.

Bouch, J. & Marshall, J. J. (2005) Suicide risk: structured professional judgement. *Advances in Psychiatric Treatment*, **11**, 84–91.

Brent, D. A., Johnson, B. A., Perper, J., *et al* (1994) Personality disorder, personality traits, impulsive violence, and completed suicide in adolescents. *Journal of the American Academy of Child and Adolescent Psychiatry*, **33**, 1080–1086.

Buck, A. (2004) Suicide and self-harm. *Practice Nurse*, **28**, 64–68.

Clarke, C. S., Bannon, F. J. & Denihan, A. (2003) Suicide and religiosity – Masaryk's theory revisited. *Social Psychiatry and Psychiatric Epidemiology*, **38**, 502–508.

Conwell, Y. & Duberstein, P. (2005) Suicide in older adults: determinants of risk and opportunities for prevention. In *Prevention and Treatment of Suicidal Behaviour* (ed. K. Hawton), pp. 221–237. Oxford University Press.

De Leo, D. & Ormsker, S. (1991) Suicide in the elderly: general characteristics. *Crisis*, **12**, 3–17.

De Leo, D., Burgis, S., Bertolote, J. M., *et al* (2004) Definitions of suicidal behaviour. In *Suicidal Behaviour: Theories and Research Findings* (eds D. De Leo, U. Bille-Brahe, A. Kerkhof & A. Schmidtke), pp. 17–40. Hogrefe & Huber.

Department of Human Services (1997) *Suicide Prevention Task Force Report 1997*. Department of Human Services, State Government of Victoria, Australia.

Dervic, K., Oquendo, M. A., Grunebaum, M. F., *et al* (2004) Religious affiliation and suicide attempt. *American Journal of Psychiatry*, **161**, 2303–2308.

Fiske, A., Gatz, M. & Hannell, E. (2005) Rural suicide rates and availability of health care providers. *Journal of Community Psychology*, **33**, 537–543.

Gajalakshmi, V. & Peto, R. (2007) Suicide rates in rural Tamil Nadu, South India: verbal autopsy of 39 000 deaths. *International Journal of Epidemiology*, **36**, 203–207.

Gask, L., Dixon, C., Morriss, R., et al (2006) Evaluating STORM skills training for managing people at risk of suicide. *Journal of Advanced Nursing*, **54**, 739–750.

Green, G. & Gask, L. (2005) The development, research and implementation of STORM (Skills-based Training on Risk Management). *Primary Care Mental Health*, **3**, 207–213.

Gunnell, D. (2005) Time trends and geographic differences in suicide: implications for prevention. In *Prevention and Treatment of Suicidal Behaviour* (ed. K. Hawton), pp. 29–52. Oxford University Press.

Gunnell, D., Harbord, R., Singleton, N., et al (2004) Factors influencing the development and amelioration of suicidal thoughts in the general population: cohort study. *British Journal of Psychiatry*, **185**, 385–393.

Harrison, A., Hillier, D. & Redman, R. (2004) Assessment of suicide risk in primary care settings. Guidance note 3. In *Integrated Care Pathway. Self-harm. Support Documents*, pp. 1–5. Avon and Wiltshire Mental Health Partnership NHS Trust & Bath Community Partnership NHS Trust.

Hawton, K., Arensman, E., Wasserman, D., et al (1998) Relation between attempted suicide and suicide rates among young people in Europe. *Journal of Epidemiology and Community Health*, **52**, 191–194.

Hegerl, U., Althaus, D., Schmidtke, A., et al (2006) The alliance against depression: 2-year evaluation of a community-based intervention to reduce suicidality. *Psychological Medicine*, **36**, 1225–1233.

Hegerl, U., Wittman, M., Arensman, E., et al (2007) The European Alliance Against Depression (EAAD): a multifaceted, community-based action programme against depression and suicidality. *World Journal of Biological Psychiatry*, **9**, 51–58.

Hegerl, U., Wittenburg, L., Gottlebe, K., et al (2009) The European Alliance Against Depression: a multilevel approach to the prevention of suicidal behavior. *Psychiatric Services*, **60**, 596–599.

Kliewer, E. (1991) Immigrant suicide in Australia, Canada, England and Wales, and the United States. *Journal of the Australian Population Association*, **8**, 111–128.

Kliewer, E. & Ward, R. (1988) Convergence of immigrant suicide rates to those in the destination country. *American Journal of Epidemiology*, **127**, 640–653.

Knox, K. L., Litts, D. A., Talcott, G. W., et al (2003) Risk of suicide and related adverse outcomes after exposure to a suicide prevention programme in the US Air Force: cohort study. *BMJ*, **327**, 1376–1380.

Krug, E. G., Dahlberg, L. L., Mercy, J. A., et al (2002) *World Report on Violence and Health*. World Health Organization.

Ladwig, K. H., Marten-Mittag, B., Formanek, B., et al (2000) Gender differences of symptom reporting and medical health care utilization in the German population. *European Journal of Epidemiology*, **16**, 511–518.

Lonnqvist, J. (2000) Psychiatric aspects of suicidal behaviour: depression. In *The International Handbook of Suicide and Attempted Suicide* (eds K. Hawton & K. Van Heeringen), pp. 107–120. Wiley.

Luoma, J. B., Martin C. E. & Pearson, J. L. (2002) Contact with mental health and primary care providers before suicide: a review of the evidence. *American Journal of Psychiatry*, **159**, 909–916.

Mackenzie, C., Gekoski, W. & Knox, V. (2006) Age, gender, and the underutilization of mental health services: the influence of help-seeking attitudes. *Aging and Mental Health*, **10**, 574–582.

Mackenzie, M., Blamey, A., Halliday, E., et al (2007) Measuring the tail of the dog that doesn't bark in the night: the case of the national evaluation of Choose Life (the national strategy and action plan to prevent suicide in Scotland). *BMC Public Health*, **7**, 146–153.

Mäkinen, I. H. (2000) Eastern European transition and suicide mortality. *Social Science and Medicine*, **51**, 1405–1420.

Mann, J. J., Apter, A., Bertolote, J., et al (2005) Suicide prevention strategies: a systematic review. *JAMA*, **294**, 2064–2074.

Maris, R. (2002) Suicide. *Lancet*, **360**, 319–326.

McAllister, M. (2003) Multiple meanings of self harm: a critical review. *International Journal of Mental Health Nursing*, **12**, 177–185.

Middleton, N., Gunnell, D., Frankel, S., *et al* (2003) Urban–rural differences in suicide trends in young adults: England and Wales, 1981–1998. *Social Science and Medicine*, **57**, 1183–1194.

Morriss, R., Gask, L., Battersby, L., *et al* (1999) Teaching front-line health and voluntary workers to assess and manage suicidal patients. *Journal of Affective Disorders*, **52**, 77–83.

Morriss, R., Gask, L., Webb, R., *et al* (2005) The effects on suicide rates of an educational intervention for front-line health professionals with suicidal patients (the STORM Project). *Psychological Medicine*, **35**, 957–960.

Neeleman, J. & Lewis, G. (1999) Suicide, religion, and socioeconomic conditions. An ecological study in 26 countries. *Journal of Epidemiology and Community Health*, **53**, 204–210.

Neeleman, J., Halpern, D., Leon, D., *et al* (1997) Tolerance of suicide, religion and suicide rates: an ecological and individual study in 19 Western countries. *Psychological Medicine*, **27**, 1165–1171.

O'Carroll, P. W., Berman, A. L., Maris, R. W., *et al* (1996) Beyond the tower of Babel: a nomenclature for Suicidology. *Suicide and Life-Threatening Behavior*, **26**, 237–252.

Packman, W. L., Marlitt, R. E., Bongar, B., *et al* (2004) A comprehensive and concise assessment of suicide risk. *Behavioral Sciences and the Law*, **22**, 667–680.

Pflanz, S. E. (2007) Air Force suicide prevention program, http://www.nrepp.samhsa. gov/programfulldetails.asp?PROGRAM_ID=68#outcomes.

Phillips, M. R., Yang, G., Zhang, Y., *et al* (2002) Risk factors for suicide in China: a national case–control psychological autopsy study. *Lancet*, **360**, 1728–1736.

Qin, P. & Mortensen, P. B. (2001) Specific characteristics of suicide in China. *Acta Psychiatrica Scandinavica*, **103**, 117–121.

Qin, P., Agerbo, E. & Mortensen, P. B. (2005) Factors contributing to suicide: the epidemiological evidence from large-scale registers. In *Prevention and Treatment of Suicidal Behaviour* (ed. K. Hawton), pp. 11–28. Oxford University Press.

Registry of Evidence-Based Suicide Prevention Programs (2005) US Air Force Program.

Rich, C. L., Fowler, R. C., Fogarty, L. A., *et al* (1988) San Diego Suicide Study. III. Relationships between diagnoses and stressors. *Archives of General Psychiatry*, **45**, 589–592.

Robins, E., Murphy, G. E., Wilkinson, R. H., Jr, *et al* (1959) Some clinical considerations in the prevention of suicide based on a study of 134 successful suicides. *American Journal of Public Health*, **49**, 888–899.

Rutz, W., von Knorring, L. & Walinder, J. (1989*a*) Frequency of suicide on Gotland after systematic postgraduate education of general practitioners. *Acta Psychiatrica Scandinavica*, **80**, 151–154.

Rutz, W., Walinder, J., Eberhard, G., *et al* (1989*b*) An educational program on depressive disorders for general practitioners on Gotland: background and evaluation. *Acta Psychiatrica Scandinavica*, **79**, 19–26.

Skegg, K. (2005) Self-harm. *Lancet*, **366**, 1471–1483.

Steele, M. M. & Doey, T. (2007) Suicidal behaviour in children and adolescents. Part 1: Etiology and risk factors. *Canadian Journal of Psychiatry*, **52**, 21S–33S.

Szanto, K., Kalmar, S., Hendin, H., *et al* (2007) A suicide prevention program in a region with a very high suicide rate. *Archives of General Psychiatry*, **64**, 914–920.

Taylor, R., Page, A., Morrell, S., *et al* (2005) Social and psychiatric influences on urban–rural differentials in Australian suicide. *Suicide and Life-Threatening Behavior*, **35**, 277–290.

US Air Force Medical Service (2002) *Air Force Suicide Prevention Program. A Population-based, Community Approach*. US Air Force.

van Tuberger, F., te Grotenhuis, M. & Ultee, W. (2005) Denomination, religious context, and suicide: neo-Durkheimian multilevel explanations tested with individual and contextual data. *American Journal of Sociology*, **111**, 797–823.

Värnik, A., Wasserman, D., Dankowicz, M., *et al* (1998*a*) Marked decrease in suicide among men and women in the former USSR during perestroika. *Acta Psychiatrica Scandinavica*, **98**, 13–19.

Värnik, A., Wasserman, D., Dankowicz, M., *et al* (1998*b*) Age-specific suicide rates in the Slavic and Baltic regions of the former USSR during Perestroika, in comparison with 22 European countries. *Acta Psychiatrica Scandinavica*, **98**, 20–25.

Wasserman, D., Värnik, A. (1998) Suicide preventive effects of Perestroika in the former USSR: the role of alcohol restriction. *Acta Psychiatrica Scandinavica*, **98**, 1–4.

WHO (1999) *Figures and Facts About Suicide*. WHO.

WHO (2002) *Suicide Prevention in Europe*. World Health Organization Regional Office for Europe Copenhagen.

WHO (2004) *Prevention of Mental Disorders. Effective Interventions and Policy Options*. Geneva: WHO.

WHO (2007*a*) *Suicide*. WHO.

WHO (2007*b*) *Suicide Prevention (SUPRE)*. WHO.

WHO (2007*c*) *Suicide Rates per 100,000 by Country, Year and Sex*. WHO.

Zhang, J., Conwell Y., Zhou, L., *et al* (2004) Culture, risk factors and suicide in rural China: a psychological autopsy case control study. *Acta Psychiatrica Scandinavica*, **110**, 430–437.

# CHAPTER 10

# Anxiety

Bruce Arroll and Tony Kendrick

Summary

This chapter describes the definition, classification and epidemiology of anxiety disorders, which are very common but often missed in primary care. Diagnosis rests on identifying triggers and cognitive symptoms. Apart from specific phobias, anxiety disorders are usually chronic and disabling but they do respond to psychological treatments and selective serotonin reuptake inhibitors. Referral for specialist care is indicated only for a small minority of persisting or complicated cases.

## Definition of anxiety

Anxiety is considered to be a universal adaptive response to a threat; this response can, however, become maladaptive. The distinction between abnormal and normal anxiety occurs when the anxiety is out of proportion to the level of threat or when there are symptoms that are unacceptable regardless of the level of threat, including recurrent panic attacks, severe physical symptoms and abnormal beliefs such as fear of sudden death. Abnormal anxiety is present when it causes 'unacceptable and disruptive problems in its own right' (House & Stark, 2002).

## Epidemiology and classification

Anxiety disorders are usually the most common mental health condition in community settings (Kessler *et al*, 2005) and are responsible for more than 50% of the diagnosable mental health conditions in international prevalence surveys (Bijl *et al*, 2003). The same is also true in primary care settings, where as many as 20% of patients have an anxiety condition based on the categories of DSM–IV (American Psychiatric Association, 2000).

In primary care, anxiety disorders overall are more common in women (26%) than in men (12%) and more common in young people than in older people (25–44 years versus 65 or older). In young women, the prevalence is as high as 35%, compared with only 8% in older women. A similar decline with age occurs in men but with lower prevalence rates (MaGPIe Research Group, 2005). Recent research has shown that about half of adults with anxiety disorders have had psychiatric problems in childhood, emphasising the scope for early diagnosis (Gregory *et al*, 2007).

## Burden of anxiety disorders

Among the various subcategories of anxiety disorders, as many as half are single phobias such as fear of spiders, fear of flying and so on, which do not interfere with functioning on a daily basis. However, generalised anxiety disorder (GAD), panic disorder, post-traumatic stress disorder (PTSD), obsessive–compulsive disorder (OCD), social phobia and agoraphobia are more pervasive and disabling conditions, which between them are as common as depression (Table 10.1).

Follow-up studies suggest that GAD, panic disorder and social phobia have a chronic clinical course, low rates of recovery and high probabilities of recurrence (Bruce *et al*, 2005). The presence of comorbid psychiatric disorders significantly lowers the likelihood of recovery from anxiety disorders. While there has been some debate about whether there has been an increase in depression over recent decades, it appears the prevalence of anxiety has remained stable over the past 40 years, at least in Stirling County in Canada (Murphy *et al*, 2004). However, there is considerable overlap between depressive and anxiety disorders in symptoms and they are frequently found together. There is even an argument that depression and anxiety are the same condition and any distinction between the two has merely been encouraged by pharmaceutical companies in order to sell more medications (Shorter & Tyrer, 2003).

**Table 10.1** Twelve-month prevalence (%) of anxiety disorders

| Condition | In primary care (*n* = 908) | In the community (*n* = 12 992) |
|---|---|---|
| Any anxiety disorder | 20.7 | 14.8 |
| Specific phobia | 11.0 | 7.3 |
| Generalised anxiety disorder | 6.6 | 2.9 |
| Post-traumatic stress disorder | 3.4 | 3.0 |
| Obsessive–compulsive disorder | 2.9 | 0.6 |
| Panic without agoraphobia | 2.0 | 1.7 |
| Social phobia | 3.7 | 5.1 |
| Agoraphobia | 0.2 | 0.6 |

Sources: MaGPIe Research Group (2003); Oakley-Browne *et al* (2006).

# Presentation in primary care

The figures in Table 10.1 are taken from a primary care study and a community study conducted in New Zealand. The two surveys were conducted over similar time periods, allowing a direct comparison of the community and primary care settings. They both used the computerised Composite International Diagnostic Interview (CIDI; World Health Organization, 1997). Most anxiety conditions were more common in primary care than they were in the community, except for social phobia and agoraphobia, both of which involve avoidance of public places like doctors' surgeries. The reason for the higher rates of the other disorders in primary care than in the community is most likely that while many people have symptoms of ill health, it is anxiety that will make them see a doctor. This was demonstrated in a study in Hong Kong where patents with irritable bowel syndrome and dyspepsia who saw a doctor, had higher levels of anxiety than those with the same symptoms who did not see their doctor (Hu *et al*, 2002).

Anxiety symptoms are often not recognised by primary care professionals, as patients may not complain of them overtly. Table 10.2 lists types of presentations of anxiety disorders that may not initially be recognised as being due to anxiety.

## Screening and case-finding

There is considerable debate about screening for common mental health disorders. A systematic review concluded that universal screening was not justified (Gilbody *et al*, 2001). However, in primary care, case-finding for anxiety may be worthwhile in groups at high risk, such as frequent

**Table 10.2** Presentations that may initially go unrecognised as being due to anxiety disorders

| Presentation | Details |
| --- | --- |
| Fatigue, insomnia, chronic pain | Consider both depression and anxiety disorders as they commonly coexist |
| Frequent attendance with multiple symptoms, despite reassurance | For example a patient with irritable bowel syndrome + headaches + back pain |
| Cardiovascular symptoms | Palpitations, chest pain, faintness, flushing, sweating |
| Respiratory symptoms | Shortness of breath, hyperventilation, dyspnoea |
| Gastrointestinal symptoms | Choking, lump in throat, dry mouth, nausea, vomiting, diarrhoea |
| Neurological symptoms | Dizziness, headache, paraesthesia, vertigo |
| Musculoskeletal symptoms | Muscle ache, muscle tension, tremor, restlessness |

After Blashki *et al* (2007).

presenters, or in specific demographic groups, such as young women or particular ethnic groups. This will clearly vary from country to country. In New Zealand, for example, Maori patients have considerably higher rates, the 12-month prevalence in Maori women being 53% and in Maori men 17%, versus 22% and 11% respectively in non-Maori patients (MaGPIe Research Group, 2005).

## Diagnosis

Physical conditions that may mimic or coexist with anxiety symptoms should be considered (House & Stark, 2002), although anxiety disorders should be positive diagnoses, made on the basis of a careful history and examination, and not diagnoses of exclusion, requiring exhaustive investigation of patients' symptoms.

Physical disorders associated with symptoms of anxiety include (House & Stark, 2002):

- thyrotoxicosis
- alcohol or drug withdrawal
- hypocapnia due to hyperventilation
- anaemia
- hypoglycaemia
- hypoxia or hypercapnia due to intermittent respiratory disorders
- poor pain control
- vertigo due to vestibular disorders.

Drugs with effects and side-effects that may commonly mimic anxiety include (House & Stark, 2002):

- bronchodilators
- insulin and oral hypoglycaemic agents
- selective serotonin reuptake inhibitor (SSRI) antidepressants
- corticosteroids
- thyroxine.

Table 10.3 lists key features of the various categories of anxiety disorders, including triggers, physical symptoms, cognitive symptoms and patients' behavioural responses to their symptoms.

## Specific diagnoses

### Generalised anxiety disorder

This may be difficult to diagnose in primary care. Patients do not experience acute panic but do feel tense and anxious most of the time and these symptoms need to be present for at least 6 months to make the diagnosis. They feel restless, tire easily, have trouble concentrating, are irritable, have increased muscle tension and initial insomnia with unrefreshing sleep. There are no specific triggers.

Table 10.3 Key features of anxiety disorders

| Category | Triggers | Physical symptoms | Cognitive symptoms | Patient behaviours |
|---|---|---|---|---|
| Generalised anxiety disorder | Non-specific day-to-day events, issues | Non-specific aches, pains, insomnia, fatigue | Constant fear and worry | Inability to carry out daily tasks |
| Panic | Initially, no specific trigger; later, associated with specific places, etc. | Rush of fear, palpitations, shortness of breath, sympathetic response | Am I dying? Am I going to pass out? Will I embarrass myself? | Paralysis in feared situation |
| Social phobia | Social situations | Milder panic | I will make a fool of myself | Avoid social situations |
| Agoraphobia | Leaving a safe place | Intense fear | Can I escape? | Avoid leaving the house |
| Specific phobia | Animals, blood, heights, etc. | Intense fear | Can I escape? | Avoid feared objects |
| Obsessive–compulsive disorder | None | None | Bothered by thoughts, impulses and images that are recurrent and do not make sense | Repetitive behaviours, checking, ruminating |
| Post-traumatic stress disorder | Started by traumatic event involving significant threat to life and limb | Any anxiety symptoms; nightmares | Detached from life; emotionally numb; flash-backs to feared situations | Avoid stimuli associated with trauma; hypervigilant that trauma will happen again |

## Panic disorder

A common presentation of panic attack is the young adult patient who presents to an emergency department with hyperventilation and tachycardia and chest pain, who gets an electrocardiograph and chest radiograph and leaves without a diagnosis of anxiety. A panic attack is a specific event, while panic disorder is a condition of recurrent attacks. The panic attacks can be triggered by specific situations but occasionally are uncued. A panic attack can include symptoms suggesting acute cardiorespiratory and neurological events, a fear of dying or passing out, and a feeling of being detached from oneself and losing self-control.

Panic disorder often occurs along with agoraphobia. Panic disorder with agoraphobia includes a change in behaviour to avoid public situations in which panic attacks may take place. Agoraphobia can be diagnosed with or without panic disorder. This involves anxiety about being in places from which escape may be difficult or where help may not be available if an unexpected panic attack or panic-like symptoms occur. Agoraphobic fears typically involve situations such as being outside the home alone, being in a crowd or standing in line, and travelling in a train, bus or car.

## Social phobia

This is a recurring fear of social performance situations that involve facing strangers or being watched by others. The patient realises that this fear is unreasonable or out of proportion to the problem. Patients under the age of 16 must have had symptoms present for 6 months or more. The distress must interfere with the person's social or occupational functioning and be more than just shyness.

## Specific phobias

These are unwarranted fears of specific objects or situations (Morrison, 1995). The most commonly recognised are phobias relating to animals, blood, heights and aeroplane travel, but can include darkness, urinating or defecating in public places, certain foods and dentistry. The resultant anxiety can present as a panic attack or GAD, but it is always directed at something specific. Patients with this condition may have a vasovagal response and faint when exposed to the object, especially blood, injury or injection. The degree of discomfort and interference with daily living is often mild, so most people do not seek professional help. Anecdotally, the presentation of specific phobias is uncommon in primary care unless asked for specifically. Onset of this condition is usually in the teens and women outnumber men, as in other anxiety disorders.

## Obsessive–compulsive disorder (OCD)

Recurrent obsessional thoughts as well as compulsive acts can occur in OCD. The recurrent thoughts, beliefs or ideas dominate a sufferer's thought content. They are almost always distressing and the patient, who is usually aware that they are unrealistic, often tries unsuccessfully to resist them.

The compulsive acts or rituals are stereotyped behaviours that are repeated again and again. They are not enjoyable, nor do they result in the completion of useful tasks. Their function is to prevent some unlikely event which, if it happened, would result in some harm, either to the patient or caused by the patient. The symptom patterns typically include a fear of contamination, which leads to excessive hand-washing, doubts, which lead to excessive checking obsessions (e.g. of locks or taps) and compulsions, which slow some patients down to the point that it can take them hours to eat breakfast.

### Post-traumatic stress disorder

Post-traumatic stress disorder (PTSD) arises as a delayed or protracted response to a stressful event or situation of an exceptionally threatening or catastrophic nature. Typical features include reliving the trauma in intrusive memories (flashbacks), dreams or nightmares occurring against the persisting background of a sense of numbness and emotional blunting, detachment from other people, unresponsiveness to surroundings, anhedonia and avoidance of activities and situations reminiscent of the trauma. The onset often follows a latency period, which may range from a few weeks to months after the traumatic event. The course is fluctuating but recovery can be expected in the majority of cases. Some individuals experience years of incapacity, however.

# Management

## General management

The guidelines produced by the UK's National Institute for Health and Clinical Excellence (NICE) on panic disorder and GAD recommend that shared decision-making should be the norm between the individual and healthcare professionals, and that patients, and where appropriate their families or carers, should be provided with information on the nature, course and treatment of anxiety disorders, including information on the use and likely side-effect profile of medications. Patients, families and carers should also be informed of self-help groups and support groups for mental health problems, in particular for anxiety disorders, and encouraged to participate where appropriate (National Institute for Health and Clinical Excellence, 2007). NICE recommends a number of steps in management.

## Step 1. Recognition and diagnosis of anxiety disorder

Relevant information should be gathered, such as personal history, self-medication, and cultural or other individual characteristics that may be important considerations in the person's care.

## Step 2. Treatment in primary care

Interventions are presented below in descending order of best evidence for effect (see Chapter 26 for more detail on the psychological treatments).

### Psychological treatments

- Cognitive–behavioural therapy (CBT) of 7–14 hours' duration has been shown to work for panic disorder, but 16–20 hours may be necessary for GAD.
- Problem-solving therapy (PST) for up to 6 hours delivered by community mental health nurses was found to be no more effective than usual general practitioner care for mild anxiety and depressive disorders (Kendrick *et al*, 2006).
- Exposure therapy for agoraphobia, if necessary in combination with drugs to relieve symptoms in feared situations.

### Drug treatments

An SSRI (sertraline, citalopram or fluoxetine rather than paroxetine, which can cause more withdrawal symptoms) is the first choice. If an SSRI is unsuitable or there is no improvement, imipramine or clomipramine may be considered.

### Guided self-help

Self-help based on CBT principles such as 'bibliotherapy' – the use of written material – or computerised self-help programmes should be used only with guidance and monitoring from a health professional.

### Other interventions

Some patients find relaxation exercises helpful and commercial relaxation tapes are available from pharmacists.

Beta-blockers may be used for performance anxiety, social phobia and specific phobias such as fear of flying.

Benzodiazepines are associated with a less good outcome in the long term and should not be prescribed for the treatment of individuals with panic disorder. They may be helpful intermittently for GAD or for specific phobias such as fear of flying, but should not usually be used beyond a few weeks, owing to the potential for tolerance and dependence.

Other drugs that are used include buspirone, hydroxyzine, pregabalin, and antipsychotic drugs such as trifluoperazine (BMJ, 2007), but the potential for serious side-effects should be weighed against the need for symptom relief.

Eye movement desensitisation may help patients with PTSD.

## Step 3. Review and offer alternative treatment

If one type of intervention does not work, the patient should be reassessed and consideration given to trying one of the other types of intervention.

## Step 4. Review and offer referral from primary care

If two primary care interventions have been provided (any combination of psychological therapy, medication or guided self-help) and the person still has significant symptoms, then referral to specialist mental health services should be offered. Referral is also indicated where the diagnosis is uncertain, or where concomitant medical problems or troublesome side-effects complicate treatment, or where hospitalisation is indicated (Blashki *et al*, 2007).

## Step 5. Care in specialist mental health services

NICE recommends that specialist mental health services should conduct a thorough, holistic reassessment of the individual, the environment and the social circumstances.

# Monitoring

NICE recommends that short, self-completion questionnaires (such as the panic subscale of the Agoraphobic Mobility Inventory (Chambless *et al*, 1985) for individuals with panic disorder) should be used to monitor outcomes wherever possible.

# Acknowledgement

Thanks to Dr Antonio Fernando III, Senior Lecturer in Psychiatry at the University of Auckland, New Zealand, for his help with the diagnostic table for anxiety conditions (Table 10.1).

Key points

- Anxiety disorders are very common: disabling, chronic disorders occur in around 10% of patients, and specific phobias occur in a further 10%.
- Anxiety disorders commonly overlap with depression.
- Anxiety disorders commonly present with physical symptoms.
- Universal screening for anxiety disorders is not recommended, but case-finding in high-risk groups may reveal many undiagnosed cases.
- Specific diagnoses are made on the basis of triggers and cognitive symptoms.
- Psychological treatments, where available, should be tried first. They include cognitive–behavioural therapy and exposure therapy for agoraphobia.
- Selective serotonin reuptake inhibitor antidepressants may also be helpful.
- Benzodiazepines should not be used for more than a few days.

# Further reading and e-resources

Bjelland, I., Dahl, A. A., Haug, T. T., *et al* (2002) The validity of the Hospital Anxiety and Depression Scale. An updated literature review. *Journal of Psychosomatic Research,* **52,** 69–77.

Kroenke, K., Spitzer, R. L., Williams, J. B., *et al* (2007) Anxiety disorders in primary care: prevalence, impairment, comorbidity and detection. *Annals of Internal Medicine,* **146,** 317–325.

National Centre for Classifications in Health (Sydney) (2004) The international statistical classification of diseases and related health problems, Tenth revision, Australian modification (ICD 10) (4th edn, Vol. 1). Sydney Australia: National Centre for Classifications in Health (Sydney).

Rubio, G. & Lopez-Ibor, J. J. (2007) Generalised anxiety disorder: a 40 year follow up study. *Acta Psychiatrica Scandinavica,* **115,** 372–379.

Sculte-Markwort, M., Marutt, K. & Riedesser, P. (2003) *Cross Walks: ICD 10 – DSM IV–TR: A Synopsis of Classifications of Mental Disorders.* Hogrefe & Huber.

Wonca (2005) *International Classification in Primary Care* (revised 2nd edn). Oxford University Press.


Centre for Evidence Based Mental Health, http://www.cebmh.com

NICE guidelines on anxiety, http://www.nice.org.uk/nicemedia/pdf/cg022appendix5_11.pdf

No Panic helpline, http://www.no-panic.co.uk

OCD Action, http://www.ocdaction.org.uk

Patient information sheets, http://www.rcpsych.ac.uk/mentalhealthinfoforall.aspx

Stress Management Society, http://www.stress.org.uk

Triumph Over Phobia, http://www.triumphoverphobia.com

WHO guide to mental and neurological health in primary care, http://www.rsmpress.co.uk/bkwhopdf.htm

# References

American Psychiatric Association (2000) *Diagnostic and Statistical Manual of Mental Disorders* (4th edn, text revision) DSM–IV–TR. APA.

Bijl, R. V., de Graaf, R., Hiripi, E., *et al* (2003) The prevalence of treated and untreated mental disorders in five countries. *Health Affairs,* **22,** 122–133.

Blashki, G., Judd, F. & Piterman, L. (2007) *General Practice Psychiatry.* McGraw-Hill Australia.

BMJ (2007) Clinical evidence: Generalised anxiety disorder. BMJ Publishing Group (http://clinicalevidence.bmj.com/ceweb/conditions/meh/1002/1002_I4.jsp?grp=1).

Bruce, S. E., Yonkers, K. A., Otto, M. W., *et al* (2005) Influence of psychiatric co-morbidity on recovery and recurrence in generalised anxiety disorder, social phobia and panic disorder. A 12 year perspective study. *American Journal of Psychiatry,* **162,** 1179–1187.

Chambless, D. L., Caputo, G. C., Jasin, S. E., *et al* (1985) The Mobility Inventory for Agoraphobia. *Behaviour Research and Therapy,* **23,** 35–44.

Gilbody, S. M., House, A. & Shledon, T. A. (2001) Routinely administered questionnaires for depression and anxiety: a systematic review. *BMJ,* **322,** 406–409.

Gregory, A. M., Caspi, A., Moffitt, T. E., *et al* (2007) Juvenile mental health histories of adults with anxiety disorders. *American Journal of Psychiatry,* **164,** 1–8.

House, A. & Stark, D. (2002) Anxiety in medical patients. *BMJ,* **325,** 207–209.

Hu, W. H., Wong, W. M., Lam, C. L., *et al* (2002) Anxiety but not depression determines health care-seeking behaviour in Chinese patients with dyspepsia and irritable bowel syndrome: a population-based study. *Alimentary Pharmacological Therapy,* **16,** 2081–2088.

Kendrick, T., Simons, L., Mynors-Wallis, L., *et al* (2006) Cost-effectiveness of referral for generic care or problem-solving treatment from community mental health nurses, compared with usual general practitioner care for common mental disorders. Randomised controlled trial. *British Journal of Psychiatry*, **189**, 50–59.

Kessler, R. C., Berglund, P., Demler, O., *et al* (2005) Lifetime prevalence and age of onset distributions of DSM–IV disorders in the national co-morbidity survey replication. *Archives of General Psychiatry*, **62**, 593–602.

MaGPIe Research Group (2003) The nature and prevalence of psychological problems in New Zealand primary healthcare: a report on mental health and general practice investigation (MaGPIe). *New Zealand Medical Journal*, **116**, 1171–1185.

MaGPIe Research Group (2005) Mental disorders among Maori attending their general practitioner. *Australian and New Zealand Journal of Psychiatry*, **39**, 401–406.

Morrison, J. R. (1995) *DSM–IV Made Easy*. Guilford Press.

Murphy, J. M., Horton, N. J., Laird, N. M., *et al* (2004) Anxiety and depression: a 40-year perspective on relationships regarding prevalence, distribution, and co-morbidity. *Acta Psychiatrica Scandinavica*, **109**, 355–375.

National Institute for Health and Clinical Excellence (2007) Anxiety. Clinical guideline (amended), at http://guidance.nice.org.uk/CG22

Oakley-Browne, M. A., Wells, J. E., *et al* (2006) *Te Rau Hinengaro: The New Zealand Mental Health Survey*. Ministry of Health, Wellington, New Zealand.

Shorter, E. & Tyrer, P. (2003) Separation of anxiety and depressive disorders: blind alley in psychopharmacology and classification of disease. *BMJ*, **327**, 158–160.

World Health Organization (1997) *Composite International Diagnostic Interview (CIDI)*. WHO.

# CHAPTER 11

# Medically unexplained symptoms

Christopher Dowrick and Marianne Rosendal

### Summary

This chapter explores the potential roles and responsibilities of the primary care team in providing care and advice for people presenting with medically unexplained symptoms (MUS). It explains how MUS can be understood from several different perspectives, and how doctors need to be careful in how they respond, in order not to make matters worse. The chapter explores the potential of a stepped-care approach, based on the principles of alliance, blame avoidance and explanation. It discusses the benefits and limitations of reattribution training for doctors, and of collaborative care approaches for severe cases.

## Concept and classification

The experience of bodily sensations is a normal phenomenon. Most people suffer from palpitations or stomach aches when they feel nervous or are exposed to stressful events. If patients start thinking of sensations as signs of illness, doctors use the term 'symptoms', and worries about symptoms may lead to visits to a general practitioner (GP). However, in general practice only a minority of physical symptoms are explained by organic pathology (Kroenke & Mangelsdorff, 1989; Toft *et al*, 2005). Most patients who present physical symptoms will have self-limiting symptoms, medically unexplained symptoms (MUS) or psychiatric disorders (Rosendal *et al*, 2007*a*).

The concept of MUS has changed in the course of time, and doctors have used many different names for this heterogeneous group of conditions, including 'somatisation', 'somatoform disorders', 'hypochondriasis', 'functional symptoms/disorders', 'multiple unexplained physical symptoms' and 'idiopathic symptoms', among others. These days a descriptive approach tends to taken, rather than a focus on aetiology. MUS are understood as a spectrum of disorders going from normal reactions through moderate conditions to chronic, disabling disorders. In general, MUS may usefully be defined as:

> conditions where the patient experiences physical symptoms that cause excessive worry or discomfort, and lead them to seek treatment, but for which no adequate organic pathology or patho-physiological basis can be found. (Fink *et al*, 2002)

Specialist care has focused on chronic presentations of MUS and classification systems such as ICD–10 (World Health Organization, 1992) and DSM–IV (American Psychiatric Association, 1994) contain specific diagnoses for conditions of long duration. In the psychiatric chapter of ICD–10, the diagnosis *somatoform disorder* requires a symptom duration of at least 6 months, while the diagnosis *somatisation disorder* requires a symptom duration of 2 years. Some chronic conditions may also be classified as syndromes (irritable bowel syndrome, chronic fatigue syndrome, etc.). Syndrome diagnoses are described in the biomedical chapters of ICD–10 and are based on a predominance of MUS from a certain organ system, but they are closely related to the broader psychiatric definitions (Fink *et al*, 2007).

The *International Classification of Primary Care* (ICPC) was developed by the World Organization of Family Doctors (Wonca, 2005) specifically for diagnoses in primary care settings Although the limited diagnostic specificity available in ICPC is problematic, it aims to include diagnoses of as yet unclarified problems and pays equal attention to the classification of symptoms not fulfilling criteria for any disease, that is, symptom diagnoses, and the classification of diseases, that is, specific diagnoses corresponding to ICD items. The episode structure of ICPC automatically accommodates mental health, biomedical comorbidity and social issues, as it simply requires the noting of all active problems at a point in time or over a specified time interval. The ICPC's substantial focus on symptom diagnoses may be used for self-limiting conditions and mild MUS, while diagnoses for chronic MUS are almost identical to those in ICD–10.

The structure of these classification systems often makes diagnoses focus on either physical disease or psychiatric disorder. Thus, only severe cases of MUS (somatisation disorder or syndromes) are diagnosed, whereas many milder conditions may be labelled with symptom diagnoses or classified as possible diseases until these are eventually ruled out. In a Danish study, GPs classified new health complaints as either physical disease or MUS. The diagnostic ratings from the participating GPs varied from 3% to 33% MUS and this variation could not be explained by differences in the patient populations (Rosendal *et al*, 2003). The large diagnostic variation may instead have been due to differences in the GPs' concept of MUS; that is, they may have diagnosed at different points in the spectrum of MUS. It may also have reflected differences in the ways in which GPs communicate with their patients.

To illustrate and explain the current uncertainty about how best to classify MUS, the (largely fictitious) cases of Kelvin, Carol and Frank are presented below. Kelvin and Carol illustrate one end of this spectrum.

Kelvin is 31. He has had intermittent stomach aches for a few weeks. At first he thought that they were just signs of an infection but he got worried that it could be something more serious – like an ulcer. Otherwise, Kelvin is healthy, of normal weight and physically active, and he usually comes to see his GP only when his children are ill. On examination, the doctor found no signs of disease, and Kelvin was reassured that the symptoms were not a sign of an ulcer or any other serious disease. When his GP saw him 6 months later, accompanying his child for vaccination, his symptoms had disappeared.

Kelvin's symptoms were mild but medically unexplained and turned out to be self-limiting.

Carol is 23. She lives in a small flat with her 4-year-old son after a divorce last year. She is unemployed but wishes to study psychology. She presents to her GP with tingling and prickly sensations in her hands and feet. The symptoms have been present for some months, and they worsen when she stays in the same position for a long time. She also has headaches at times, and often feels tired. Carol has seen another doctor in the practice a couple of times. He thoroughly investigated her symptoms. The paraesthesiae were symmetrical and did not follow the innervation areas, her biochemical profile was normal and a previous examination by the neurologist excluded neurological disease.

Carol has multiple MUS but she has been ill for only a short while and she is not (yet) a chronic case.

At the other end of the spectrum are patients with a higher degree of chronicity, such as Frank:

Frank consults his GP about his stomach pain. He finds it hard to pin down exactly where it is. 'It starts with my tummy button but spreads all over one side.' It has been off and on for about 18 months. It lasts around a day at a time, sometimes longer. He finds it hard to get to sleep because he has to try to lie in a way that eases the pain. When it flares up he feels very low, thinking 'Oh no, this is starting again'. When it is not happening he feels anxious that it might start again.

He has found himself noticing other problems lately. He is aware how busy the doctor is today, and is unsure whether she will want to hear about them all, as well as his stomach complaint. He had a migraine the other day. He used to get them a lot but has been free of them for a few years. He has also had bad acne for about 3 months. Whatever he does, the spots will not go away. He has a mole on his arm which might have grown a little over the past few months. He sometimes has throbbing in his leg at night. He is worried about what it all might be.

He has missed several weeks of work recently, and often finds it too much trouble to socialise with his friends at weekends. He used to enjoy painting wildlife scenes with oils and acrylics, and gained several local commissions, but has not picked up his brush in the past 2 years.

Frank has tried to work out what the cause of his stomach pain is. It does not seem to be linked to diet. He has talked to people about it. A previous doctor suggested he had bruised his ribs. Another doctor suggested gall-stones. This is his ninth consultation this year. Over the past 2 years, he has had blood tests and scans of his gall-bladder and liver but these were all normal. Friends have suggested it could be his appendix, and his grandmother thinks it is probably his 'nerves'. He had flu last year and is wondering if he might have a lingering virus. He also wonders if stress might be involved. His wife had an affair 3 years ago but they have moved house since then and are trying to put those problems behind them. 'But the pain is horrible', he says, 'so it can't just be stress'.

# Psychiatric perspectives

If Frank were interviewed by a psychiatrist, he might well be considered to have a DSM–IV 'somatoform disorder'. He has symptoms which:

- are not fully explained by a general medical condition
- are not the direct effect of drugs or another mental disorder
- cause him clinically significant distress
- lead to impairment of social, occupational and other areas of functioning.

He does not fulfil DSM–IV criteria for full somatisation disorder, however: for this he would need to complain of at least 12 different symptoms from a list of 37, and to have experienced them over many years. He does meet diagnostic research criteria for 'abridged somatisation disorder' (Escobar *et al*, 1998), since he presents at least four somatic symptoms. These criteria are gender specific: women need to present at least six relevant physical symptoms before they can be offered this diagnosis, because of the apparent frequency of gynaecological symptoms from which men are exempt!

Frank might also be a candidate for a diagnosis of a functional somatic syndrome, such as irritable bowel syndrome, functional dyspepsia or chronic fatigue. Barsky & Borus (1999) characterise these syndromes by the commonality of the symptoms, suffering and disability they generate, rather than by demonstrable tissue abnormality. Suffering is exacerbated by self-perpetuating cycles in which somatic symptoms are incorrectly attributed to serious abnormality, reinforcing patients' belief that they have a serious disease. However, Frank does not fully fit this picture, since he does not have a fixed view about a pathological aetiology of his symptoms. He is prepared to entertain a wide variety of physical, social and psychological factors as possible causes.

It is likely that Frank meets current diagnostic criteria for an anxiety disorder, and possibly also for major depression. He describes himself as feeling low, and he certainly worries a lot. Symptom amplification – the tendency to attribute greater intensity or significance to physical symptoms than appears to be warranted by the available clinical evidence – is commonly the result of psychological distress (Ferrari, 2004). There is now a considerable amount of empirical evidence suggesting that MUS frequently coexist with mood or anxiety disorders. This coexistence may be cross-sectional, when all these symptoms appear together at the same time (de Waal *et al*, 2004); or it may be longitudinal, in the sense that one set of symptoms is followed closely in time by another (Creed & Barksy, 2004).

It may be possible to persuade Frank that his main problems are psychological, and to offer him treatment for anxiety and depression. This is the basic premise behind the IMPACT programme, where patients with evidence of symptom amplification in a range of chronic conditions were screened for depression and then offered either antidepressant medication or problem-solving treatment (Harpole *et al*, 2005). However, many patients with unexplained symptoms do not accept the assertion that their problems are primarily psychological (Stone *et al*, 2002). As Frank says, 'the pain is horrible, so it can't just be stress'. Doctors must be careful to avoid shoehorning patients' problems into categories that make life easier for themselves while failing to address patients' real concerns (Dowrick, 2004).

## Primary care perspectives

In the ICPC, Frank would be categorised in the same way as described above and classification would include the same problematic issues. However, the previous cases of Kelvin and Carol would be difficult to fit into the classification system in a clinically useful way. Kelvin's diagnosis could be a symptom diagnosis (abdominal pain), which would be inactivated when his symptoms disappeared. Carol, on the other hand, would be labelled with several symptom diagnoses at different times: tingling fingers and toes, headache, weakness/tiredness general and maybe a work problem. These diagnoses do not clearly separate the cases, and reflect the problem of MUS.

There is currently no agreed diagnosis for the broad category of MUS seen in primary care. Furthermore, it is widely acknowledged among specialists in the field that the diagnosis 'somatoform disorder' used in specialised care has failed as a diagnostic grouping (Mayou *et al*, 2005; Engel, 2006). There is a need to develop the current classification systems in primary care as well as in specialised care, in order to include MUS in a way that makes this patient group visible and helps the clinician to avoid iatrogenesis and to make appropriate decisions about care.

## The impact of healthcare

The ways in which Frank experiences and describes his symptoms are not exclusively the product of his own mind and/or body. They are also affected by his interactions with healthcare professionals, as well as other individuals, including family and friends. Across the world, patients vary considerably in the extent to which they report somatic symptoms in relation to depression, for example. This variation is strongly dependent on the healthcare systems with which they interact. In a study of psychological problems in general healthcare in 15 countries (Simon *et al*, 1999), somatic presentations were significantly more likely in centres where patients lacked an ongoing relationship with a primary care physician, compared with those primary care centres where most patients had a personal physician.

The presentation of physical symptoms also depends on the characteristics and attitudes of physicians. GPs are not always very keen on patients like Frank. They express symptoms which are difficult to characterise and manage within the parameters of general practice, and also consult often. Doctors tend to be wary about their motives for presentation, and doubt the legitimacy of their symptoms (Wileman *et al*, 2002). Frank seemed to be aware of this tension, since he was uncertain how many of his current problems he should mention.

Doctors often try to contain the situation by *normalisation*, that is, stressing to the patient that there is no serious disease, that symptoms are likely to be benign or self-limiting and that there is no need for healthcare intervention. While this approach may be effective for Kelvin and Carol – provided that the explanations given are tangible, non-blaming and involve the patient – the same tactic may simply exacerbate the situation with patients like Frank, prompting them to provide further evidence of the importance of their problems (Dowrick *et al*, 2004; Salmon *et al*, 2007).

Although patients like Frank tend to present with a complex variety of problems and cues, GPs are much more likely to pay attention to patients' physical symptoms than to their manifest psychological or social problems (Salmon *et al*, 2004). GPs are also more likely than their patients to recommend investigations, somatic treatments or referrals. In a real sense, therefore, it is GPs who are encouraging – perhaps even creating – somatisation in their patients (Ring *et al*, 2005).

The issue for the patient therefore becomes (Hodgson *et al*, 2005) 'How can I make sure that my suffering and concerns are taken seriously?' The issue for the doctor becomes 'How can I contain this patient?' This can all too easily develop into a spiral of confusion, conflict and even hostility. With no exit point in sight, the doctor–patient relationship itself risks becoming a chronic problem (Chew-Graham *et al*, 2004).

# Epidemiology

In spite of the problems of MUS classification, there is a fairly good picture of the prevalence of these symptoms (Fig. 11.1). Bodily symptoms are common in the general population (National Institue of Public Health, 2003); in fact, many of the patients in the GP's waiting room will have MUS (Kroenke & Mangelsdorff, 1989). However, less than 10% of patients presenting in primary care will have persistent MUS for which they wish to receive treatment (de Waal *et al*, 2004; Toft *et al*, 2005).

Patients with somatoform disorders risk long-term illness: 30–50% still have symptoms after 2 years (Craig *et al*, 1993; Barsky *et al*, 1998; de Waal *et al*, 2004). We know very little about patients with short-term MUS in general practice. Some of the factors that are associated with persistence of

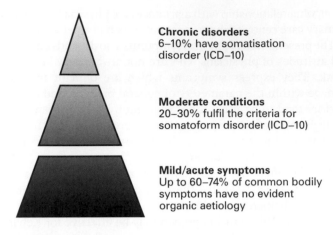

**Chronic disorders**
6–10% have somatisation
disorder (ICD–10)

**Moderate conditions**
20–30% fulfil the criteria for
somatoform disorder (ICD–10)

**Mild/acute symptoms**
Up to 60–74% of common bodily
symptoms have no evident
organic aetiology

**Fig. 11.1** The prevalence of medically unexplained symptoms in general practice.

symptoms are: number of physical symptoms; poor social networks; severe social problems; and frequent attendance in primary care (Lieb *et al*, 2002; Jackson *et al*, 2006). After long-term follow-up, less than 10% of patients with MUS eventually have an organic disease diagnosed (Wilson *et al*, 1994; Crimlisk *et al*, 1998; Carson *et al*, 2003).

# Aetiology

The aetiology behind MUS is unknown and probably multi-factorial. We may usefully divide the aetiological factors into:

- *Predisposing factors.* These include genetics (Kato *et al*, 2006), childhood traumas and role models. Predisposing factors make the individual vulnerable in terms of a biological hypersensitivity, increased illness worry and a lack of coping strategies. Biological mechanisms have been demonstrated in patients with severe somatisation disorders. These patients may have little or no inhibition of afferent stimuli from bodily sensations, resulting in a conscious experience of multiple symptoms (Miller, 1984).
- *Triggering/activating factors.* These include physical traumas, disease, social strain (Theorell *et al*, 1999) and emotional conflicts (Hatcher & House, 2003).
- *Maintaining factors.* These include illness perception (Frostholm *et al*, 2005a,b), iatrogenic factors (Salmon *et al*, 1999; Fink *et al*, 2002; Ring *et al*, 2005) and neurophysiological changes (Rief *et al*, 1998). Patients' illness behaviour is determined by their perceptions, symptom evaluations and interpretations (Mechanic, 1962). Thus, cognitive and emotional factors may provide the motivation for a given behaviour. As

described above, the healthcare system can also influence the course of the patient's illness.

# Treatment

Patients with MUS should be offered the same professional treatment as any other patient seeking healthcare. Some will have only self-limiting symptoms, others will have persisting MUS and a few will be chronically ill and disabled by their symptoms. Depending on the severity, the patient may benefit from different treatment approaches (Henningsen *et al*, 2007) (Fig. 11. 2).

## *Mild conditions and general treatment aspects*

In mild and potentially self-limiting conditions (as in the case of Kelvin), it is important that the doctor takes a balanced bio-psychosocial approach to the patient's symptoms and considers all three aspects from the beginning of the consultation. A narrow focus on the exclusion of physical disease will result in negative feedback to the patient and the patient may interpret a subsequent focus on psychological or social issues as a rejection of the perceived illness (Salmon, 2006). Furthermore, a narrow biomedical focus may increase the patient's illness worry and reinforce illness behaviour (maintaining factors) (Kendrick *et al*, 2001; Fink *et al*, 2002; Dowrick *et al*, 2004).

### Avoiding iatrogenic communication

A crucial starting point is to acknowledge that the problems of patients with MUS do not necessarily – or completely – lie within themselves, and

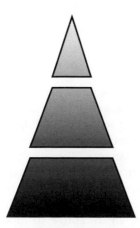

**Chronic disorders**
Management principles
Specific treatment methods
(e.g. cognitive–behavioural therapy)
Liaison models/collaborative care

**Moderate conditions**
Primary care psychosocial intervention
(e.g. reattribution models)

**Mild/acute symptoms**
Avoid iatrogenesis
Reassurance/normalisation
Bio-psychosocial approach

**Fig. 11.2** Treatment of medically unexplained symptoms.

that their interaction with healthcare also plays its part. It is also important to be aware of what patients with MUS want or expect from their doctors. They do not generally have high expectations of cure. They are often aware that their problems are complex, and that medicine is limited in what it can do to overcome them. Instead, they may merely be looking for an acknowledgement of suffering, for emotional support and for explanations that enable them to make sense of their problems (Salmon *et al*, 2005).

Peters *et al* (1998) have identified three key elements of successful consultations, as seen from the perspective of patients with persistent unexplained symptoms. The first element is *alliance*, the sense that doctor and patient are in this together. The second element is *exculpation*, the ability to absolve the patients from blame for their current predicament, something that the powerful status of the family doctor still enables. And the third element is a *convincing explanation*. To be convincing, the explanation needs to be presented within the context of a tangible – usually physical – mechanism, which validates the bodily nature of the patient's symptoms. It should be also grounded in the patient's own concerns and illness perceptions (Dowrick *et al*, 2004).

Below is a genuine example of such a convincing explanation, provided by a doctor for a female patient concerned about an abdominal pain. The doctor makes deliberate and elegant use of the ambiguous meaning of the word 'nerves' in order to bring physical and psychosocial problems together:

> Dr: The only thing that fits is, it's the sort of pain you get with shingles because it comes around in that pattern.
>
> P: Yes, yes.
>
> Dr: And that's sometimes irritation of the nerve endings.
>
> P: That's what somebody else, me Nan, says, 'It could be your nerves'.
>
> Dr: I don't mean your emotional nerves, your actual physical nerves that come round your body – but it could be made worse by stress and things like that.
>
> P: I mean I'm obviously one of them people that are highly strung anyway, I know that. I'm not, I'm not you know a 'come day go day' like, laid-back person, I'm quite like, you know, everything's got to be done at that day, at that time.

## Encouraging self-help

General practitioners have learned much about curing physical symptoms when a biomedical aetiology is present. However, when it comes to MUS there is no biomedical cure and the doctor will have to shift the paradigm from 'the doctor as the expert' to 'the patient as the expert' on illness perception, meaning and behavioural changes. Whenever possible, GPs' explanations should provide patients with the opportunity to do something themselves about the problems they face. GPs should be aiming to build up the patient's sense of *personal agency* (Dowrick, 2004). Patients with irritable bowel syndrome, for example, are receptive to models of self-care that acknowledge the intensity of their bodily experiences and that stress physical as well as psychological dimensions, the disruption that the symptoms cause to their to social and domestic roles, and the consequent loss of control (Kennedy *et al*, 2003).

By taking an approach based on facilitated self-management, GPs can help patients with MUS to acquire the skills and confidence to manage their own illness (Chew-Graham, 2005). At the same time, they can reduce the burden of expectation on themselves. If they can be reassured that patients with MUS do not expect them to cure their problems, they may feel less of a failure, and so become less defensive in their dealings with them. They may then be more able to respond empathically to these patients' need for emotional support and understanding, and to think with them about what steps they can take to make life better for themselves.

## Managing moderate conditions

In moderate conditions, the bio-psychosocial approach and effective normalisation may be supplemented by brief psychological interventions. Several psychosocial and cognitive-oriented interventions exist. During the past 20 years, the focus has been on the *reattribution model* and different versions of this model have been applied throughout Europe. These models have all been designed for general practice and include basic interviewing skills.

The reattribution model used in the MUST trial (Morriss *et al*, 2006) contains four key elements:

1   *Feeling understood.* The doctor elicits physical symptoms, psychosocial problems, mood state, beliefs held by patient about the problem, relevant physical examination and investigations.
2   *Broadening the agenda.* The doctor summarises the physical and psychosocial findings, and negotiates these findings with the patient.
3   *Making the link.* The doctor then gives an explanation relating the physical symptoms to psychosocial problems of lifestyle in terms of a link in time or physiology.
4   *Negotiating further treatment.* The doctor arranges follow-up or treatment of symptoms, psychosocial problems or mental disorder.

Another example is the 'extended reattribution and management model' (TERM; Fink *et al*, 2002). The central elements of this model are:

•   making the patient feel understood and securing the doctor–patient relationship
•   gaining insight into the patient's illness understanding and expectations
•   maintaining a bio-psychosocial approach throughout the consultations
•   ensuring the diagnosis of significant psychiatric disorders.

The model makes a clear demarcation between the patient's part of the consultation and the GP's part:

•   When the patient history has been fully taken, the GP must express their own expertise explicitly.

- The reality of the patient's symptoms must always be acknowledged.
- A new and common way of symptom understanding is negotiated between the GP and the patient.
- The agreements are reinforced and further appointments may be negotiated.

Results from trials of reattribution models have shown positive effects on GPs' interviewing skills (Kaaya *et al*, 1992), attitudes (Rosendal *et al*, 2005) and diagnoses of MUS (Rosendal *et al*, 2003), as well as improved patient satisfaction with care (Morriss *et al*, 1999; Frostholm *et al*, 2005a). There are also indications that reattribution models may have a positive impact on patients' healthcare-seeking behaviour (Morriss *et al*, 1998; Blankenstein, 2001).

However, trials evaluating patient health outcomes from reattribution models show less promising results. While a Dutch trial indicated positive effects on patient functioning (Blankenstein, 2001), three randomised controlled trials, from Denmark (Rosendal *et al*, 2007b), Germany (Larisch *et al*, 2004) and the UK (Morriss *et al*, 2007), have demonstrated few sustained, significant positive effects on patient health or functional status. Indeed, the UK trial suggests a possible negative impact of reattribution training on patients' psychological status. We consider that there is a need for greater specificity with regard to the patients and circumstances in which the techniques of reattribution may successfully be applied.

## Severe conditions: management and collaborative care

In patients with severe and persistent MUS, the aim is often containment, support and prevention of iatrogenic harm, rather than cure. We speak of 'management' rather than of 'treatment'.

Efforts should focus on:

- reducing anxiety and distress emanating from the symptoms and their associated impact
- avoiding unwarranted diagnostic and therapeutic procedures and medications
- preventing serious psychiatric complications of chronic invalidism and/or drug dependence (Bass, 1990; Fink *et al*, 2002; Blumenfield & Strain, 2006).

A precondition for good management is a strong doctor–patient relationship and general practice provides good opportunities for this because of the continuity of care. There is evidence that this can lead to improved outcomes for patients with MUS, when combined with mixed cognitive–behavioural and pharmacological treatments provided by trained family physicians. The principles for management are set out in Box 11.1. These principles may be part of collaborative care, where the specialised psychiatric service works together with primary care in a stepped-care model (Smith *et al*, 2006).

**Box 11.1** Principles for the management of patients with persistent MUS in primary care (chronic conditions)

*Physical*

1   Make a brief physical examination, focusing on the organ system from which the patient has (new) complaints.
    - Look for signs of disease instead of symptoms.
    - Avoid tests and procedures, unless indicated by objective signs of disease or a well-defined (new) clinical illness picture.
2   Reduce unnecessary drugs, do not use on-demand prescriptions and avoid habit-forming medication.

*Psychological*

3   Make the diagnosis and inform the patient that the disorder is known and has a name when you are dealing with a chronic disorder (e.g. 'somatisation disorder').
4   Acknowledge the reality of the patient's symptoms.
5   Be direct and honest with the patient about the areas you agree on and those you do not agree on, but be careful not to make the patient feel ignorant or not respected.
6   Be stoical; do not expect rapid changes or cure.
7   Reduce expectations of cure and aim at containment and (iatrogenic) damage limitation.
8   Perceive worsening of symptoms or new symptoms as emotional communication rather than as a manifestation of a new disease.
9   Apply a specific therapeutic technique (e.g. reattribution or TERM-model).
10  Consider referral to specialised treatment and motivate the patient to receive such treatment.

*Psychopharmacological*

11  Consider treatment with psychoactive medication (usually an antidepressant).
12  Choose non-habit-forming medication and, if possible, choose medication that can be serum monitored.
13  Start with a smaller dosage than usual and increase slowly (be stoical about side-effects).
14  Treat any coexisting psychiatric disorders according to usual guidelines.

*Administrative*

15  Be proactive rather than reactive. Agree on a course with fixed, scheduled appointments with 2–6-week intervals and avoid consultations on demand.
16  If the patient has a job, avoid giving sick leave if at all possible.
17  Try to become the patient's only physician and minimise the patient's contact with other healthcare professionals, doctors on call and alternative therapists.
18  Inform your colleagues of your management plans and develop contingency plans for when you are not accessible.
19  Inform the patient's nearest relative and try to co-opt a relative as a therapeutic ally.
20  If necessary, arrange support or supervision for yourself.

One step in a collaborative care model may be a psychiatric assessment, with subsequent consultation letters, including treatment recommendations for the GP. This approach has been evaluated in US trials, which provided evidence that psychiatric consultation letters may improve the patient's physical functioning and reduce healthcare costs (Rost *et al*, 1994; Smith *et al*, 1995). These models focus on the management of chronic patients and are of low cost to the healthcare system.

Finally, most patients with chronic MUS may benefit from specialised treatment (Arnold *et al*, 2006). The possibilities of referral depend on the services available in the local area and there is often a shortage of specialists providing treatment for patients with MUS. Referral may be easier to introduce if the first specialist assessment of the patient is made in the primary care clinic, within a stepped-care model. When specialised therapy is available, psychodynamic/interpersonal psychotherapy and cognitive–behavioural therapy may be effective (Kroenke & Swindle, 2000; Escobar *et al*, 2007).

Pharmacological treatment may also be part of care if the disorder is chronic. Only a few studies of pharmacological treatment with psychoactive drugs for MUS have been conducted. They indicate that antidepressants may be effective (O'Malley *et al*, 1999). Although tricyclic medication seems to be most effective, selective noradrenaline reuptake inhibitors or selective serotonin reuptake inhibitors are often preferred, owing to the perception of fewer side-effects. Patients with MUS may be very sensitive to side-effects, and treatment should be started with the minimum dosage ('start low, go slow').

# Conclusion

The management of patients with MUS in primary care is often complex, sometimes frustrating and only occasionally rewarding. By definition, MUS involve high levels of uncertainty in diagnosis and treatment, which can be a source of stress for both GP and patient. Yet GPs are characterised – in contrast to their hospital colleagues – by a preference for, even an enjoyment of, uncertainty. Patients with MUS provide important challenges to GPs' existing store of knowledge and skills. They give all professionals the opportunity to reflect on their attitudes to illness and healthcare; indeed, they can enable professionals to move beyond the comfort (and tedium) of routinised delivery of medical care.

Next time you meet a patient like Frank, perhaps you could spend a few minutes asking him about his perceptions and expectations – and his strengths. As well as providing your diagnostic expertise, and offering him a choice of the best available medical interventions, you might also ask him about his wildlife paintings, and encourage him to pick up his paint brush once again.

Key points

- Patients commonly present medically unexplained symptoms (MUS) in primary care.
- MUS can be understood from different perspectives, including as psychiatric disorders, as functional somatic problems, and as difficulties arising from dysfunctional doctor–patient communication and entrenched cultural beliefs about the relationship of mind and body.
- Many presentations of MUS are simple and self-limiting.
- It is important for doctors to avoid communication and intervention strategies that exacerbate or perpetuate MUS.
- For patients with persistent MUS, a stepped-care approach can offer practical solutions.
- Successful primary care consultations with patients with MUS contain three key elements: alliance, exculpation, and convincing explanation.
- Training in reattribution enhances GP skills in doctor–patient communication, and increases patient satisfaction with care; however, it is unclear whether reattribution leads to improved health or functional outcomes for patients with persistent MUS.
- Collaborative models of care, including targeted psychological and pharmacological interventions, can be effective in severe cases.

# Further reading and e-resources

Morriss, R., Gask, L., Dowrick, C., *et al* (2007) Primary care: management of persistent medically unexplained symptoms. In *Handbook of Liaison Psychiatry* (eds G. Lloyd & E. Guthrie), pp. 847–870. Cambridge University Press.

Useful information and materials may be downloaded from the Research Clinic for Functional Disorders and Psychosomatics in Denmark, http://www.ki.au.dk/forskningsenheder/forskflpuk

A video of the reattribution model is available from the University of Manchester, http://www.medicine.manchester.ac.uk/psychiatrytrainingvideos/

# References

American Psychiatric Association (1994) *Diagnostic and Statistical Manual of Mental Disorders* (4th edn) (DSM–IV). APA.

Arnold, I. A., de Waal, M. W., Eekhof, J. A., *et al* (2006) Somatoform disorder in primary care: course and the need for cognitive–behavioral treatment. *Psychosomatics*, **47**, 498–503.

Barsky, A. J. & Borus, J. F. (1999) Functional somatic syndromes. *Annals of Internal Medicine*, **130**, 910–921.

Barsky, A. J., Fama, J. M., Bailey, E. D., *et al* (1998) A prospective 4- to 5-year study of DSM–III–R hypochondriasis. *Archives of General Psychiatry*, **55**, 737–744.

Bass, C. (1990) Assessment and management of patients with functional somatic symptoms. In *Somatization: Physical Symptoms and Psychological Illness* (ed. C. Bass), pp. 40–72. Blackwell Scientific.

Blankenstein, A. H. (2001) Somatising patients in general practice. Reattribution, a promising approach. PhD thesis. Vrije Universiteit, Amsterdam.

Blumenfield, M. & Strain, J. J. (2006) *Psychosomatic Medicine*. Lippincott Williams & Wilkins.

Carson, A. J., Best, S., Postma, K., *et al* (2003) The outcome of neurology outpatients with medically unexplained symptoms: a prospective cohort study. *Journal of Neurology Neurosurgery and Psychiatry*, **74**, 897–900.

Chew-Graham, C. (2005) Why do doctors feel pressurised? (Commentary.) *Journal of Psychosomatic Medicine*, **59**, 261–262.

Chew-Graham, C. A., May, C. M. & Roland, M. O. (2004) The harmful consequences of elevating the doctor–patient relationship to be the primary goal of the general practice consultation. *Family Practice*, **21**, 229–231.

Craig, T. K., Boardman, A. P., Mills, K., *et al* (1993) The South London Somatisation Study. I: Longitudinal course and the influence of early life experiences. *British Journal of Psychiatry*, **163**, 579–588.

Creed, F. & Barsky, A. J. (2004) A systematic review of the epidemiology of somatisation disorder and hypochondriasis. *Journal of Psychosomatic Research*, **56**, 391–408.

Crimlisk, H. L., Bhatia, K., Cope, H., *et al* (1998) Slater revisited: 6 year follow up study of patients with medically unexplained motor symptoms. *BMJ*, **316**, 582–586.

de Waal, M. W. M., Arnold, I. A. & Eekhof, J. A. H. (2004) Somatoform disorders in general practice : prevalence, functional impairment and comorbidity with anxiety and depressive disorders. *British Journal of Psychiatry*, **184**, 470–476.

Dowrick, C. (2004) *Beyond Depression: A New Approach to Understanding and Management*. Oxford University Press.

Dowrick, C. F., Ring, A., Humphris, G. M., *et al* (2004) Normalisation of unexplained symptoms by general practitioners: a functional typology. *British Journal of General Practice*, **54**, 165–170.

Engel, C. C. (2006) Explanatory and pragmatic perspectives regarding idiopathic physical symptoms and related syndromes. *CNS Spectrums*, **11**, 225–232.

Escobar, J. I., Gara, M., Silver, R. C., *et al* (1998) Somatisation disorder in primary care. *British Journal of Psychiatry*, **173**, 262–266.

Escobar, J. I., Gara, M. A., Diaz-Martinez, A., *et al* (2007) Effectiveness of a time-limited cognitive behavior therapy-type intervention among primary care patients with medically unexplained symptoms. *Annals of Family Medicine*, **5**, 328–335.

Ferrari, R. (2004) The clinical relevance of symptom amplification. *Pain*, **107**, 276–277.

Fink, P., Rosendal, M. & Toft, T. (2002) Assessment and treatment of functional disorders in general practice: the extended reattribution and management model – an advanced educational program for nonpsychiatric doctors. *Psychosomatics*, **43**, 93–131.

Fink, P., Toft, T., Hansen, M. S., *et al* (2007) Symptoms and syndromes of bodily distress. An explorative study among 978 internal medical, neurological and primary care patients. *Psychosomatic Medicine*, **69**, 30–39.

Frostholm, L., Fink, P., Christensen, K. S., *et al* (2005*a*) The patient's illness perceptions and the use of primary health care. *Psychosomatic Medicine*, **67**, 997–1005.

Frostholm, L., Fink, P., Oernboel, E., *et al* (2005*b*) The uncertain consultation and patient satisfaction: the impact of patients' illness perceptions and a randomized controlled trial on the training of physicians' communication skills. *Psychosomatic Medicine*, **67**, 897–905.

Harpole, L. H., Williams, J. W. Jr, Olsen, M. K., *et al* (2005) Improving depression outcomes in older adults with comorbid medical illness. *General Hospital Psychiatry*, **27**, 4–12.

Hatcher, S. & House. A. (2003) Life events, difficulties and dilemmas in the onset of chronic fatigue syndrome: a case–control study. *Psychological Medicine*, **33**, 1185–1192.

Henningsen, P., Zipfel, S. & Herzog, W. (2007) Management of functional somatic syndromes. *Lancet*, **369**, 946–955.

Hodgson, P., Smith, P., Brown, T., *et al* (2005) Stories from frequent attenders: a qualitative study in primary care. *Annals of Family Medicine*, **3**, 318–323.

Jackson, J., Fiddler, M., Kapur, N., *et al* (2006) Number of bodily symptoms predicts outcome more accurately than health anxiety in patients attending neurology, cardiology, and gastroenterology clinics. *Journal of Psychosomatic Research*, **60**, 357–363.

Kaaya, S., Goldberg, D. & Gask, L. (1992) Management of somatic presentations of psychiatric illness in general medical settings: evaluation of a new training course for general practitioners. *Medical Education*, **26**, 138–144.

Kato, K., Sullivan, P. F., Evengard, B., *et al* (2006) Premorbid predictors of chronic fatigue. *Archives of General Psychiatry*, **63**, 1267–1272.

Kendrick, D., Fielding, K., Bentley, E., *et al* (2001) Radiography of the lumbar spine in primary care patients with low back pain: randomised controlled trial. *BMJ*, **322**, 400–405.

Kennedy, A., Nelson, E., Reeves, D., *et al* (2003) A randomised controlled trial to assess the impact of a package comprising a patient-orientated, evidence-based self-help guidebook and patient-centred consultations on disease management and satisfaction in inflammatory bowel disease. *Health Technology Assessment*, **7**, 1–113.

Kroenke, K. & Mangelsdorff, A. D. (1989) Common symptoms in ambulatory care: incidence, evaluation, therapy, and outcome. *American Journal of Medicine*, **86**, 262–266.

Kroenke, K. & Swindle, R. (2000) Cognitive–behavioral therapy for somatization and symptom syndromes: a critical review of controlled clinical trials. *Psychotherapy and Psychosomatics*, **69**, 205–215.

Larisch, A., Schweickhardt, A., Wirsching, M., *et al* (2004) Psychosocial interventions for somatizing patients by the general practitioner: a randomized controlled trial. *Journal of Psychosomatic Research*, **57**, 507–514.

Lieb, R., Zimmermann, P., Friis, R. H., *et al* (2002) The natural course of DSM–IV somatoform disorders and syndromes among adolescents and young adults: a prospective-longitudinal community study. *European Psychiatry*, **17**, 321–331.

Mayou, R., Kirmayer, L. J., Simon, G., *et al* (2005) Somatoform disorders: time for a new approach in DSM–V. *American Journal of Psychiatry*, **162**, 847–855.

Mechanic, D. (1962) The concept of illness behaviour. *Journal of Chronic Disease*, **15**, 189–194.

Miller, L. (1984) Neuropsychological concepts of somatoform disorders. *International Journal of Psychiatry in Medicine*, **14**, 31–46.

Morriss, R., Gask, L., Ronalds, C., et al (1998) Cost-effectiveness of a new treatment for somatized mental disorder taught to GPs. *Family Practice*, **15**, 119–125.

Morriss, R. K., Gask, L., Ronalds, C., *et al* (1999) Clinical and patient satisfaction outcomes of a new treatment for somatized mental disorder taught to general practitioners. *British Journal of General Practice*, **49**, 263–267.

Morriss, R., Dowrick, C., Salmon, P., *et al* (2006) Turning theory into practice: rationale, feasibility and external validity of an exploratory randomized controlled trial of training family practitioners in reattribution to manage patients with medically unexplained symptoms (the MUST). *General Hospital Psychiatry*, **28**, 343–351.

Morriss, R., Dowrick, C., Salmon, P., *et al* (2007) Better doctor–patient communication did not improve clinical outcome: results of a randomised controlled trial of training practices in reattribution to manage patients with medically unexplained symptoms (MUST). *British Journal of Psychiatry*, **191**, 536–542.

National Institute of Public Health (2003) SUSY: Sundheds-og sygelighedsundersøgelsen 2000. http://www.si-folkesundhed.dk/susy/

O'Malley, P. G., Jackson, J. L., Santoro, J., *et al* (1999) Antidepressant therapy for unexplained symptoms and symptom syndromes. *Journal of Family Practice*, **48**, 980–990.

Peters, S., Stanley, I., Rose, M., *et al* (1998) Patients with medically unexplained symptoms: sources of patients' authority and implications for demands on medical care. *Social Science and Medicine*, **46**, 559–565.

Rief, W., Shaw, R. & Fichter, M. M. (1998) Elevated levels of psychophysiological arousal and cortisol in patients with somatization syndrome. *Psychosomatic Medicine*, **60**, 198–203.

Ring, A., Dowrick, C., Humphris, G., *et al* (2005) The somatizing effect of clinical consultation: what patients and doctors say and do not say when patients present medically unexplained physical symptoms. *Social Science and Medicine*, **61**, 1505–1515.

Rosendal, M., Bro, F., Fink, P., *et al* (2003) Diagnosis of somatisation: effect of an educational intervention in a cluster randomised controlled trial. *British Journal of General Practice*, **53**, 917–922.

Rosendal, M., Bro, F., Sokolowski, I., *et al* (2005) A randomised controlled trial of brief training in assessment and treatment of somatisation: effects on general practitioners' attitudes. *Family Practice*, **22**, 419–427.

Rosendal, M., Fink, P., Falko, E., *et al* (2007a) Improving the classification of medically unexplained symptoms in primary care. *European Journal of Psychiatry*, **21**, 25–36.

Rosendal, M., Olesen, F., Fink, P., *et al* (2007b) A randomized controlled trial of brief training in assessment and treatment of somatisation in primary care: effects on patient outcome. *General Hospital Psychiatry*, **29**, 364–373.

Rost, K., Kashner, T. M., Smith, R. G., Jr (1994) Effectiveness of psychiatric intervention with somatization disorder patients: improved outcomes at reduced costs. *General Hospital Psychiatry*, **16**, 381–387.

Salmon, P. (2006) The potentially somatizing effect of clinical consultation. *CNS Spectrums*, **11**, 190–200.

Salmon, P., Peters, S. & Stanley, I. (1999) Patients' perceptions of medical explanations for somatisation disorders: qualitative analysis. *BMJ*, **318**, 372–376.

Salmon, P., Dowrick, C. F., Ring, A., *et al* (2004) Voiced but unheard agendas: qualitative analysis of the psychosocial cues that patients with unexplained symptoms present to general practitioners. *British Journal of General Practice*, **54**, 171–176.

Salmon, P., Ring, A., Dowrick, C., *et al* (2005) What do general practice patients want when they present medically unexplained symptoms? *Journal of Psychosomatic Research*, **59**, 255–260.

Salmon, P., Humphris, G., Ring, A., *et al* (2007) Primary care consultations about medically unexplained symptoms: the role of patients' presentations and doctors' responses in leading to somatic interventions. *Psychosomatic Medicine*, **69**, 571–577.

Simon, G. E., VonKorff, M., Picinnelli, M., *et al* (1999) An international study of the relationship between somatic symptoms and depression. *New England Journal of Medicine*, **341**, 1329–1335.

Smith, G. R. Jr, Rost, K. & Kashner, T. M. (1995) A trial of the effect of a standardized psychiatric consultation on health outcomes and costs in somatizing patients. *Archives of General Psychiatry*, **52**, 238–243.

Smith, R. C., Lyles, J. S., Gardiner, J. C., *et al* (2006) Primary care clinicians treat patients with medically unexplained symptoms: a randomized controlled trial. *Journal of General Internal Medicine*, **21**, 671–677.

Stone, J., Wokcik, W., Durrance, D., *et al* (2002) What should we say to patients with symptoms unexplained by disease? The 'number needed to offend'. *BMJ*, **325**, 1449–1450.

Theorell, T., Blomkvist, V., Lindh, G., *et al* (1999) Critical life events, infections, and symptoms during the year preceding chronic fatigue syndrome (CFS): an examination of CFS patients and subjects with a nonspecific life crisis. *Psychosomatic Medicine*, **61**, 304–310.

Toft, T., Fink, P., Oernboel, E., *et al* (2005) Mental disorders in primary care: prevalence and co-morbidity among disorders. Results from the Functional Illness in Primary care (FIP) study. *Psychological Medicine*, **35**, 1175–1184.

Wileman, L., May, C. M. & Chew-Graham, C. A. (2002) Medically unexplained symptoms and the problem of power in the consultation: a qualitative study. *Family Practice*, **19**, 178–182.

Wilson, A., Hickie, I., Lloyd, A., *et al* (1994) Longitudinal study of outcome of chronic fatigue syndrome. *BMJ*, **308**, 756–759.

Wonca (2005) *International Classification of Primary Care* (2nd edn) (ICPC–2–R). Oxford University Press.

World Health Organization (1992) *International Classification of Diseases* (10th revision) (ICD–10). WHO.

# CHAPTER 12

# Mental health problems in older people

## Carolyn Chew-Graham and Robert Baldwin

### Summary

This chapter discusses the primary care management of the commonest mental health problems in older people. These are the four 'D's: delirium, depression, dementia and delusions. We present cases drawn from practice, clinical presentations and management within primary care and liaison with secondary care. Useful tools for use by the primary care team are suggested and how they are integrated into clinical practice is discussed. The management of patients is discussed largely with reference to UK primary care systems and policy, but the international readership should find parallels within their own healthcare systems.

This chapter is divided into four main sections, presenting, in turn, the primary care management of the commonest mental health problems in older people: delirium, depression, dementia and delusions (the first three of these are compared in Table 12.1). The presentation and management of a typical case are illustrated for each. Although the discussion largely refers to the UK context and the general practitioner (GP), the majority of it will apply internationally and to primary care physicians (and indeed other professionals) more generally.

## Delirium

### Clinical presentation

Delirium is a syndrome comprising disturbance of consciousness (often manifest as impaired attention or concentration), cognitive deficits (such as memory, orientation or language problems), disturbed sleep–wake cycle, associated features such as delusions or hallucinations (especially visual) and behavioural disturbances (such as agitation or apathy) and alterations in affect, notably fear (Table 12.1).

**Table 12.1** Differentiating delirium, depression and dementia

|  | Delirium | Depression | Dementia |
| --- | --- | --- | --- |
| Onset | Acute | Variable | Insidious |
| Duration | Days | Variable | Months to years |
| Course | Fluctuates | Possible diurnal variation (worse in morning) | Slowly progressive (though may be step-wise) |
| Consciousness | Impaired and fluctuating | Unimpaired | Clear at onset |
| Attention and memory | Inattentive Poor memory | Poor concentration, sometime complaining of poor memory | Poor memory but without inattention |
| Affect | Variable | Depressed, loss of interest and pleasure in usual activities | Variable |

The onset is often sudden (hours or days) and fluctuation is a hallmark. A useful mnemonic is the four 'I's (Crausman, 2004):

1  intermittent impairment of cognition
2  inattention
3  incoherent thought
4  impaired consciousness.

Delirium is synonymous with 'acute confusional state' (see Chapter 16).

### Case 1. Delirium: Marjorie

The GP is called to see an 83-year-old lady, Marjorie, who lives in a residential home and who has quickly become confused, withdrawn and irritable. She has wandered out of her room, awake, for the past three nights.

She has a history of diabetes, ischaemic heart disease, peptic ulcer and recurrent urinary tract infections.

Her medication comprises gliclazide, digoxin, aspirin, ramipril, atorvastatin, thyroxine, omeprazole and paracetamol.

The nurse in charge has asked the GP to see her because Marjorie is being disruptive.

What does the GP need to consider in relation to assessment, diagnosis and management?

Two main presentations are recognised:

- *hyperactive delirium* (hallucinations, delusions, agitation and disorientation)
- *hypoactive delirium* (cognitive impairment with apathy or withdrawal, less often accompanied by hallucinations and delusions).

The latter form can easily be overlooked in older patients.

Usually, delirium is triggered by an underlying physical disorder such as an infection (Boxes 12. 1 and 12.2), but those with pre-existing cognitive impairment or dementia are at increased risk (Box 12.1). As age is a risk factor, those in nursing and residential homes and intermediate care are at increased risk. Factors frequently combine, for example a person with both dementia and severe constipation who has recently developed a viral illness. Delirium is common in end-of-life care and poor management will contribute to a poor death and distress for carers.

The differential diagnosis includes depression (Table 12.1), which can be associated with agitation or withdrawal and 'confusion' (see section below on depression), and mania. The latter rarely presents *de novo* in old age but when it does it has some overlap with delirium and is usually triggered by a somatic disorder, for example a stroke.

---

**Box 12.1** Risk factors for delirium

**Socio-economic**
- Advanced age
- Male gender
- Little contact with relatives
- Institutional care

**Physical**
- Parkinson's
- Previous stroke
- Constipation

**New physical**
- Any infection but particularly urinary tract infection (UTI) or lower respiratory tract infection (LRTI)
- Fracture, dehydration

**Mental health**
- Pre-existing dementia

**Medications**
- Hypnotics, analgesics
- Anti-Parkinson disease drugs
- Drug interactions and polypharmacy
- Side-effects causing electrolyte disturbances

**Sensory impairment**
- Visual impairment
- Hearing impairment (lost hearing aid)

**Functional impairment and disability**
- Malnutrition
- Dehydration

---

**Box 12.2** Precipitants of delirium

- Medication
  - Benzodiazepines
  - Opioid analgesics
  - Anti-Parkinson agents
  - Tricyclic antidepressants
  - Steroids
  - Beta-blockers
  - Anti-arrhythmics
- Alcohol and substance misuse
  - Intoxication and withdrawal
- Severe or acute illness
  - Urinary tract infection, chest infection, silent myocardial infarction
- Metabolic
  - Hyper- or hypo-glycaemia
  - Hyper- or hypo-calcaemia
  - Thyrotoxicosis
  - Adrenal insufficiency
- Organ failure
  - Hepatic, renal, respiratory
- Shock
- Anaemia
- Neurological
  - Subdural haematoma
  - Stroke
  - Malignancy
- Pain
- Surgery and anaesthesia
- Sleep deprivation
- Change in circumstances
  - Accommodation, ward

## Diagnosis

The diagnosis is made on the history from patient and carers, plus a physical examination to look for physical cause. Investigations in primary care will include: Mid-stream specimen of urine (MSU), full blood count (FBC), urea and electrolytes (U&Es), liver function tests (LFTs), C-reactive protein, thyroid function tests (TFTs) and blood glucose, and the practitioner should consider the need for other investigations, such as electrocardiogram (ECG) and chest X-ray (CXR). If more intensive investigation is thought necessary (such as blood gases and blood cultures), then admission to hospital should be arranged.

It is important to assess cognitive function, both as a baseline and to assess fluctuation. This is discussed more fully in the section below on dementia. The Abbreviated Mental Test Score (Box 12.3) is a quick test.

**177**

---

**Box 12.3** Abbreviated Mental Test Score (AMT)

The patient is asked the following and given one point for each correct response:

1  Age
2  Time (to nearest hour)
3  Address for recall at end of test (42 West St)
4  Year
5  Name of hospital
6  Recognition of 2 persons (e.g. doctor, nurse)
7  Date of birth
8  Year of First World War
9  Name of present monarch
10 Count backwards from 20 to 1 (this also tests attention)

A score of less than 8/10 suggests confusion.

---

More detailed assessment is possible with the Confusion Assessment Method (Inouye *et al*, 1990).

## Principles of management

There are two treatment principles: to treat the underlying disorder and to ameliorate symptoms. The latter can be subdivided into: non-pharmacological strategies and medical management.

*Non-pharmacological approaches* help keep the patient in touch with reality and therefore less likely to become distressed and agitated. There are two key aspects:

- *managing the environment*, by avoiding sensory deprivation (e.g. a windowless room) or sensory overload (e.g. a noisy environment), ensuring day–night variation in the environment is preserved, providing a large clock, avoiding unnecessary room changes and trying to have some familiar objects around the patient
- *ensuring the patient's safety*, by anticipating and taking steps to prevent complications such as pressure sores, falls, further infections, constipation and reduction in mobility.

*Pharmacological (medical) interventions* aim to reduce symptoms that distress the patient or add to risk. They are targeted at specific symptoms, for example pain, psychotic phenomena or agitation. Psychotropic medications should be reserved for older persons in distress or with psychotic symptoms, to prevent them endangering themselves or others. The use of psychotropic medication to manage wandering is *not* advocated.

Antipsychotic medications ('major tranquillisers') are often the pharmacological treatment of choice. Haloperidol is most frequently used because it has few anticholinergic side-effects, few active metabolites and only a small chance of causing sedation and hypotension. Vigilance is needed for side-effects such as excessive sedation, extrapyramidal side-effects and akathisia (motor restlessness), which may arise suddenly after several days, so sedative medication should never be prescribed without an arrangement for review.

## Mental capacity

Patients with delirium may not possess mental capacity. The GP needs to assess whether the patient has the capacity to consent to treatment. In the UK, the Mental Capacity Act 2005 enshrines in statute current best practice and common law principles concerning people who lack mental capacity and those who take decisions on their behalf. It sets out a single clear test for assessing whether a person lacks capacity to take a particular decision at a particular time. A person lacks capacity if he or she is unable to do any of the following:

- to understand the information relevant to the decision
- to retain that information
- to use or weigh that information as part of the process of making the decision
- to communicate that decision (whether by talking, using sign language or any other means).

It is a 'decision-specific' test, in this case whether to accept either treatment for a medical condition underlying delirium or a drug to treat its effects. Everything that is done for or on behalf of a person who lacks capacity must be in that person's *best interests*. The Act provides a checklist of factors that decision-makers must work through in deciding what is in a person's best interests, such as known prior wishes, prior verbal or written statements, and the views of those caring for them. General practitioners should be aware of Deprivation of Liberty Safeguards introduced in 2008 under an amendment to the 2005 Mental Capacity Act. These apply if a person must be deprived of their liberty in a care home in order to receive care and treatment (http://www.dh.gov.uk/en/SocialCare/Deliveringadultsocialcare/MentalCapacity/MentalCapacityActDeprivationofLibertySafeguards/index.htm).

### Management of Case 1

The GP needs to take a careful history from Marjorie, as far as possible, and from the carers and staff. The GP might consider contacting Marjorie's relatives to obtain further details about when she was last well, whether she normally has cognitive impairment and whether she complained of any particular symptoms before she became confused.

The GP needs to review her medication chart and ask about other tablets (over-the-counter and complementary) taken and use of alcohol.

The GP needs to carefully examine Marjorie, check whether a urine dipstick analysis has been carried out and temperature measured, and assess her cognitive function. If the GP feels that Marjorie's symptoms can confidently be attributed to a treatable cause, then appropriate management of that problem (e.g. urinary tract infection, new medication, chest infection) can be instituted in the residential home. Advice to staff should be given about carefully orienting Marjorie, managing her distress and minimising risks. Medication for the confusion should be avoided if possible and the risks of prescribing (if that is what the residential home staff request) outlined. Arrangements should be made to review the patient within the next 48 hours or when requested by the staff.

If the cause of Marjorie's confusion is unclear, then admission to hospital should be discussed with carers and relatives.

## Referral and liaison

Ideally, patients with delirium should be treated in their usual environment, but if confusion and wandering are not controlled and they are at risk or if dehydration is developing, then admission to hospital may be needed. Intermediate care may be an alternative (Department of Health, 2000, 2004).

# Depression

## Epidemiology

Population studies have demonstrated that depression severe enough to warrant intervention is one of the commonest mental health problems facing older people, affecting around one in ten older people in the community (Copeland *et al*, 1999). However, the majority of people with depression are not detected and treated by their GPs (Age Concern England, 2007). The early identification and monitoring of 'sub-syndromal' symptoms is important and have been included within influential clinical guidelines (National Institute for Health and Clinical Excellence, 2004). Major depression is a recurring disorder and older people are more at risk of recurrence (Mitchell & Subramaniam, 2005) (see Chapter 8 on depression).

### Case 2. Depression: Mr Y
The GP first saw Mr Y 6 weeks ago. He had become withdrawn, miserable, was not looking after himself and had lost weight after the death of his wife 3 months earlier. He had scored 16 on the Patient Health Questionnaire (PHQ-9 – see below and Chapter 8) at that consultation.

The GP had carried out some investigations to exclude a physical illness and discussed with him the possibility that he might be depressed. Mr Y had disagreed with this but agreed to return a week later for a further discussion. At this consultation he had agreed that he would try antidepressants and the GP started him on citalopram.

Mr Y now returns to say that the tablets were no good and he still can't eat anything.

What should the GP do?

## Diagnosing depression in older people

Age of itself is not a risk factor for depression but comorbidity from physical disorder or poor cognition do contribute to depression in later life. Somatic preoccupation, hypochondriasis and the morbid fear of illness are more common presentations than the complaint of low mood or sadness. This can cause problems for the physician, as patients' hypochondriacal complaints (in the context of depression) can be quite different from the bodily symptoms one might expect from a knowledge of their medical history. Subjective memory disturbance may be a prominent symptom and lead to a differential diagnosis of dementia, but true cognitive disturbance is also common in late-life depression.

Anxiety is a common presenting or accompanying symptom and may mask underlying depression. Dementia may alter the presentation of depression and primary care clinicians should be aware that sustained irritable disruptive outbursts in patients with dementia may signify comorbid depression. Apathy and withdrawal are not uncommon symptoms and it is thought that apathetic presentations in later life with executive dysfunction may be due to vascular disease of the brain, to which older people are prone. Late-onset alcohol misuse is often linked to depression.

Bereavement is naturally common in later life and many of the features overlap with depression, especially in the early months (Clayton, 2004). Besides the failure of earlier symptoms to resolve after a few weeks, those that suggest depression rather than bereavement are: suicidal thoughts or wishing oneself dead, pervasive guilt (not merely remorse over what more might have been done to prevent death), retardation, marked feelings of worthlessness or hopelessness, 'mummification' (maintaining grief by keeping everything the same) and psychomotor retardation. Antidepressants are effective in bereavement-induced major depression (Reynolds *et al*, 1999*a*).

## Detection/screening

Some clinicians use validated schedules to assist in the diagnosis of depression with patients in whom they already have a high index of suspicion. As described in Chapter 8, the PHQ-9, Hospital Anxiety and Depression Scale (HAD) and Beck Depression Inventory are now included in the Quality and Outcomes Framework (QOF) of the new General Medical Services contract in England and Wales.

The Geriatric Depression Scale (GDS) (Box 12.4) is widely used to screen for depression in later life. False positives mean that its use in entire practice populations of older people is not justified, but opportunistic screening or screening of at-risk groups (Box 12.5) may be useful, although there is little evidence to support this. The GDS has the advantage of having a comprehensive website (http://stanford.edu/~yesavage/GDS.html), which gives short and long versions in a variety of languages, many of which have demonstrated cross-cultural validity (Rait *et al*, 1999).

**181**

**Box 12.4** Geriatric Depression Scale

Patients are instructed to choose the best answer for how they have felt over the past week, and are presented with 'yes/no' response options. The answers that score 1 (rather than 0) are indicated below (in italic). Phrases in parentheses are alternative ways of expressing the questions. The following 30 items comprise the long form. There is also a 15-item short form, comprising questions 1–4, 7–10, 12, 14, 15, 17, 21–23.

1   Are you basically satisfied with your life? *No*
2   Have you dropped many of your activities and interests? *Yes*
3   Do you feel your life is empty? *Yes*
4   Do you often get bored? *Yes*
5   Are you hopeful about the future? *No*
6   Are you bothered by thoughts you can't get out of your head? *Yes*
7   Are you in good spirits most of the time? *No*
8   Are you afraid something bad is going to happen to you? *Yes*
9   Do you feel happy most of the time? *No*
10  Do you often feel helpless? *Yes*
11  Do you often get restless and fidgety? *Yes*
12  Do you prefer to stay at home, rather than going out and doing new things? *Yes*
13  Do you frequently worry about the future? *Yes*
14  Do you feel you have more problems with your memory than most? *Yes*
15  Do you think it is wonderful to be alive now? *No*
16  Do you often feel down-hearted and blue (sad)? *Yes*
17  Do you feel pretty worthless the way you are? *Yes*
18  Do you worry a lot about the past? *Yes*
19  Do you find life very exciting? *No*
20  Is it hard for you to start on new projects (plans)? *Yes*
21  Do you feel full of energy? *No*
22  Do you feel that your situation is hopeless? *Yes*
23  Do you think most people are better off (in their lives) than you are? *Yes*
24  Do you frequently get upset over little things? *Yes*
25  Do you frequently feel like crying? *Yes*
26  Do you have trouble concentrating? *Yes*
27  Do you enjoy getting up in the morning? *No*
28  Do you prefer to avoid social gatherings (get-togethers)? *Yes*
29  Is it easy for you to make decisions? *No*
30  Is your mind as clear as it used to be? *No*

Cut-off scores for possible depression are 11 or more on the long version (GDS-30) or 5 or more on the short version (GDS-15).

## Principles of management

Treatment should be multimodal (employing somatic, psychological and environmental/social dimensions) and often multidisciplinary, possibly drawing on the skills of nurses, social care agencies, a podiatrist, a physiotherapist and so on (Baldwin *et al*, 2003). The treatment goals are to

---

**Box 12.5** Indicators of at-risk groups of older people who might be targeted for depression screening in primary care

- Recent (<3 months) major physical illness or hospital admission
- Chronic illness
- In receipt of high levels of home care
- Recent bereavement
- Social isolation
- Persistent complaints of loneliness
- Persistent complaints of sleep problems

---

treat the whole person, to reduce risk, to achieve remission of depressive symptoms (because partial recovery is associated with later risk of relapse and chronicity), to prevent relapse and recurrence, and to help the person achieve optimum function (Chew-Graham *et al*, 2008).

## Collaborative care

Most elderly people with depression in the UK will be managed in primary care and the lead clinician will be the GP. The collaborative care model (see Chapter 27) may be more effective, with components such as a protocol or care pathway and a depression care manager (usually a nurse, psychologist or social worker) who coordinates the care, including medication concordance and regular dialogue between the primary care team and the specialist psychiatric services. The model is effective in the management of depression in older people (Unützer *et al*, 2002; Chew-Graham *et al*, 2007).

## Clinical evaluation

The GP should cover five areas in the primary care consultation when suspecting depression: history, mental state, risk assessment, focused physical examination and appropriate investigations. The risk of self-harm must be established. Even seemingly medically trivial attempts at self-harm in older people cannot be ignored. *All* should be assumed to be due to depression unless proven otherwise. It is important to check carefully for delusional ideas, as the assessment and treatment of such patients require early referral for specialist input.

## Initiating treatment with an antidepressant

The prescribing principles with older people are to 'start low and go slow' with respect to dosage and to tailor the antidepressant to the patient, taking account of anticipated effects and side-effects. Although they are effective, tricyclic antidepressants have too many potentially serious adverse effects to be justified as first-line treatments in primary care.

If, at 4 weeks, there has been little or no response to an antidepressant given in adequate dosage, it is best to change it to a drug from a different class. Non-response after the trial of a second antidepressant should prompt referral to a specialist.

## Psychological interventions

Cognitive–behavioural therapy (CBT), interpersonal psychotherapy (IPT), problem-solving therapy (PST) and psychodynamic psychotherapy are the most widely researched forms of psychotherapy in later-life depression (Gatz *et al*, 1998; Pinquart & Sorensen, 2001) and, where available, can be offered as an alternative to an antidepressant for depression of moderate severity. For a moderate to severe (non-psychotic) depressive episode, combining antidepressant medication with a psychological intervention such as CBT or IPT can improve outcomes further (Reynolds *et al*, 1999b).

Anxiety management can be a highly effective adjunctive treatment for patients with depression, especially where patients who are recovering from it are left with residual anxiety, low confidence or phobic avoidance, which can undermine functional improvement.

Exercise and activity are important. 'Behavioural activation' can overcome the withdrawal and apathy that often feature in late-life depression. It works by helping the patient develop a schedule of activities, agreed with the patient, and with or without a written diary to support implementation. The GP can use some of these techniques within the primary care consultation, particularly advising about diet, exercise and alcohol, encouraging behaviour change and goal-setting, challenging negative thinking and teaching relaxation techniques. Most GPs have access to self-help leaflets, which can be given to patients to reinforce the content of their discussion within consultations.

Family work is important: the patient may unconsciously use the family to foster invalidism, which the family may then unwittingly reinforce. The unconscious goal may be to live under the same roof as one's children. More positively, the family is often critical in ensuring a successful outcome in treatment, for example by reinforcing messages about treatment concordance, exercise and activity, and goal-setting, and the primary care team should work with the family as well as with the individual patient.

### Management of Case 2

At this consultation, the GP needs to explore Mr Y's concerns about the tablets. Is he still taking them or has he stopped them? Do they have side-effects? Has a member of his family told him not to take them? The GP should ask specific questions about the biological symptoms of depression (mood and diurnal variation, sleep, appetite, concentration) and whether Mr Y thinks that life is worth living since the death of his wife.

The GP should particularly enquire about thoughts of self-harm. It is vital to assess the risk of suicide in this high-risk situation. If Mr Y expresses thoughts of self-harm, then whether he has made plans and what would stop him harming himself should be explored. If the GP considers that he is at risk of suicide, a referral to old age psychiatry is indicated (with a view to admission if he has made active plans, or an urgent out-patient appointment if this is more appropriate and the GP feels there is family or other support).

The GP needs again to ask the patient what he feels his symptoms are due to and how the GP can help. Hypochondriasis can be a presenting feature with older people who are depressed, but an older person can present with depressive symptoms associated with an underlying physical illness. The GP needs to decide whether any investigation of Mr Y's gastrointestinal tract is indicated (if only to reassure him that everything is normal).

The GP should explore with Mr Y what he previously enjoyed doing, before the death of his wife, and sensitively enquire about alcohol consumption.

The GP also needs to ascertain what support Mr Y has at home, if any, and ask whether he would like any of his family to be involved in future consultations.

Mr Y's own views about his depression should be explored with 'sign-posting' to a self-help group or CRUSE Bereavement Care (see www.crusebereavementcare.org.uk).

The GP should discuss with Mr Y whether he wishes to continue to try a tablet for his symptoms. It may be appropriate to continue the citalopram or change to a different class if Mr Y had side-effects. If insomnia is a problem, then a more sedating antidepressant, such as mirtazepine or trazodone, could be prescribed. The GP needs to encourage Mr Y to resume activities he enjoyed before the death of his wife. If a service exists, the GP could refer Mr Y to the primary care mental health team (according to the stepped-care approach). A review appointment should be offered in a couple of weeks.

## Referral and liaison

Most older people with depression will be managed within primary care. Specialist referral is indicated (Box 12.6) when the diagnosis is in doubt, when depression is severe (with active suicidal intent, an urgent referral is indicated) and when the patient has failed to respond to trials of at least two different antidepressants.

---

**Box 12.6** When to refer a patient with depression for specialist opinion or care

- When the diagnosis is in doubt (e.g. is this dementia?)
- When depression is severe, as evidenced by:
  - psychotic depression
  - severe risk to health because of failure to eat or drink
  - suicide risk
- Complex therapy is indicated (e.g. in cases with medical comorbidity)
- When the patient has not responded to two adequate trials of antidepressants from different classes

See: Baldwin *et al* (2003); National Institute for Health and Clinical Excellence (2004); Chew-Graham *et al* (2008).

---

# Dementia

## Classification

Dementia is a syndrome, a cluster of symptoms, and not a diagnosis in its own right. In later life the main causes (Box 12.7) are neurodegenerative or vascular. Pure forms are unusual: most are mixed (e.g. Alzheimer's plus vascular). This section will deal with the non-reversible causes of dementia.

> **Case 3. Dementia: Mrs G**
>
> The GP's next patient is an 82-year-old woman, Mrs G, who has lived alone in sheltered accommodation since the death of her husband 2 years ago. She is brought in by her niece, who lives nearby.
>
> Her niece complains that she is increasingly forgetful and is not eating properly. Once or twice she has got lost when out shopping, and last week could not find her car in the car park.
>
> What should the GP do in that consultation?

According to ICD–10 (World Health Organization, 1992), dementia is defined as:

> a syndrome due to disease of the brain, usually of a chronic or progressive nature, in which there is disturbance of multiple higher cortical functions, including memory, thinking, orientation, comprehension, calculation, learning capacity, language, and judgement. Consciousness is not clouded. Impairments of cognitive function are commonly accompanied, and occasionally preceded, by deterioration in emotional control, social behaviour, or motivation.

## Epidemiology

The prevalence of dementia increases dramatically with age (Table 12.2), to as much as a quarter among those aged over 80. The risk factors are

---

**Box 12.7** Causes of dementia

*Main primary causes in later life:*

- Alzheimer's disease
- Vascular (cortical, subcortical and mixed)
- Lewy-body disease (including Lewy-body dementia and dementia in Parkinson's disease)

*Potentially reversible:*

- Vitamin $B_{12}$ deficiency, hypothyroidism, HIV, alcoholic dementia, tumour, normal-pressure hydrocephalus, neurosyphilis, severe depression.

*Other, rarer causes:*

- Fronto-temporal dementia (including Pick's disease), vasculitides, Huntington's disease, Wilson's disease

---

highly influential. For example, higher rates have been found in the UK in the African–Caribbean population than in the White, and this may because of the increased prevalence of cardiovascular disease, hypertension and diabetes in the former. Vascular disease is the most important risk factor for *both* vascular dementia and Alzheimer's disease.

Genetic predisposition is strong in young-onset familial cases. Among older people, a double dose of the allele ε4 confers an increased risk.

## Diagnosis

This is made on the history from patient and carers (family and carers in residential accommodation). It is *vital* to have some corroborative history, as a core feature of dementia is loss of insight.

The presenting symptom is normally deteriorating memory. The GP should ask the patient or family member to give an example of specific problems resulting from a memory lapse. However, poor memory alone is insufficient for a diagnosis. Some basic familiarity with brain structure helps with questioning. For example, in Alzheimer's disease the pathology starts in the mid-to-back parts of the brain, often in the temporal lobe, hence the memory deficits. In vascular dementia, the precise area of cortical damage will determine the symptoms and signs. In subcortical dementia, the problem is mental inefficiency, leading to sluggish memory and apathy. In frontal dementia (more common in mid-life), apathy or disinhibition syndromes predominate, whereas memory is relatively intact.

The GP should also explore details of the patient's home circumstances, ability to cope with activities of daily living and to handle more complex tasks (e.g. dealing with money, driving) and enquire about support from family. A home visit is often more informative in relation to risk assessment (Box 12.8), as it will allow the GP to gauge the state of hygiene, repair, odours, evidence of alcohol, and environmental risks, including driving (see below on driving).

The physical examination focuses on physical risk factors (pulse, blood pressure, peripheral pulses), neurological examination (facial expression, gait, abnormal movements, fundi and visual fields, primitive reflexes) and a mental state examination, especially a test of cognition (some key tests are described below).

**Table 12.2** Prevalence of dementia

| Age range (years) | Prevalence rates (per 100 population) |
|---|---|
| 31–60 | 0.1 |
| 61–70 | 1.5 |
| 71–80 | 5.0 |
| 81–90 | 25 |
| 91+ | 35 |

---

**Box 12.8** Risk assessment

A patient with dementia, especially one who lives alone, is at risk and this should be assessed by the GP in relation to:

- self-neglect – malnutrition, dehydration, food poisoning, hypothermia
- misuse of household appliances – fire, flooding, electrocution
- falls
- robbery
- exploitation (e.g. by tradespeople)
- abuse – emotional and sexual abuse by carers is a real risk that the clinician should be aware of and alert to.

---

The GP may also be able to diagnose the type of dementia the patient has. There are clues specific to each of the main forms of dementia encountered in later life, and these are presented next.

## Clues in the history to type of dementia

### Alzheimer's disease

Patients commonly present or are presented with memory loss, initially for recent events. Language impairment and a decline in complex motor skills (which can affect driving) may be reported by carers. There is a loss of recognition skills, as well as disorientation.

### Mixed dementia

Alzheimer's disease and vascular dementia overlap to a considerable degree and because Alzheimer's disease is common, mixed dementia is more common than pure vascular dementia. It is difficult to determine the diagnosis because many of the features are shared.

### Vascular dementia

Patients with vascular dementia may have a step-wise deterioration in both physical and cognitive function, for example in the context of a stroke. Neurological signs and symptoms are determined by the site of cortical damage and brain imaging is helpful. Parkinsonism may occur as a result of vascular damage to the basal ganglia or the motor projections to the frontal premotor cortex. Where the subcortical structures are primarily affected ('small-vessel disease'), the cognitive deficits are more of the executive type and memory is patchily affected.

### Lewy-body disease

Other than progressive cognitive decline, dementia with Lewy bodies is characterised by three further features: fluctuating alertness and attention, visual hallucinations and Parkinsonism. Affected patients may stare into space for long periods and be unresponsive to changes in the environment.

At other times they may be able to participate in normal conversation. Arousal also fluctuates, sometimes from stupor to normal levels of vigilance and responsiveness. Patients are often excessively sensitive to antipsychotic drugs, such that very small doses may cause profound sedation, worsening Parkinsonism and even death. Some patients with idiopathic Parkinson's disease, especially those with an onset in later life, may progress to a clinical picture indistinguishable from Lewy-body dementia.

### Korsakoff's psychosis

Patients with Korsakoff's psychosis usually have a history of alcohol misuse and also show confabulation. It is this feature that has attracted the label of 'psychosis' to this disorder, but true psychotic symptoms do not occur.

### Frontotemporal dementia

Frontotemporal dementia refers to a group of conditions in which behavioural or language impairments predominate and there is a relative preservation of memory. Patients often present with disinhibition and other behavioural impairments, or marked deterioration in language out of proportion to other cognitive deficits. There is often a family history and onset is generally earlier than with Alzheimer's disease (mean age is 60).

## Cognitive testing and cognitive screening

Cognitive tests are diagnostic aids rather than definitive tests and must be interpreted in the light of knowledge of the patient, the testing environment and the limitations of the tests.

The Mini-Mental State Examination (MMSE; Folstein et al, 1975, and http://www.minimental.com) covers orientation, registration, attention, calculation and language, and takes about 10 minutes. The instrument is copyrighted. Useful information is provided the Alzheimer's Society (2008a). The MMSE is used in secondary care to determine whether specific drug treatments can be offered (National Institute for Health and Clinical Excellence, 2006). The MMSE can be purchased from PAR Inc (http://www.parinc.com).

The six-item Orientation–Memory–Concentration (OMC) test (Katzman et al, 1983 (Table 12.3), adapted by Brooke & Bullock (1999) to form the Cognitive Impairment Test (CIT), has been validated in community samples. A score of 8 or above indicates likely significant confusion.

The clock-drawing test has been proposed as a quick and easy method, in primary care, of confirming the presence of dementia; patients with dementia tend to fill in the numbers by working clockwise from the number 12 or 1 and spacing between the figures is uneven and inaccurate. Unimpaired individuals start by writing 12, 3, 6 and 9 at the four quadrants before completing the clock (for a review see Shulman, 2000). A practical guide to cognitive testing can be found on http://www.patient.co.uk/showdoc/40002381 and Cullen et al (2007) give a scientific overview of tests. Either the MMSE or the CIT is appropriate for use in primary care.

**Table 12.3** The six-item CIT test[a]

| Question | Maximum number of errors | Initial score | Weighting | Weighted score |
|---|---|---|---|---|
| 1. What year is it now? | 1 | | 4 | |
| 2. What month is it now? | 1 | | 3 | |
| Repeat this phrase: John Brown, 42 Market Street, Chicago or (UK): John Brown, 42 West Street, Gateshead | | | | |
| 3. About what time is it? | 1 (within an hour) | | 3 | |
| 4. Count backwards from 20 to 1 | 2 | | 2 | |
| 5. Say the months in reverse order | 2 | | 2 | |
| 6. Repeat the phrase just given | 5 | | 2 | |

a. This generates a total error score out of a possible total of 28.

### Differential diagnosis

The main differentials are delirium (short history, consciousness affected; see Table 12.1), depressive disorder (often 'don't know' answers more than true forgetfulness or low effort) and anxiety (poor concentration, absent minded).

### Investigations

In primary care, FBC, U&Es, cholesterol, LFTs, C-reactive protein, TFTs, $B_{12}$ and folate, blood glucose (and HbA1C if diabetic), MSU and CXR may be indicated. Although hypothyroidism and $B_{12}$ deficiency can cause dementia – and it is suggested that all patients have these tests done before considering referral to secondary care – it is unusual for any of these tests to be abnormal.

If dementia is suspected, most patients are referred to a specialist (an old age psychiatrist, neurologist or geriatrician) who can then advise on treatment and arrange more specialised tests, such as neuroimaging.

## Dementia and driving

Dementia is a condition likely to impair driving and in the UK the patient must be told to inform the Driving and Vehicle Licensing Agency (DVLA) as this is a legal requirement. In dementia, where insight may be impaired, this advice may not be followed, so carers must also be involved. Where patients refuse either to report themselves or to allow others to do so, breaching confidentiality by directly approaching the medical advisers of the DVLA (contact details at http://www.direct.gov.uk/en/Motoring/DriverLicensing/MedicalRulesForDrivers/DG_4022415) is entirely appropriate. The DVLA may then arrange a test of driving skills.

Not all patients with dementia are unfit to drive and patients with early dementia may be fit to drive if they keep to familiar routes, do not drive at busy times and have someone accompanying them.

The Alzheimer's Society (2008b) gives useful information for patients and relatives.

## Management

Once a firm diagnosis has been made (usually in secondary care) and information imparted to patient and carer (e.g. leaflets and the contact number for the local Alzheimer's Society group), the general aims of management include: ruling out reversible causes of dementia; attending to factors likely to magnify the effects of dementia (e.g. poorly controlled heart failure, constipation or sensory problems); arranging for a risk assessment; treating behavioural and psychological symptoms; and supporting carers.

### Psychological treatments

Psychological support (provided by the local authority, specialist old age psychiatry services or the independent sector) may include general support via day centres or more specific therapies – such as reality orientation (which aims to improve patients' orientation and awareness of the environment), validation therapy (recognising the importance of patients' feelings and their attempts to express them, rather than correcting patients' mistakes) or reminiscence therapy (encouraging the patient to recollect details or events in an individual's life). Specific stress management and coping skills training may also help caregivers.

### Drug treatments

As discussed above, depressive disorder frequently accompanies dementia (and is also common among carers). Since depression adversely affects cognition, it is usual to give a course of an antidepressant prior to considering specific drug treatment for the dementia for any patient with at least moderate depression and then readminister a cognitive test. There is no evidence that one antidepressant is any more effective than another.

Three drugs are currently licensed in England and Wales for the *specific treatment of cognitive decline and associated functional impairment* in Alzheimer's disease. Memantine (Ebixa), a glutamatergic modulator, was withdrawn after a review by the National Institute for Health and Clinical Excellence (2006). The three licensed drugs are all cholinesterase inhibitors: donepezil (Aricept), rivastigmine (Exelon) and galantamine (Reminyl). They can be given only to patients with moderate Alzheimer's disease, suggested by an MMSE score of 10–20. Their administration must be initiated by a specialist (i.e. an old age psychiatrist, neurologist or geriatrician) and monitored. Most areas have an arrangement for the transfer of prescribing to primary care after a specified time. There is good evidence that these drugs slow the rate of cognitive decline, but less good evidence of their effects on function and quality of life.

Side-effects include nausea, vomiting, headaches and dizziness. These drugs aggravate cardiac conduction defects, and patients with pre-existing heart disease, a dysrhythmia or a pulse rate below 60 beats/min indicate the need for an ECG before treatment is started.

There is no place for the indiscriminate use of drugs merely to sedate an older person with dementia. Except where the patient is clearly distressed, non-pharmacological approaches should be used. Furthermore, in England, in 2004 the Committee on Safety of Medicines (CSM) issued guidance to avoid the use of risperidone and olanzapine in the treatment of behavioural problems in dementia because of an increased risk of stroke (http://www.mhra.gov.uk/Safetyinformation/Generalsafetyinformationandadvice/Product-specificinformationandadvice/Antipsychoticdrugs/index.htm). It is unlikely that this effect is confined to two drugs only.

### Management of Case 3

Mrs G has been brought by her niece; it is important for the GP to check with her that, as the patient, she is comfortable with her niece coming in to this appointment with her. The GP needs to try to find out whether Mrs G feels she has any problems; it is particularly important to enquire about biological symptoms of depression, such as poor attention and concentration, as these cause apparent short-term memory loss. The GP needs to allow time for the niece to outline her concerns and to note how Mrs G behaves during this discussion: whether she is irritable and upset by her niece's narrative, confabulates to cover up her niece's concerns, or agrees that there have been problems.

Careful questioning is necessary to exclude fluctuating consciousness and hallucinations, as this may require urgent referral to secondary care, to exclude dementia with Lewy bodies or delirium.

A brief family history is needed (especially for evidence of neurodegenerative disorder) and discussion of alcohol and smoking status is necessary, with an explanation of why this is important. A review of any physical problems such as diabetes or hypertension and medication review to check compliance are important.

A focused physical examination to look for signs of Parkinson's disease and vascular disease is vital. A cognitive test such as the MMSE (which may be available as a computer template) or the CIT should be conducted, along with initial investigations, particularly blood tests, to look for reversible causes of memory loss.

It is vital to assess whether this patient is at risk and whether a home visit is necessary to assess this further. Risk to others should also be considered and the GP needs to inform the niece and Mrs G that she should not drive until the cause of her memory loss has been elicited, and that she may need to inform the DVLA if a diagnosis of dementia is made. The GP should document that discussion in the notes.

Note should also be made of the niece's telephone number for future contact and agreement from Mrs G obtained that her niece can be contacted in this way, assuming Mrs G has capacity to give this consent.

Arrangements should then be made for follow-up to discuss the blood test results and agreement of a management plan. If it seems that a diagnosis is likely of an irreversible dementia due to Alzheimer's disease or vascular dementia or a mixed picture, then discussion of referral to old age psychiatry should be undertaken at this or future consultations, explaining why such a referral is being made. It is helpful to carry out an ECG if a cholinesterase inhibitor might be prescribed.

If a firm diagnosis of dementia is made, then the GP will have a vital role in supporting Mrs G and her carers (in this case, her niece) as the disease progresses, liaising with secondary care and prescribing cholinesterase inhibitors according to a shared care protocol if appropriate. The GP needs to ensure that an assessment of capacity is made at each contact, and to be astute to the potential risks that this patient may present to herself or others (e.g. when driving) as well as be aware that she is vulnerable to neglect or even abuse.

The QOF requires that practices develop a register of patients with dementia and review care every 15 months. It does not, though, stipulate what review should entail. However, the following are suggested:

- appropriate review of physical comorbidities
- review of mental health (MMSE, screening questions for depression)
- review of medication
- review of smoking status
- review of alcohol consumption
- assessment of carers
- review of communication with secondary and social care, with a note of key workers/case managers
- end-of-life discussion if appropriate.

## Mild cognitive impairment

Mild cognitive impairment (MCI) denotes a condition of measurable cognitive deficit, notably involving memory, but without other features to suggest dementia. A proportion of these patients will go on to develop dementia. These patients, along with others who may have early dementia, are difficult to diagnose and arrangements should be made for assessment via a specialist. The Alzheimer's Society (2008c) has a fact sheet on MCI.

# Delusions

Delusions in later life generally arise in the context of schizophrenia and delusional disorder. In principle the presentation and management are the same as for younger adults but there are some nuances and the differential diagnosis, especially where onset is new, should always include consideration of an organic (medical) cause, delirium, a drug or an early dementia.

### Case 4. Delusions: Diane R

A patient, Diane R, is discharged from hospital to a local nursing home and is registered by the staff with the local general practice. Her discharge letter states that she was admitted to hospital from a local residential home with a chest infection and that the previous home refused to take her back because of 'difficult behaviour'. Discharge medication is risperidone, temazepam, lansoprazole, ramipril and bendrofluazide.

Her old general practice records arrive, in which it is noted that she has 'chronic schizophrenia'.

**193**

The day after discharge, the nurse in charge of the home rings the new practice and asks for an urgent visit because Diane is reported to be aggressive, has urinated in another person's room and is talking to herself.

What should the GP do?

Delusional disorders range from highly circumscribed persecutory delusions, through the presence of both delusions and hallucinations, to a full-blown schizophrenia-like presentation. Whether these conditions are distinct from schizophrenia is unresolved. Aetiological factors include a genetic component, sensory deprivation (particularly deafness) and long-standing social isolation. Treatment is often difficult because of lack of insight, but response to antipsychotics is usually good, especially if they are given as a long-acting 'depot' preparation.

As older people are at particular risk of tardive dyskinesia, atypical antipsychotics may be appropriate. In view of the risk of stroke, vascular risk factors should be considered as a caution, but unless these risks are major or poorly controlled, atypical drugs should still be considered first-line treatment. Impaired glycaemic control is also a caution.

### Management of Case 4

The GP needs to take a careful history from the nurse over the telephone and obtain key information about symptoms and details of carers, social services and key workers within the community mental health team (CMHT), and to assess whether a visit is required today.

The GP needs to contact the family if possible to obtain a picture of how Diane was before discharge and whether her condition has deteriorated. A discussion with the social services key worker who placed the women in the nursing home would be helpful, as would contact with the community psychiatric nurse to gain a picture of her mental state and function.

At a home visit, the GP should review her medication chart and ask about other tablets (over-the-counter and complementary) and use of alcohol.

The GP needs to carefully examine Diane, particularly exploring delusions and hallucinations, looking for evidence of extrapyramidal signs, and assessing risk to self and to other residents. The GP should ask whether a urine dipstick has been carried out and temperature measured, and assess her cognitive function. If it seems that Diane has developed an acute confusion (delirium) on top of the schizophrenia, and the cause can confidently be attributed to a treatable cause, then appropriate management of that problem (e.g. change of environment, urinary tract infection, new medication started, chest infection) can be instituted in the nursing home. Advice to staff should be given about carefully orienting Diane and managing her distress and minimising risks. Medication for the confusion should be avoided if possible and the risks of prescribing (if that is what the residential home staff request) outlined. Arrangements should be made to review the patient within the next 48 hours or when requested to by the staff.

If it seems that Diane has been distressed during discharge (and at the previous residential home), then the GP should discuss with the community psychiatric nurse and old age psychiatrist the need for a Care Programme Approach review and review of medication and the development of a new management plan that will enable her to be supported in this new nursing home.

# Conclusion

Primary care is a key provider of care for older people with mental health problems. The GP has a key role in diagnosis and initial management and has an ongoing role in providing good-quality proactive physical and mental healthcare. Other members of the primary care team need to be aware particularly of the risk of depression in older people with chronic physical conditions, and the increasing prevalence of dementia with increasing patient age. Members of the primary care team need to remember that they are supporting not just an individual but their wider family and carers (paid and unpaid), as they come to terms with the diagnosis and support the patient.

---

**Key points**

- Members of the primary care team are important partners in providing good-quality holistic care for older people with mental health problems, both at the point of diagnosis and in the longer term.
- Recognition by the primary care physician (PCP) or general practitioner (GP) of early changes, clinical intuition and acting on family worries are vital in the early detection of mental health problems in older people.
- An awareness of the increased risk of depression in older people with co-morbid physical conditions is vital.
- Appropriate referral and good liaison and collaboration between primary and secondary care are vital in the management of older people with mental health problems.
- The primary care team needs to remember that they are supporting not just an individual, but also their wider family, as they come to terms with the diagnosis and support the patient.

---

# Further reading and e-resources

## Delirium

The British Geriatric Society has online guidance which, although more geared towards hospital practitioners, is relevant for reference by primary care professionals: http://www.bgs.org.uk/Publications/Clinical%20Guidelines/clinical_1-2_fulldelirium.htm

## Depression

*A Collective Responsibility to Act Now on Ageing and Mental Health: A Consensus Statement* (http://www.mentalhealthequalities.org.uk/silo/files/consensus-statement-august.pdf). Issued by key organisations integral to the care, support and treatment of mental health in later life.

Baldwin, R., Anderson, D., Black, S., *et al* (2003) Guideline for the management of late-life depression in primary care. *International Journal of Geriatric Psychiatry*, **18**, 829–838. For those with access rights (e.g. some forms of Athens passwords) this can be downloaded in pdf format.

The Geriatric Depression Scale website is http://stanford.edu/~yesavage/GDS.html

The National Institute for Health and Clinical Excellence (2004) has issued a clinical guideline – *Depression: Management of Depression in Primary and Secondary Care*. NICE guidance CG23, which includes guidance for older people, downloadable from http://www.nice.org.uk/guidance/cg23

The Old Age Psychiatry Faculty of the Royal College of Psychiatrists has published guidance specifically for older people.

## Dementia

The National Institute for Health and Clinical Excellence in 2006 published extensive guidance for the management of dementia. It emphasises person-centred care and the use of individual care plans, and makes evidence-based recommendations for the diagnosis and management of patients with dementia, including the role of care managers and the need for integrated health and social care: http://www.nice.org.uk/guidance/cg42

The National Service Framework for Older People (2001) recommends specialist training for those working in primary care on the diagnosis and management of dementia. The Framework suggests that primary and secondary care should work together to draw up protocols and guidelines for the identification and appropriate referral pathways for patients, including the use of rating scales: http://www.dh.gov.uk/en/Publicationsandstatistics/Publications/PublicationsPolicyAndGuidance/DH_4003066

# References

Age Concern England (2007) *Improving Services and Support for Older People with Mental Health Problems*. Second Report from the UK Inquiry into Mental Health and Wellbeing in Later Life. Age Concern England.

Alzheimer's Society (2008a) *How Dementia is Diagnosed*. Fact sheet 436. Downloadable from http://www.alzheimers.org.uk/factsheet/436

Alzheimer's Society (2008b) *Driving and Dementia is Diagnosed*. Fact sheet 439. Downloadable from http://www.alzheimers.org.uk/factsheet/439

Alzheimer's Society (2008c) *Driving and Dementia is Diagnosed*. Fact sheet 470. Downloadable from http://www.alzheimers.org.uk/factsheet/470

Baldwin, R., Anderson, D., Black, S., *et al* (2003) Guideline for the management of late-life depression in primary care. *International Journal of Geriatric Psychiatry*, **18**, 829–838.

Brooke, P. & Bullock, R. (1999) Validation of the 6 item Cognitive Impairment Test. *International Journal of Geriatric Psychiatry*, **14**, 936–940.

Chew-Graham, C. A., Lovell, K., Roberts, C., *et al* (2007) A randomised controlled trial to test the feasibility of a collaborative care model for the management of depression in older people. *British Journal of General Practice*, **57**, 364–370.

Chew-Graham, C., Baldwin, R. & Burns, A. (2008) *The Integrated Management of Depression in the Elderly*. Cambridge University Press.

Clayton, P. J. (2004) Bereavement and depression. In *Late-Life Depression* (eds R. P. Roose & H. A. Sackeim), pp. 107–114. Oxford University Press.

Copeland, J. R., Beekman, A. T., Dewey, A. T., *et al* (1999) Depression in Europe. Geographical distribution among older people. *British Journal of Psychiatry*, **174**, 312–321.

Crausman, R. S. (2004) The four 'I's of delirium (letter). *Journal of the American Geriatrics Society*, **52**, 645.

Cullen, B., O'Neill, B., Evans, J. J., *et al* (2007) A review of screening tests for cognitive impairment. *Journal of Neurology, Neurosurgery and Psychiatry*, **78**, 790–799.

Department of Health (2000) *The NHS Plan: A Plan for Investment, a Plan for Reform*. The Stationery Office.

Department of Health (2004) *The NHS Improvement Plan.* Cm 6268. The Stationery Office.

Folstein, M. F., Folstein, S. E. & McHugh, P. R. (1975) 'Mini-Mental State': a practical method for grading the cognitive state of patients for the clinician. *Journal of Psychiatric Research,* **12,** 185–198.

Gatz, M., Fiske, A., Fox, L. S., *et al* (1998) Empirically validated psychological treatments for older adults. *Journal of Mental Health and Aging,* **4,** 9–46.

Inouye, S. K., van Dyck, C. H., Alessi, C. A., *et al* (1990) Clarifying confusion: the confusion assessment method. A new method for detection of delirium. *Annals of Internal Medicine,* **113,** 941–948.

Katzman, R., Brown, T., Fuld, P., *et al* (1983) Validation of a short Orientation–Memory Concentration Test of cognitive impairment. *American Journal of Psychiatry,* **140,** 734–739.

Mitchell, A. J. & Subramaniam, H. (2005) Prognosis of depression in old age compared to middle age: a systematic review of comparative studies. *American Journal of Psychiatry,* **162,** 1588–1601.

National Institute for Health and Clinical Excellence (2004) *Depression: Management of Depression in Primary and Secondary Care.* NICE clinical guideline CG23. NICE. Downloadable from http://www.nice.org.uk/guidance/cg23

National Institute for Health and Clinical Excellence (2006) *Dementia: Supporting People with Dementia and Their Carers in Health and Social Care.* NICE clinical guideline 42. NICE. Downloadable from http://www.nice.org.uk/guidance/cg42

Pinquart, M. & Sorensen, S. (2001) How effective are psychotherapeutic and other psychosocial interventions with older adults? A meta-analysis. *Journal of Mental Health and Aging,* **7,** 207–243.

Rait, G., Burns, A., Baldwin, R., *et al* (1999) Screening for depression in older Afro-Caribbeans. *Family Practice,* **16,** 591–595.

Reynolds III, C. F., Miller, M. D., Pasternak, R. E., *et al* (1999a) Treatment of bereavement-related major depressive episodes in later life: a controlled study of acute and continuation treatment with nortriptyline and interpersonal psychotherapy. *American Journal of Psychiatry,* **156,** 202–208.

Reynolds III, C. F., Frank, E., Perel, J. M., *et al* (1999b) Nortriptyline and interpersonal psychotherapy as maintenance therapies for recurrent major depression: a randomized controlled trial in patients older than 59 years. *JAMA,* **281,** 39–45.

Shulman, K. I. (2000) Clock-drawing: is it the ideal cognitive screening test? *International Journal of Geriatric Psychiatry,* **15,** 548–561.

Unützer, J., Katon, W., Callahan, C. M., *et al* (2002) Collaborative care management of late-life depression in the primary care setting: a randomized controlled trial. *JAMA,* **288,** 2836–2845.

World Health Organization (1992) *International Classification of Diseases* (10th revision) (ICD–10). WHO.

**197**

# CHAPTER 13

# Perinatal mental health

Debbie Sharp

### Summary

This chapter covers the definition of perinatal mental health, the classification of disorders in the postnatal period, risk factors, and the identification and treatment of postnatal depression, including both psychosocial and drug treatments.

The term 'perinatal mental health' covers mental health problems that occur in women during pregnancy and the first postnatal year. There has been a great deal written about postnatal depression, the most common postnatal mental health problem, during the past two decades but much less about the mental health problems that occur during pregnancy. It is only recently that research has revealed how prevalent and important these are, particularly in terms of their relationship to postnatal disorders and their subsequent effect on both the mother's and the infant's health and well-being (Evans *et al*, 2001; O'Connor *et al*, 2002; O'Keane, 2006).

Although the range of mental health problems occurring at these times is not dissimilar to those affecting all adults, their nature, treatment and effects are different in several ways. For example, stopping psychotropic medication abruptly in a pregnancy owing to concerns about teratogenicity can worsen or precipitate an episode of mental illness. In women with, for example, bipolar illness, the risk of relapse is higher in the immediate postpartum period. When considering the diagnosis and treatment of perinatal mental health problems, there is often more than one patient to consider. An acute psychotic episode after the birth may place the infant as well as the mother at risk. A lengthy postnatal depression may have long-term adverse effects on the child's development and the marital relationship (Cooper & Murray, 1998). The Confidential Enquiry into Maternal and Child Health (2004) reported that, overall, the leading cause of maternal death was suicide, with more than half of the women who died having an underlying history of mental illness. Many of these women had had regular contact with healthcare professionals. The need to prevent, identify as early as possible and treat such potentially life-threatening conditions optimally is clear.

# Classification

In the two major systems, the *International Classification of Diseases, Tenth Revision* (ICD–10; World Health Organization, 1992) and the *Diagnostic and Statistical Manual of Mental Disorders, Fourth Edition* (DSM–IV; American Psychiatric Association, 1994), perinatal mental disorders have only just been categorised separately, but both require certain qualifications to be met that limit their use: ICD–10 categorises mental disorders that occur postpartum as 'puerperal', but only if they cannot otherwise be classified, and DSM–IV allows 'postpartum onset' to be specified for mood disorders starting within 4 weeks of delivery. Currently there are no separate descriptors for antenatal mental health problems. The World Health Organization's *Guide to Mental and Neurological Health in Primary Care* (also known as ICD–10–PHC) does classify postnatal disorders separately (F53), and offers guidance concerning diagnosis and management to primary care health professionals in the UK (World Health Organization, 2004).

# Epidemiology

There are still unanswered questions as to whether there is an increased relative risk of depression within a given time after the birth of a child, what these time limits might be, whether there are any characteristic clinical features that distinguish postnatal depression from any other kind of depression, and whether (aside from the coincidence with childbirth) there are any pathognomonic aetiological factors associated with it. The most recent controversy surrounding postnatal depression concerns the timing of its onset and the question of whether it is an extension of antenatal depression or a totally different entity. Recent studies reveal an equally high or higher level of antenatal depression, and problems with recall bias in retrospective interview-based studies (see Chapter 30 on research in primary care mental health) call into question the supremacy of postnatal depression over antenatal depression in terms of predicting adverse sequelae for mother and child (Evans *et al*, 2001).

The mental health problems seen during pregnancy are for the most part very similar to those seen in the non-pregnant population. Common mental disorders characterised by anxiety and depression in different proportions constitute the vast majority of (new) illnesses. Patients with known psychotic and the rarer neurotic illnesses such as obsessive–compulsive disorder may well relapse. There has been very little research on anxiety disorders (see Chapter 10 on anxiety disorders). The best epidemiological data, from the Avon Longitudinal Study of Parents and Children (ALSPAC), revealed a high prevalence of anxiety symptoms in pregnancy, 14.6% at 18 weeks, falling to 8% at 8 weeks after the birth (Heron *et al*, 2004). A meta-analysis (Gavin *et al*, 2005) has estimated the point prevalence of depression in pregnancy as 3.8% at the end of the first trimester, 4.9% at the end of the second and 3.1% at the end of the third. This contrasts with ALSPAC, which found 13.5% at 32 weeks of pregnancy. This discrepancy may be due to methodological differences: the meta-analysis included only studies in which depression had been diagnosed according to recognised criteria, whereas ALSPAC used self-report questionnaires. However, most people now accept that there are three well-defined disorders in the postpartum period: 'baby blues', the most common of the three, puerperal psychosis and postnatal depression.

## Baby blues

The 'baby blues' affects as many as 50% of women in the first week after childbirth. The condition is characterised by tearfulness and emotional lability. It usually responds to simple reassurance, is self-limiting and is most likely to have a hormonal aetiology (Stein, 1982).

## Puerperal psychosis

In a very few instances, emotional lability after childbirth may herald the onset of a much rarer disorder, puerperal psychosis. This very serious illness affects only 1–2 women per 1000 and has its onset in the first month after the birth (Kendell *et al*, 1987). It is a florid disorder which may manifest with signs of either mania or depression. Alternatively, there may be overt psychotic phenomena, with disordered thinking, paranoia and confusion, and women may even have ideas of harming themselves or the baby. It is likely to have a hormonal aetiology and occurs more often in younger women, primiparae, women with a personal or family history of psychosis and possibly after a Caesarean section.

## Postnatal depression

In terms of severity, postnatal depression sits somewhere between the blues and puerperal psychosis, but from a public health perspective, owing to its high prevalence, it is probably the most important adverse psychological outcome of childbirth. A meta-analysis of 59 studies (with a total of 12 810 women, mainly from high-income countries) found an average prevalence of postnatal depression of 13% (95% confidence interval 12.3–13.4%) (O'Hara & Swan, 1996). This meta-analysis included studies in which the diagnosis was made using validated psychiatric interviews and self-report questionnaires. The prevalence varied depending on the method of assessment, the differing inclusion criteria for the studies and the length of the follow-up. The incidence was highest in the first 3 months postpartum and the peak time of onset was in the first 4–6 weeks. This depression may be the start of a chronic relapsing illness or a relatively short-lived episode never to be repeated. In either case the consequences for the woman herself, both at home and at work, for her partner and the quality of their relationship, and for her family and friends may be irrevocable. Postnatal depression can also have particularly adverse effects on the mother–infant relationship and subsequently on child behaviour and intellectual development (Sharp *et al*, 1995).

There are varying reports of the prevalence of postnatal depression in different ethnic groups (Kumar, 1994). There are studies that show that women are protected in some cultures from postnatal depression while they maintain their sociocultural practices, but others show the same prevalence in very diverse countries. It may be that 'depression' is a Western construct of a disease not culturally recognised in other parts of the world. Women may be at greater risk after immigration, when it is not so easy to maintain their usual rituals around the time of childbirth.

# Prediction

Pregnancy and the postnatal period are times of profound psychological adjustment for women. Mental illness at this time has an impact not only on the mother but on friends, family, partners and the child, possibly both before birth and throughout childhood. Although this mental illness may be no different in terms of phenomenology to that occurring at other times in the woman's life, the regular contact with health professionals offers an unrivalled opportunity for detection and treatment.

## Screening

Until recently, the most frequently debated issue in perinatal mental health concerned the case for or against screening for postnatal depression and the instrument to be used. The final word on this matter was had by the National Screening Committee, which decided that screening for postnatal depression using the Edinburgh Postnatal Depression Scale (EPDS; Cox *et al*, 1987) did not meet its stringent criteria (Shakespeare, 2001). The agenda has now moved on, and guidance from the National Institute for Health and Clinical Excellence (2007) is couched in terms of the prediction (of those at high risk) and detection of these disorders.

When considering whether a disorder is amenable to prediction, there has to be good evidence that the presence of certain risk factors increases the likelihood of that disorder, and the ability of health professionals to ascertain these factors has to be robust. To date, the evidence base is really sufficient only to offer guidance for the prediction of postnatal depression. Puerperal psychosis is too rare to have provided a sufficient body of evidence; and post-partum anxiety has only infrequently been studied, as have disorders during pregnancy.

## Risk factors

Although there are three good reviews of the risk factors for postnatal depression, they are difficult to reconcile, as they have included different studies (Box 13.1).

For puerperal psychosis, there are no good reviews, but high-quality individual studies report the major risk factors to be a history of psychiatric illness, especially bipolar disorder and schizophrenia, as well as a previous episode of puerperal psychosis. There is less good evidence for some psychosocial factors, such as age at delivery, marital status and family history of puerperal mental illness.

In terms of providing health professionals with a tool or tools to use during antenatal healthcare contacts that might have sufficiently good psychometric characteristics to be incorporated into the care pathway, Austin & Lumley (2003) concluded in their review that there was no one instrument that met the necessary criteria. The current recommendations are thus for health professionals to include questions about past and present personal symptoms of mental illness, their severity, as well as any family history of mental illness at the first contact for antenatal care and at an appropriate time soon after the baby is born.

# Detection and diagnosis

Research on the detection of perinatal mental health problems has concentrated on postnatal depression, with many studies reporting the usefulness or otherwise of a wide variety of instruments, both generic and those specifically developed for the puerperium. A review by Boyd *et al* (2005) considered eight self-report scales, including the EPDS. For most scales there were very few studies, with only the EPDS being the subject of a sufficient number to draw robust conclusions, which were that, despite its high sensitivity, its low specificity and thus poor positive predictive value meant it could not be recommended for routine use. It should be noted that the Patient Health Questionnaire (PHQ-9) (Spitzer *et al*, 1999), a scale currently favoured by many UK general practitioners (GPs) when

---

**Box 13.1** Risk factors for postnatal depression

- Depression during pregnancy
- Anxiety during pregnancy
- Poor social support
- Adverse life events
- Past history of depression
- Past history of anxiety

measuring the severity of depression prior to treatment (see Chapter 8), was not included in this review.

An alternative to self-report questionnaires is the use of case-finding with 'interview questions'. There is now reasonable evidence, in terms of sensitivity and specificity, from general populations, to support the use of a two-question screen which asks about recent low mood and about recent loss of pleasure (Whoolley et al, 1997). The addition of a third question (Arroll et al, 2005), 'Do you need help?', improves the specificity (see Chapter 8 for more detail of the questions). Despite the lack of any research evidence in the perinatal period, these questions are now recommended for use by health professionals early in pregnancy and after the birth in order to facilitate the detection of depression (National Institute for Health and Clinical Excellence, 2007). Self-report questionnaires such as the EPDS or PHQ-9 can be used as a follow-up with those who respond positively on the two- or three-question screen.

# Principles of management

Early detection and possible prevention have been dealt with in the previous section. The imperative for such action is the potential for reducing harm, both to the mother and to the infant, by timely intervention. In line with other common mental disorders in the primary care setting, a significant proportion of perinatal mental illness goes undetected. In the case of postnatal illness, there is often reluctance on the part of mothers to disclose symptoms, in order to reduce the possibility of statutory involvement in the care of the baby. Pregnant and postnatal women need care from health professionals who have developed good communication skills, to reduce the possibility of non-disclosure. Once a diagnosis has been made, the full involvement of the woman (and her partner or family where appropriate) is mandatory. Only when a woman is suffering from psychotic illness and requires compulsory admission should her views be secondary.

The principles of management are similar to those for depression in a non-perinatal population (see Chapter 8). However, when considering the risk–benefit ratio of treatment, the needs of the fetus or child also need to be taken into account. Discussion of treatment needs to be based on clear, up-to-date and comprehensible information, with written documents available in languages relevant to the local population. Sufficient time to make decisions about treatment and reassurance that decisions are not irrevocable (that is, if one approach does not work, then another can be substituted or added) are important aspects of consultations.

## Psychological approaches to prevention and treatment

Despite evidence that anxiety disorders and depression are common in pregnancy, most research has focused on evaluating treatments for depression in the postnatal period. The treatments that have been evaluated include various types of psychotherapy, for example cognitive–behavioural therapy (CBT) and interpersonal psychotherapy (IPT), counselling, and other (less well-defined) psychosocial interventions, such as social support. Some studies have focused on the prevention the development of mental health problems and others on the treatment of actual disorder; both have separately considered women with risk factors and those without.

## Prevention

For women with risk factors, for whom the potential benefits of screening may be substantial, although the timing of treatment and the therapeutic approach employed vary by study, it seems that treatment, especially for those women with subthreshold symptoms in the postnatal period, is beneficial. Social support interventions, either individual or group based, for women who have not had a previous episode of anxiety or depression and structured psychological short-term treatments, CBT or IPT, when they have a previous history, are recommended (Dennis & Hodnett, 2007).

For those women who have no identifiable risk factors, a review of 16 studies using a variety of psychological therapies in both the antenatal and the postnatal period to prevent the development of postnatal depression concluded that there was no one treatment that could be recommended (National Institute for Health and Clinical Excellence, 2007).

## Treatment

There is more evidence when it comes to looking at the actual treatment of postnatal depression. The types of studies that have been undertaken comprise those where a psychological treatment has been compared with standard care or a waiting-list control, and those where two treatments have been compared. With regard to the former, CBT, IPT, psychodynamic psychotherapy and non-directive counselling (see Chapter 26) all show an effect (National Institute for Health and Clinical Excellence, 2007; Box 13.2).

The healthcare professionals best placed to detect postnatal depression and to offer psychological support are health visitors, since they are in

---

**Box 13.2** Psychosocial treatments for postnatal depression

- Six sessions of counselling are more effective than one.
- Individual counselling is more effective than counselling in a group.
- Exercise may also be effective.
- Group exercise is superior to social support.
- Interpersonal therapy (IPT) appears more effective than psycho-education.
- Psycho-education with a partner is more effective than for the woman alone.

Source: National Institute for Health and Clinical Excellence (2007).

---

regular contact with women throughout the first postnatal year. The detection of postnatal depression by health visitors was first studied in the mid-1980s (Briscoe, 1986) and the first controlled trial of counselling by health visitors for women with postnatal depression in general practice took place in the early 1990s (Gerrard et al, 1993). A trial of eight weekly non-directive counselling sessions provided by trained health visitors demonstrated improvements in depressive symptoms. After 3 months, 18 of the 26 women in the treatment group (69%) had fully recovered, compared with nine (38%) of the 24 in the control group (Holden et al, 1989). Non-directive counselling has been widely taken up by health visitors and is the intervention most likely to be routinely implementable in the service setting.

In addition to developing the evidence base for treating maternal depression, another therapeutic focus has been the mother–infant relationship, with the hope that improving this interaction might improve maternal symptoms and thus reduce any adverse effect on the infant's development. Six studies have each used a different intervention, so there are no overall conclusions as to which elements of the mother–infant interaction are most amenable to change. In general, these interventions did have some impact on the mother–child relationship, but it is not clear if this was mediated by an improvement in maternal mental symptoms (National Institute for Health and Clinical Excellence, 2007).

## Pharmacological approaches

The main alternative to psychological therapies is, as is the case in the non-pregnant and postpartum population, a pharmacological approach. Psychotropic medication may be required for ongoing treatment of a disorder, especially at the more severe end of the spectrum, such as bipolar disease or schizophrenia, or the treatment for a new disorder, such as psychosis or depression.

### Risks

During pregnancy and when breastfeeding, the potential risks to the developing fetus must be balanced against the benefits to the mother. It should not be assumed that avoiding medication is always to be preferred, as poorer obstetric outcomes are associated with depressive illness (Misri & Kostaras, 2002; Bonari et al, 2004) and in the case of schizophrenia and bipolar illness there is an increased risk of suicide (Jablensky et al, 2005). Furthermore, there is some evidence of poorer long-term outcomes for the developing infant associated with mental illness during pregnancy (Nulman et al, 2002). Of overriding importance in any of these situations is that, as far as is possible, the responsible clinician supports the woman and her family in making the best decision.

Assessing the data on risk during pregnancy and breastfeeding is hindered by the difficulty in attributing causal effect to a drug in the presence of a relatively high background rate of congenital abnormalities, as well as the difficulty of undertaking controlled trials and thus the relative paucity of data, especially relating to new drugs. The conclusions that can be drawn are that in pregnancy paroxetine is not advised, fluoxetine is the safest drug and tricyclic antidepressants have fewer risks than the selective serotonin reuptake inhibitors but have a higher fatal toxicity index (Box 13.3).

With regard to breastfeeding, citalopram and fluoxetine are present at relatively high levels in breast milk, while imipramine, nortriptyline and sertraline are present at relatively low levels. Benzodiazepines should not be prescribed in pregnancy except for the short-term treatment of severe anxiety or agitation. Antipsychotics may affect a woman's ability to conceive. Clozapine is associated with agranulocytosis in the fetus or infant (if breast-fed), olanzapine is associated with gestational diabetes and depot medications may result in extrapyramidal side-effects in the infant.

Overall, there is clearly a quantifiable risk to taking certain psychotropic medications in all women of childbearing age, particularly as some groups of women, despite being on drugs associated with these risks such as valproate and lithium, may not be using adequate contraception. For pregnant and breastfeeding women, previous response to treatment should help guide future treatment, the lowest effective dose of the safest drug should be used, and psychological therapies may be more appropriate, at least in the short term. In all cases, it is important to discuss the risks and benefits to mother and child at an individual level so that any decision is safe, informed and personalised,

---

**Box 13.3** Principles of antidepressant treatment for postnatal depression

- Fluoxetine is the selective serotonin reuptake inhibitor (SSRI) with the lowest known risk during pregnancy.
- Tricyclic antidepressants have lower known risks during pregnancy than other antidepressants.
- Imipramine, nortriptyline and sertraline are present in breast milk at relatively low levels.
- SSRIs taken after 20 weeks' gestation may be associated with an increased risk of persistent pulmonary hypertension in the neonate.
- Paroxetine taken in the first trimester may be associated with fetal heart defects.
- Venlafaxine may be associated with increased risk of high blood pressure at high doses, higher toxicity in overdose than SSRIs and some tricyclic antidepressants, and increased difficulty in withdrawal.
- All antidepressants carry the risk of withdrawal or toxicity in neonates; in most cases the effects are mild and self-limiting.

Source: National Institute for Health and Clinical Excellence (2007).

## Drug treatment of postnatal depression

The lack of specific trials of psychotropic drugs in pregnant and postnatal women means that to some extent extrapolation from more general samples is required, while recognising that women's physical and psychological state may influence their attitude and thus adherence to medication, as well as their physiological response. There are surprisingly few good trials of antidepressants for postnatal depression. Fluoxetine has been most studied (with counselling), with some evidence for efficacy (Appleby et al, 1997). A Cochrane review concluded that there was insufficient evidence and that more trials were needed to investigate the effectiveness of antidepressants and their place in treatment of postnatal depression, particularly in breastfeeding women (Hoffbrand et al, 2001). In searching for evidence to support a hormonal aetiology for postnatal depression, one trial found some evidence in favour of oestrogen treatment compared with placebo (Gregoire et al, 1996).

## Pharmacological prophylaxis of severe mental disorder

There have been studies of the use of psychotropic drugs in populations with a diagnosis of bipolar disorder, schizoaffective disorder and depression. There is some evidence, although of low quality, that prophylactic medication can reduce the risk of relapse in the postnatal period. The same holds true for women with a history of depression who are prescribed an antidepressant in the early postnatal period to prevent relapse (Howard et al, 2005).

## Conclusion

To summarise, the risk–benefit ratio to both mother and fetus or child must be considered before a drug is withdrawn or a new one begun. Substituting a drug being prescribed for mild or moderate depression with a self-help approach (c-CBT, exercise) or a brief psychological treatment (counselling, CBT, IPT) can, with careful monitoring, reduce the risks. In the case of severe depression, changing to a safer drug is recommended.

# Organisation of care

A GP in the UK with an average list size of 1800 patients can expect somewhere between 15 and 27 births a year. The National Service Framework for Mental Health (Department of Health, 1999) identified very specific actions for pregnant and postnatal women in the primary care setting. Between 8% and 15% of women will experience some form of common mental disorder associated with their pregnancy, most of whom will receive all their care in primary care and very few (less than 2%) will be referred to specialist mental health services or be admitted (National Institute for Health and Clinical Excellence, 2007).

Women developing a first onset or new episode of a psychotic disorder (about 2 in a 1000 births) will usually require admission to a specialist mother and baby unit, not only for their own care but also for the safety and care of the baby. This very rare occurrence makes planning services rather difficult, as providing a local resource is not usually cost-effective. This has led in some cases to the provision of very intensive outreach services, whereby the woman and her baby are cared for round the clock at home (Royal College of Psychiatrists, 2000).

The vast majority of women with a mild-to-moderate disorder that presents during pregnancy or the postnatal period must rely on the observational and diagnostic skills of their midwife, health visitor and GP. Hospital staff, including obstetricians and paediatricians, also need to be aware of the prevalence and presentations of these disorders. Communication between primary and secondary care teams for the optimum care of these women and their families is critical. As the provision of mental health services in general has become the responsibility of primary care trusts and their provider units, the skills of community-based psychologists, counsellors and primary care mental health workers can all be called into play. Understanding the local care pathways, especially for those women needing referral to specialist mental health services, is a prerequisite for the training of all staff involved in the care of pregnant and postnatal women.

A stepped-care approach for perinatal mental illness is now favoured, as for most other common mental disorders (see Chapter 27), and, depending on the precise structure of services, a managed clinical network model is proposed (National Institute for Health and Clinical Excellence, 2007). With an identified manager, a clear mission statement and a system that has an inclusive approach, the benefits should be effective and cost-effective care for women and their families across the range of morbidity.

---

**Key points**

- Perinatal mental health covers pregnancy and the first postnatal year.
- Treating perinatal mental disorders should take into account the needs of both mother and baby (fetus).
- There are three main postnatal disorders: the baby blues, puerperal psychosis and postnatal depression.
- Screening all women for postnatal depression is not recommended; identifying women at high risk is.
- A variety of psychological approaches, similar to those used to treat non-perinatal common mental disorders, are effective in both pregnancy and the postnatal year.
- Pharmacological approaches need careful consideration of the risk–benefit ratio for mother and baby (fetus).
- Perinatal mental health is mainly the responsibility of the primary care team but effective liaison with specialist services to deliver stepped care is required for women with more severe illnesses.

# Further reading and e-resources

National Institute for Health and Clinical Excellence (2006) *Postnatal Care: Routine Postnatal Care of Women and Their Babies*. NICE. Downloadable from http://www.nice.org.uk

National Institute for Health and Clinical Excellence (2007) *Antenatal and Postnatal Mental Health*. British Psychological Society and Gaskell.

World Health Organization (2004) *Guide to Mental and Neurological Health in Primary Care: A Guide to Mental and Neurological Ill Health in Adults and Children and Adolescents* (2nd edn). RSM Press. Downloadable from http://www.mentalneurologicalprimarycare.org

# References

American Psychiatric Association (1994) *Diagnostic and Statistical Manual of Mental Disorders* (4th edn) (DSM–IV). APA.

Appleby, L., Warner, R., Whitton, A., *et al* (1997) A controlled study of fluoxetine and cognitive–behavioural counselling in the treatment of postnatal depression. *BMJ*, **314**, 932–936.

Arroll, B., Goodyear-Smith, F., Kerse, N., *et al* (2005) Effect of the addition of a 'help' question to two screening questions on specificity for diagnosis of depression in general practice: diagnostic validity study. *BMJ*, **331**, 884.

Austin, P. & Lumley, J. (2003) Antenatal screening for postnatal depression: a systematic review. *Acta Psychiatrica Scandinavica*, **107**, 10–17.

Bonari, L., Pinto, N., Ahn, E., *et al* (2004) Perinatal risks of untreated depression during pregnancy. *Canadian Journal of Psychiatry*, **49**, 726–735.

Boyd, R. C., Le, H. N. & Somberg, R. (2005) Review of screening instruments for postpartum depression. *Archives of Women's Mental Health*, **8**, 141–153.

Briscoe, M. (1986) Identification of emotional problems in postpartum women by health visitors. *BMJ*, **292**, 932–936.

Confidential Enquiry into Maternal and Child Health (2004) *Why Mothers Die: Report on Confidential Enquiries into Maternal Deaths in the UK 2000 to 2002*. RCOG Press.

Cooper P. J. & Murray, L. (1998) Postnatal depression. *BMJ*, **316**, 1884–1886.

Cox, J. L., Holden, J. M. & Sagovsky, R. (1987) Detection of postnatal depression: development of the ten-item Edinburgh Postnatal Depression Scale. *British Journal of Psychiatry*, **150**, 782–786.

Dennis, C.-L. & Hodnett, E. (2007) Psychosocial and psychological interventions for treating postpartum depression. *Cochrane Database of Systematic Reviews*, (**4**), CD006116.

Department of Health (1999) *National Service Framework for Mental Health: Modern Standards and Service Models*. HMSO.

Evans, J., Heron, J., Francomb, H., *et al* (2001) Cohort study of depressed mood during pregnancy and after childbirth. *BMJ*, **323**, 257–260.

Gavin, N., Gaynes, B., Lohr, K., *et al* (2005) Perinatal depression: a systematic review of prevalence and incidence. *Obstetrics and Gynaecology*, **106**, 1071–1083.

Gerrard, J., Holden, J., Elliott, S., *et al* (1993) A trainer's perspective of an innovative programme teaching health visitors about the detection, treatment and prevention of postnatal depression. *Journal of Advanced Nursing*, **18**, 1825–1832.

Gregoire, A., Kumar, R., Everitt, B., *et al* (1996) Transdermal oestrogen for treatment of severe postnatal depression. *Lancet*, **347**, 918–919.

Heron, J., O'Connor, T., Evans, J., *et al* (2004) The course of anxiety and depression through pregnancy and the postpartum in a community sample. *Journal of Affective Disorder*, **80**, 65–73.

Hoffbrand, S., Howard, L. & Crawley, H. (2001) Antidepressant treatment for post-natal depression. *Cochrane Database of Systematic Reviews*, (**2**), CD002018.

Holden, J., Sagovsky, R. & Cox, J. (1989) Counselling in a general practice setting: a controlled study of health visitor intervention in the treatment of postnatal depression. *BMJ*, **298**, 223–226.

Howard, L. M., Hoffbrand, S., Henshaw, C., *et al* (2005) Antidepressant prevention of postnatal depression. *Cochrane Database of Systematic Reviews*, (**2**), CD004363.

Jablensky, A., Morgan,V., Zubrick, S., *et al* (2005) Pregnancy, delivery and neonatal complications in a population cohort of women with schizophrenia and major affective disorders. *American Journal of Psychiatry*, **162**, 79–91.

Kendell, R., Chalmers, J. C. & Platz, C. (1987) Epidemiology of puerperal psychoses. *British Journal of Psychiatry*, **150**, 662–673.

Kumar, R. (1994) Postnatal mental illness: a transcultural perspective. *Social Psychiatry and Psychiatric Epidemiology*, **29**, 250–264.

Misri, S. & Kostaras, X. (2002) Benefits and risks to mother and infant of drug treatment for postnatal depression. *Drug Safety*, **25**, 903–911.

National Institute for Health and Clinical Excellence (2007) *Antenatal and Postnatal Mental Health*. British Psychological Society and Gaskell.

Nulman, I., Rovet, J., Stewart, D., *et al* (2002) Child development following exposure to tricyclic antidepressants or fluoxetine throughout fetal life: a prospective controlled study. *American Journal of Psychiatry*, **159**, 1889–1895.

O'Connor, T. G., Heron, J. & Glover, V. (2002) Antenatal anxiety predicts child behavioural/emotional problems independently of postnatal depression. *Journal of the American Academy of Child and Adolescent Psychiatry*, **41**, 1470–1477.

O'Hara, M. W. & Swan, A. M. (1996) Rates and risk of postpartum depression – a meta-analysis. *International Review of Psychiatry*, **8**, 37–54.

O'Keane, V. (2006) Mood disorder during pregnancy: aetiology and management. In *Psychiatric Disorders and Pregnancy* (eds V. O'Keane, M. Marsh, G. Seneviratne, *et al*), pp. 69–105. Taylor & Francis.

Royal College of Psychiatrists (2000) *Perinatal Maternal Mental Health Services*. Council report CR88. Royal College of Psychiatrists.

Shakespeare, J. (2001) *Evaluation of Screening Instruments for Postnatal Depression Against the National Screening Committee Handbook Criteria*. National Screening Committee.

Sharp, D., Hay, D. F., Pawlby, S., *et al* (1995) The impact of postnatal depression on boys' intellectual development. *Journal of Child Psychology and Psychiatry*, **36**, 1315–1336.

Spitzer, R. L., Kroenke, K. & Williams, J. (1999) Validation and utility of a self report version of PRIME-MD: the PHQ primary care study. Primary care evaluation of mental disorders, Patient Health Questionnaire. *JAMA*, **282**, 1737–1744.

Stein, G. (1982) The maternity blues. In *Motherhood and Mental Illness* (eds I. F. Brockington & R. Kumar), pp. 119–154. Academic Press.

Whoolley, M., Avins, A., Miranda, J., *et al* (1997) Case finding instruments for depression. Two questions are as good as many. *Journal of General Internal Medicine*, **12**, 439–445.

World Health Organization (1992) *International Classification of Diseases* (10th revision) (ICD–10). WHO.

World Health Organization (2004) *Guide to Mental and Neurological Health in Primary Care: A Guide to Mental and Neurological Ill Health in Adults and Children and Adolescents* (2nd edn). RSM Press.

# CHAPTER 14

# Child and adolescent mental health

Tami Kramer and Elena Garralda

Summary

Epidemiological evidence shows that although most children and adolescents present to primary care with physical symptoms, many will have concurrent psychiatric difficulties or disorders, particularly anxiety and depression. Currently, limited intervention takes place within primary care. Evidence on interventions that could be implemented is reviewed. Specialist child and adolescent mental health services are scarce and unable to meet need. Ways to improve capacity within primary care to address unmet need are discussed, although the evidence base to support these in this context is underdeveloped. The chapter discusses the role of primary care in the identification and management of disorder, referral to specialist services and promotion of mental health. It also describes the varied service structure of primary healthcare across countries and the implications for service provision.

Epidemiological research has shown that mental health problems and psychiatric disorder are common in childhood and adolescence. They are associated with suffering and impairment, and continue into adult life. Even in countries where specialist child and adolescent mental health services have been developed, access remains a problem owing to scarcity of resources. As evidence for the effectiveness of some interventions accumulates, the role of primary healthcare in child and adolescent mental health is evolving.

## Common presentations and epidemiology

Many children and adolescents, particularly in higher-income countries, have regular contact with primary healthcare services. Within the UK, over 90% of pre-school children and about two-thirds of 5- to 14-year-olds will consult primary care at least once a year (Office of Population

Censuses and Surveys, 1995). Over 50% of 13- to 17-year-olds registered with a large London inner-city practice attended in 1 year (Kramer *et al*, 1997) and comparable results are reported in other countries (Veit *et al*, 1995; Frankenfield *et al*, 2000). When primary care services are already in contact with young people, there is a clear opportunity for such services to be involved in addressing mental health.

Surveys across countries have documented that the majority of children and adolescents present to primary care with overtly physical complaints. Only 2–10% of those attending present primarily for psychological problems, for example anxiety, behavioural problems, overactivity, educational or social problems (Jacobson *et al* 1980; Starfield *et al*, 1980; Garralda & Bailey, 1986, 1989; Kramer & Garralda, 1998). Despite low levels of emotional or behavioural presentations in attenders, research interviews have demonstrated psychiatric disorders in one-tenth to one-quarter (Giel *et al*, 1981; Garralda & Bailey, 1986; Costello *et al*, 1988; Gureje *et al*, 1994), with higher rates in adolescents (40%) (Kramer & Garralda, 1998) and in schoolchildren attending hospital paediatric out-patient departments (28%) (Garralda & Bailey, 1989). In contrast to population surveys, emotional disorders predominate over conduct disorders (Garralda & Bailey, 1986: Kramer & Garralda, 1998), suggesting a specific role for primary care in identifying and managing anxiety and depressive disorders. The relatively increased rates of psychiatric disorders in attenders in relation to community surveys, in conjunction with increased primary care use among those with a disorder (Offord *et al*, 1987; Monck *et al*, 1994; Lavigne *et al*, 1998), suggest that the presence of psychiatric disorder increases the likelihood of attendance with somatic complaints.

# The role of psychosomatic symptoms

A proportion of young people present with recurrent unexplained functional physical symptoms (e.g. abdominal pains, vague aches and pains, fatigue). These may be an expression of the somatisation of distress and are often seen in conjunction with psychiatric disorders. Campo *et al* (1999) reported frequent complaints of aches and pains with no organic diagnosis in 2% of 11- to 15-year-old paediatric primary care attenders, and occasional complaints in 11%, with a ratio of two girls to one boy. In about half the children – significantly more than in children attending with other complaints – doctors and parents identified psychosocial problems and impairment caused by the symptom, and about a third were described as frequent users of health services. In 8- to 15-year-olds with recurrent abdominal pain attending primary care, Campo *et al* (2004) identified a comorbid anxiety disorder in as many as 79% and a depressive disorder in 43%, as well an excess of temperamental harm avoidance and functional impairment. The close links between emotional and functional physical symptoms in children is further supported by indications that parental anxiety in the first year of the child's life, as well as irregular feeding and sleeping habits, can predict recurrent abdominal pains in childhood (Ramchandani *et al*, 2006).

### A case of unexplained physical symptoms

An 8-year-old girl has repeated presentations to general practice with recurrent abdominal pains (RAP); there are no indications from the history that there is a likely medical cause for her symptoms. It would be helpful for the doctor to conduct a full physical examination, to confirm the lack of evidence suggestive of a medical disorder. The doctor might ask whether the family is concerned about any particular disorder and reasons for this.

The doctor might then explain that there is nothing in the history or physical examination suggestive of a medical disorder (and might list the most common ones, along with the reasons why they are unlikely to be present). This helps the child and family see that the symptom has been taken seriously. The doctor can explain: that recurrent 'functional' abdominal pains are common in the general population (about one in ten children) and are often associated with other 'functional' symptoms such as headaches or tiredness; that children who suffer from RAP are more sensitive to abdominal bodily sensations and discomfort than other children; and that there is evidence that situations of stress particularly bring on discomfort and pain in these children. This tends to run in families, and may reflect family susceptibility

Many children with RAP are sensitive to stress generally, are prone to worry and often experience feelings of anxiety. It is therefore important to find out whether there are any particular stresses in the child's life at present (most commonly worry about school, exams, teacher or friends, or about stresses at home) and see whether the stress can be relieved in some way. Many children also experience anxiety disorders and their identification and treatment can help substantially. On the whole, it is helpful for parents not to show their concern about the physical symptom to the child, and for them to encourage coping through distraction and the child's involvement in everyday activities (as opposed to withdrawal from these).

A further important group of children presenting with physical complaints are those in whom psychosocial problems and psychiatric disorders adversely affect their physical health. When doctors are asked to note any physical presentation with associated or contributing psychological factors, for example asthma exacerbated by stress, such presentations are recorded for about a fifth of schoolchildren attending primary care and for as many as half in out-patient paediatric clinics, indicating a high degree of sensitivity and vigilance by many clinicians to these issues (Bailey *et al*, 1978; Garralda & Bailey, 1987, 1990). Presenting symptoms in these cases tend to be those regarded traditionally as having psychosomatic components (e.g. aches and pains, incontinence, asthma and blackouts), although virtually all physical complaints are featured. These children have an excess of emotional and behavioural symptoms, including mood changes and relationship problems. However, most do not have a psychiatric disorder. For such children, the mother's stress over parenting and concerns over schooling have particularly been noted in primary care settings, suggesting a need for the primary care practitioner to address family stress as part of a holistic intervention.

Primary care professionals could maximise the effect of their contact with children and adolescents if they were alert to emotional and behavioural difficulties and recognised the links with physical presentation (Box 14.1).

# Diagnosis

Rates of recognition of psychiatric disorder within primary care have been shown to be poor (Costello & Eddelbrock, 1985; Garralda & Bailey 1986; Chang *et al*, 1988; Kramer & Garralda, 1998; Glazebrook *et al*, 2003; Sayal & Taylor, 2004), with poor sensitivity but high specificity (Brugman *et al*, 2001). Most affected children fail to receive any mental health services (Burns *et al*, 1995; Verhulst & van der Ende, 1997; Rushton *et al*, 2002). Recognition has been linked to severity of disorders, age (recognition is best with 7- to 14-year-olds), male gender, presence of social difficulties (being on welfare, broken home), presenting symptoms (chronic conditions, digestive problems and ill-defined problems), type of consultation (well child clinics rather than acute care visits), clinician relationship with the child and parental perception of difficulty (Goldberg *et al*, 1984; Horwitz *et al*, 1992; Kramer & Garralda, 1998; Martinez, 2006) (Box 14.2).

---

**Box 14.1** Recognising emotional and behavioural problems

The primary care physician should be especially alert in the following presentations, which can all be deemed warning signs of the presence of emotional and behavioural problems in a child presenting with a physical condition:

- children with chronic paediatric problems (such as asthma) where symptoms seem to be reactive to family or school stresses
- children who appear anxious, dejected or withdrawn at the surgery
- children whose parents report the child's reluctance to attend school
- children with hyperactive, oppositional behaviour
- children whose parents appear especially concerned about their children
- children with frequent primary care visits or known family stress.

The primary care physician should, in such presentations:

- consider seeing adolescents alone
- ask parents about any stress with regard to parenting their children
- use a transitional question to shift the focus of the consultation from the physical to the emotional or behavioural (e.g. 'Other than John's asthma, how has he been getting on?')
- ask one or two general questions about adjustment at home and school (e.g. 'Any worries about his behaviour, development or school progress?').

If the parents or child do have any concerns, the primary care physician should clarify the nature of any symptoms and the impact on function (e.g. 'How long has John been displaying difficult and defiant behaviour? How is this affecting life at home and progress at school?').

---

> **Box 14.2** Factors found to be associated with identification by primary care doctors of psychological problems in children
>
> - Age (recognition is highest in 7- to 14-year-olds)
> - Male gender
> - Social difficulties (such as being on welfare, broken home)
> - Presenting symptoms (chronic conditions, digestive problems ill-defined problems)
> - Type of consultation (well child clinics rather than acute care visits)
> - Severity of disorder
> - Clinician relationship with the child
> - Parental perception of difficulty
> - Parental expression of concern

Sayal & Taylor (2004) demonstrated that parental expression of concern during consultation increased the sensitivity of doctor recognition of mental health problems. In children of 11–39 months, Ellingson et al (2004) demonstrated that parental discussion with the primary care provider was associated with parental worry, perceived low socio-emotional competence in the child, and disruption to family routines. Even though many parents believe it is appropriate to express concerns about child behaviour to a primary care provider, few parents who have concerns do so (Dulcan et al, 1990; Horwitz et al, 1998; Ellingson et al, 2004; Sayal & Taylor, 2004). Similarly, many adolescents are reluctant to raise emotional difficulties even when aware of these (Martinez, 2006). Thus, education that enables young people and parents to identify their own or their children's needs, express these within the consultation and understand the potential for intervention is an important first step in promoting identification within the primary care setting. Such education should alert parents and young people to the nature and consequences of common disorders, and the potential for effective early intervention; it should point out specifically the role of primary care in accessing help (Table 14.1).

The use of screening questionnaires has been considered as a potentially quick and easy method to improve the identification in primary care of mental health conditions, for a wide range of ages (Borowsky et al, 2003; Briggs-Gowan et al, 2004; Luby et al, 2004) (see Box 14.3 for examples). However, questionnaires alone are likely to indicate too many children requiring further assessment and may be best used as guide to when psychological, behavioural and psychosocial routes of enquiry should be followed.

## Management

The role of primary care in managing child and adolescent mental health has been highlighted in relation to the significant numbers of children and adolescents presenting with physical complaints but who have concurrent

**Table 14.1** Educating parents and young people

| Topics | Methods |
| --- | --- |
| Postnatal depression and early behaviour problems (e.g. sleep difficulties, feeding difficulties, overactivity) | Posters, leaflets, liaison with health visitors, discussion within the consultation, broader public health campaigns: highlight the signs and point out that these are common problems and amenable to intervention following early identification |
| Childhood headaches and tummy aches | See case example in text (p. 216) |
| Adolescent depression | Leaflets, discussion within consultation: highlight signs and indicators of severity, point out that depression is common in adolescence and usually resolves, and that help is available (with ideas for self-help in milder cases – see Box 14.4) |
| Adolescent health-risk behaviours (smoking, drinking, substance use, sex) | Leaflets, screening questions for young people at risk – 'Do you smoke', 'Have you ever tried alcohol (how much, how often?), cannabis (how often?), or any other drugs?', 'Are you worried about your drinking of alcohol or taking drugs?', 'Would you like some help with this?' (If so, introduce to the team's substance misuse service worker) |
| The role of primary care in accessing help | This should be publicised, so that parents and young people understand that emotional and behavioural difficulties are the concern of primary care practitioners and are amenable to help |

---

**Box 14.3** Screening questionnaires

For pre-school behaviour difficulties:

- Early Years Behavioural Checklist (Barnes & Richman, 2003) (suitable for nurseries and teachers)

For childhood and adolescent emotional/behavioural difficulties:

- Strengths and Difficulties Questionnaire (SDQ; Goodman, 1997)

For childhood/adolescent depression and anxiety:

- Hospital Anxiety and Depression Scale (White *et al*, 1999)
- Moods and Feelings Questionnaire (MFQ; Angold *et al*, 1987)
- Children's Depression Inventory (CDI; Kovacs, 1992)

For adolescent health risks see screening questions in Table 14.1

---

emotional difficulties. Even where child mental health services are well developed, only a small proportion of young people with a psychiatric disorder currently access these services (Rushton *et al*, 2002) and specialist mental health services are already often working to capacity, with long waiting lists for treatment (US Public Health Service, 2000). Primary care is viewed by service users as more accessible and less stigmatising than mental health services, and primary care practitioners have the advantage of knowing young people and their families over time.

Potentially, the role of primary care clinicians (Box 14.4), following the identification of mental health conditions in young people, would include delivery of simple treatments – including psycho-education, supportive

---

**Box 14.4** Core activities in primary care

**Preschool behaviour problems**

Community-based group parenting programmes addressing child behavioural difficulties have been shown to improve parenting practices, parent–child interactions and child behaviour (Webster Stratton *et al*, 1989, 2001; Scott *et al*, 2001; Sonuga-Barke *et al*, 2001; Turner & Sanders, 2006). Implementation by health visitors or primary mental health workers within the primary care setting could improve access for parents and contribute to prevention of more serious behaviour problems in older children, which are more costly to manage.

**Recurrent somatic complaints in school-age children**

Children seen in specialist paediatric services with recurrent abdominal pains are helped by family cognitive–behavioural therapy involving:

- discussion of investigations, rationale for pain management
- self-monitoring of pain
- reinforcement of 'well behaviour' (and reduced attention to symptoms), promotion of distracting activities, ignoring non-verbal pain behaviours, avoidance of modelling the sick role and discrimination of serious symptoms
- coping skills (e.g. relaxation, positive self-talk, distraction, positive imagery skills)
- problem-solving for future pain
- encouragement to participate in routine activities.

These principles should also be of help in the primary care setting.

**Mild to moderate depression in adolescents**

Brief intervention by general practitioners for mild to moderate depression within the ordinary consultation should include psycho-education (that depression is common in adolescents, typical features and impairments, likely resolution, need to get help if persistent or worsens), promotion of self-help, and advice about coping strategies such as finding someone to confide in, gradually increasing activity and reflecting positively on any efforts made (Gledhill *et al*, 2003). For some cases this could be coupled with brief cognitive–behavioural therapy or psychological support delivered by a practice nurse or primary care mental health worker. Such approaches will contribute to the alleviation of suffering and may prevent future episodes and impairment. Adolescents with more severe or persistent symptoms, including those with suicidal impulses or severe impairment of functioning or relationships, should be referred for specialist assessment.

counselling, brief cognitive–behavioural therapy and psychotropic medication (Box 14.5) – parenting support, support for those with chronic conditions, referral of severe and complex cases, and mental health promotion and prevention (Table 14.2).

However, studies of the current contribution of primary care mental health are limited in number and of variable quality. Wren *et al* (2005) documented the practice of 395 primary care clinicians in consultation with 20 861 consecutive attenders aged 4–15 years in the USA, Puerto Rico and Canada. Children identified as having a mood or anxiety syndrome were no more likely to be counselled than those with other psychosocial problems and – unless that condition was accompanied by a comorbid behavioural syndrome – they were offered fewer follow-up appointments. Rates of antidepressant or anti-anxiety prescribing were higher for the mood/anxiety groups but uncommon (6.7%), and they were more likely to be referred to mental health services. Thus, even when identified, active management by primary care was uncommon. This may reflect

---

**Box 14.5** Medication issues

**Use of antidepressants for adolescent depression**

Although there is evidence that fluoxetine, a selective serotonin reuptake inhibitor (SSRI), is efficacious in the treatment of depression in adolescents, it is also apparent that in a minority of adolescents the use of SSRIs is associated with agitation and an increase in suicidal symptoms. This has led to recommendations that psychological therapies be used as first-line treatments (the evidence supports efficacy of cognitive–behavioural treatments in mild to moderate depression), and that fluoxetine be used as a second-line treatment. It would follow that SSRIs should not be started as a matter of course in primary care, but rather following consultation with child psychiatrists.

**Use of medication for children with hyperkinetic syndrome or attention deficit hyperactivity disorder (ADHD)**

There is good research evidence for the efficacy of medication such as methylphenidate or dexamphetamine in hyperkinetic syndrome or ADHD. However, concerns have been expressed about its use, given that treatment is often continued throughout childhood and adolescence. The institution of medical treatment is therefore best carried out in specialist clinics, after a careful diagnostic work-up, where other (behavioural) treatments are also available as alternatives to or complementary to the use of medication, and with regular follow-up to assess whether continuation of treatment is required. Some parents disagree with the notion of using medication for a disorder with behavioural manifestations, and it is important to discuss with them fully their concerns and to offer alternatives (e.g. behavioural attention training exercises, where available). Against this concern is the fact that hyperkinetic syndrome is associated with biological and cognitive anomalies and that the use of medication can greatly improve a child's performance and adjustment.

**Table 14.2** Range of primary care interventions

| Interventions | Practical examples |
|---|---|
| Mental health promotion | Home visiting by health visitors or community nurses for vulnerable mothers; well child visits (include discussion of behaviour, nutrition, child safety, etc.); postnatal screening for depression |
| Psycho-education | Applicable in adolescent depression, anxiety, medically unexplained physical symptoms |
| Supportive counselling | For mild depression, adjustment to stress (e.g. exams) or bereavement |
| Brief cognitive/behavioural therapy | Applicable in adolescent depression, anxiety, medically unexplained physical symptoms |
| Psychotropic medication | Shared care in ADHD, psychoses |
| Parenting support | Behaviour difficulties, ADHD |
| Support for those with chronic conditions and referred severe complex cases | Psychosis or suspected psychosis, severe depression, eating disorders, emotional or behavioural difficulties in the context of serious family difficulties or breakdown, autistic spectrum disorders with comorbid psychiatric disorders |

primary care clinicians feeling more responsible for recognising than for treating child and adolescent depression. In another survey (Olson *et al*, 2001) rates of intervention were higher: respondents reported providing brief interventions to almost 80% of young people with depression and prescribing medication to approximately 20%, and they also reported referring a similar proportion to mental health professionals. However, the low response rate suggested that this may have been a biased sample. Few paediatricians and family physicians routinely screen adolescent patients for suicide risk (Frankenfield *et al*, 2000) and while a 1-day training course for general practitioners (GPs) in Australia enhanced detection rates of adolescent psychological distress and suicidal ideation, it failed to lead to changes in patient management (Pfaff *et al*, 2001).

In a systematic review, Bower *et al* (2001) identified six studies of treatment actually offered by the primary care team, comprising a variety of interventions (e.g. parenting support, behaviour therapy and education) for different problems across the age spectrum. Of four controlled studies, only the study by Cullen (1976) and Cullen & Cullen (1996), of preventive interviews with parents of pre-school children, demonstrated significantly improved objective outcomes.

More recently, Asarnow *et al* (2005) carried out the most rigorous and comprehensive study of the treatment of adolescent depression in primary care. This randomised controlled trial of a 'quality improvement' intervention, compared with usual care, included the following treatment options: cognitive–behavioural therapy (CBT), medication, combined CBT with medication, care manager follow-up, or specialist referral. After 6 months, patients in the quality improvement intervention group reported significantly fewer depressive symptoms, higher quality of life and greater satisfaction with mental healthcare. They also received significantly higher rates of mental healthcare and psychotherapy or counselling. However, almost a third of these patients continued to show severe depressive symptoms. Increased use of combined psychotherapy and medication might have led to improved outcomes (March *et al*, 2004). Screening and recruitment resulted in loss of many young people to the study, indicating that this approach may benefit only a select group and longer-term benefits require further study. Nevertheless, the study demonstrated improved quality of care, increased access to evidence-based treatments and favourable outcomes in naturalistic settings.

This is in line with adult studies in the field of the primary care treatment of depression, which demonstrate that simple educational strategies for staff or passive dissemination of guidelines to improve the recognition and management of depression have minimal effect. Multifaceted programmes that integrate improvements in detection, treatment and follow-up, and that include combinations of clinician and patient education, nurse case management, enhanced support from specialist services and monitoring of medication, are most effective (Katon *et al*, 1999; Pignone *et al*, 2002; Gilbody *et al*, 2003; World Health Organization, 2004).

# Specialist clinics

A systematic review by Bower *et al* (2001) identified, in addition to direct interventions offered by the primary care team, interventions offered by specialist mental health professionals based in primary care (often referred to as 'shifted out-patient clinics'). Interventions described were brief (6–12 sessions) and included a variety of techniques: CBT, family therapy, non-directive counselling, dynamic therapy, psychiatric evaluation and guidance, parent education and counselling, group work and child education. Studies consisted largely of simple before–after designs without control groups and often lacked details on the process of treatment delivery. Two large-scale studies that used randomisation failed to demonstrate a marked effect on child health outcomes (Nicol *et al*, 1993; Cooper & Murray, 1997). Conclusions about effectiveness are therefore tentative. Moreover, provision of comprehensive coverage of this nature by specialist staff would require marked expansion of specialist services, is unlikely to be cost-effective and may not be achievable.

# Mixed-care models

For chronic problems such as hyperkinetic disorder (which has high levels of comorbidity) a comprehensive model of care could include long-term monitoring within the primary care setting, with intermittent involvement of specialist services, as appropriate for medication review or adjuvant behaviour therapy (Box 14.6). However, GPs have been shown to be sceptical about hyperkinetic disorder as a diagnostic entity (Klasen & Goodman, 2000). Many believe that attention-deficit hyperactivity disorder (ADHD) is overdiagnosed, report lack of knowledge and confidence in diagnosing and managing the disorder, and believe multidisciplinary team involvement in making the diagnosis is necessary (Shaw et al, 2002). There is also concern about the longer-term outcomes with medication for ADHD in childhood, as yet unanswered by long-term follow-up studies. The same scepticism is likely to apply to other mental health problems in children and young people. Adequate training and ongoing support would be necessary if such a model of joint working were to be developed, and may require more complex, service-level interventions.

# Referral to specialist services

Primary care practitioners are a consistent source of referrals to specialist child and adolescent mental health services. Referral of schoolchildren has been found to be linked to severity of the child's disorder, male gender, the presence of antisocial symptoms and relationship problems, and psychosocial disadvantage (i.e. family stress, unemployment) (Garralda & Bailey, 1988; Lavigne et al, 1998; Laclave & Campbell, 2006). Parental request remains a central determinant for referral, with GPs and paediatricians tending to remain more passive (Bailey & Garralda, 1989; Briggs-Gowen et al, 2000; Sayal et al, 2002). In a Dutch study, referral to a service offering a highly developed preventive child health system (90% of children and adolescents received three or four preventive assessments) was related to information regarding the mental health of the child per se, rather than socio-demographic factors (Brugman et al, 2001). This may indicate practice that is more directly focused on specific mental health need rather that on associated

---

**Box 14.6** Shared care of children and adolescents with ADHD

- Specialist services should complete full diagnostic assessment, initiation and stabilisation of medication, and attend to comorbid difficulties or disorders.
- Primary care then has an important role in ongoing prescription of medication, with monitoring of height, weight and blood pressure (approximately 6 monthly) and monitoring for any other medication side-effects.
- The emergence of side-effects or of other difficulties (such as oppositional or conduct disorder symptoms) should trigger review by child mental health specialists, who would otherwise usually review the young person less frequently.
- Specific details of such arrangements for shared care should be formalised within protocols formulated jointly by primary care and specialist services.

psychosocial risks. Although research indicates that psychiatric referrals by primary care doctors are generally appropriate, protocols refining the criteria for severity, psychosocial complexity and likely response to treatment would support primary care clinicians in decision-making about whom to refer, particularly if their role in identification were to increase.

# Prevention

Primary care professionals are already engaged with public health programmes relevant to primary prevention of mental distress and disorder in young people, by targeting risk and resilience factors. Examples include family planning programmes, prenatal care, promotion of adequate nutrition, child safety information and home visiting programmes. Dissemination of information on child health, development, behaviour and positive parenting within these programmes could realistically be achieved.

A pioneering Australian study of preventive GP consultations during a child's first 4 years demonstrated favourable outcomes at 6 years and 20 years later (Cullen, 1976; Cullen & Cullen, 1996). However, it is unlikely that many GPs or paediatricians would be able to invest the time required for such an intervention. It may be more practical and cost-effective to implement prenatal and infancy home visiting by trained nurses with mothers at high risk of difficulties.

Three such large randomised controlled trials have demonstrated benefits for young, low-income, unmarried mothers and their children, including improved parental care of the child, with fewer injuries and accidents, fewer emergency visits and less use of punishment in the first 4 years (Olds *et al*, 1997, 1998, 2004; Olds, 2002). In one trial, the programme also produced longer-term effects on the number of arrests, convictions, emergent substance use and promiscuous sexual activity of 15-year-olds. Another programme promoting psychosocial well-being and prevention of problems was implemented across five European countries (Puura *et al*, 2002). Primary care workers were trained to conduct interviews with all prospective mothers before and after childbirth, with ongoing counselling for mothers in need. Early evaluation revealed user satisfaction in some countries. Impact on the children and families is still being evaluated. Prior attempts at training primary care community nurses or health visitors to promote parenting to reduce behavioural problems in young children have reported inconsistent or equivocal results, and this area requires further exploration (Bower *et al*, 2001). It is important to establish which elements of such interventions are the minimum required to achieve mental health gains for children.

Secondary prevention, aimed at early detection and diagnosis, could be implemented by professionals in a range of primary care settings across different countries. For early behaviour difficulties, community-based group parenting programmes should be offered. These have been shown to improve parenting practices, parent–child interactions and child behaviour in independently replicated, randomised controlled trials (Webster-Stratton *et al*, 1989, 2001; Scott *et al*, 2001). A study of such a group offered by health visitors based in primary care in the UK, to children scoring highly on screening questionnaires, demonstrated significant improvements in child behaviour scores (Patterson *et al*, 2002). In low- and middle-income countries, where most of the healthcare is delivered by the primary or general healthcare team, the detection of developmental delays and epilepsy is also relevant. However, research is required to ascertain whether systematic early detection by primary care would lead to better outcomes in the medium to long term.

# Barriers

Similar barriers to the provision of mental health interventions for children and adolescents by primary care clinicians have been reported across different countries (Blum & Bearinger, 1990; Veit *et al*, 1995; Stiffman *et al*, 1997; Jacobson *et al*, 2002; Shaw *et al*, 2002; Kang *et al*, 2003) and include: time constraints, financial constraints (new primary care services will have to be provided and subsequent savings on specialist services, which are usually in different budgets, will not materialise immediately); a lack of training, which will also be expensive initially; and a lack of confidence in detecting and managing disorders.

A range of training initiatives have addressed this (Hughes *et al*, 1995; de Jong, 1996; Bernard *et al*, 1999; Bower *et al*, 2001; Luk *et al*, 2002; Gledhill *et al*, 2003; Leaf *et al*, 2004; Dogra *et al*, 2005; Sanci *et al*, 2005; Omigbodun *et al*, 2007) and evaluation has demonstrated increased skills and confidence of primary care staff who receive training. However, some practitioners have concerns about medicalising distress in children and adolescents (Iliffe *et al*, 2004) and for primary care practitioners exposure to training in child and adolescent mental health remains limited (Levav *et al*, 2004).

# Service organisation and complex interventions

Primary healthcare services for children and adolescents across different countries vary widely in terms of setting, staffing and funding (in terms of both source and level relative to the size of the population), and are delivered by a range of physicians (GPs, family physicians, general and community paediatricians) and non-physicians (nurses, health visitors, public health workers). They are based in primary care clinics, health centres, child health clinics, school medical services, emergency departments and ambulatory hospital/out-patient departments. Funding may be private, on the basis of insurance, or part of centrally organised national or regional health services.

More specifically, Katz *et al* (2002) found that 35% of European countries (12/34) reported a system of paediatric primary care provided by paediatricians, 18% (6/34) by GP/family doctor systems and the remainder by mixed systems (47%; 16/34). Within the USA, both paediatricians and family physicians provide paediatric primary care; however, increasingly over the past 20 years, these services have been provided by paediatricians (Freed *et al*, 2004). In Canada, paediatric primary care is provided largely by GPs and public health units. Within Australia, most young people receive primary care services from general practice as well as more recently established community health centres, which provide a range of free services for non-acute problems, mental health, sexual health and drug and alcohol problems (Kang *et al*, 2003). In many low- and middle-income countries, public health workers provide the point of first contact with health services and paediatricians provide specialised Western-type medical care (Cheng, 2004). Thus, globally, the differences in level of provision, structure of services and competencies of personnel delivering the services are important and likely to affect the potential to provide mental health services for children and adolescents within the primary care setting.

Although organisation and level of provision for child and adolescent mental health within primary care (and other sectors) differ markedly across countries, all face the problem of lack of both capacity and skilled personnel. Attempts to address this have required the development of complex interventions which require alteration to models of service delivery, in conjunction with improved training. A number of national policy initiatives have addressed this directly (Health Advisory Service, 1995; US Public Health Service, 2000; Australian Health Ministers, 2003), although the majority of countries still lack any specific child and adolescent mental health policy (Shatkin & Belfer, 2004).

## Interface between primary care and specialist mental health services

Within the UK, policy aimed at improving access to child and adolescent mental health services led to the development of primary care mental health workers (PCMHWs) to work with both primary and specialist child and adolescent mental health services in order: to consolidate skills of existing workers in primary services; to provide training and education; to support recognition of disorders and referral to specialist services; and to assess and treat some individuals (Department of Health, 2004). This approach has been shown to bridge the gap between primary care and specialist mental health services (Macdonald *et al*, 2004). Within the USA, Campo *et al* (2005) have described a service model with similar features, where an advanced practice nurse (APN) assesses young people after identification of difficulties by primary care clinicians, following which young people are triaged to care by primary care clinicians or mental health practitioners. They found that the vast majority of cases were treatable by the primary care clinician with APN support.

Both of these approaches incorporate consultation liaison, where the mental health specialists act to support management by primary care rather than take responsibility for individual patients themselves (Gask *et al*, 1997). Consultation liaison has traditionally been viewed as a means to increase the capacity of primary care clinicians to offer mental health services, partly through improving their skills and knowledge. However, there has been little systematic study of the patient outcomes following consultation liaison interventions and this model would apply only in those countries with more developed specialist services. Patel *et al* (2007) have argued that, in low-resource settings, the integration of mental health programmes into general youth health and welfare programmes (such as education and sexual health) would be a way forward.

# Future developments

Future developments within primary healthcare should include coordination of provision by the range of professionals already in contact with children and adolescents (including pre-school, education, welfare and juvenile justice) across sectors and agencies. It makes sense to conceptualise a stepped provision, starting with improved primary care recognition, followed by advice and treatment within primary care of the less complex and less severe difficulties, with referral of more complex and more severe cases to specialist child mental health services, where these are available. This will require improved professional knowledge, skills and attitudes (incorporating innovative roles for new workers similar to those described above), changes to service delivery systems following locally determined, culturally sensitive needs assessment (Rahman *et al*, 2000) and public education.

To support these developments, renewed research efforts should be directed at pragmatic evaluations of primary care. These should include the evaluation of: appropriate, broadly disorder-specific management techniques for child and adolescent mental health problems presenting to primary care; new bridging or interface services between primary and specialist care; and initiatives aimed at increasing awareness of child and adolescent mental health problems at the primary care level.

---

Key points

- Psychiatric disorders are common in children and adolescents attending primary care.
- Primary care interventions are appropriate for children and adolescents with disorders of mild to moderate severity.
- Early evaluation of interventions within primary care demonstrate promising results.
- To increase capacity of primary care to manage these difficulties, considerable attention to developing appropriate attitudes and skills is crucial.

---

# Further reading and e-resources

Garralda, M. E. & Hyde, C. (eds) (2003) *Managing Children with Psychiatric Problems* (2nd edn). BMJ Publishing.

National Institute for Health and Clinical Excellence (2005) *Depression in Children and Young People: Identification and Management in Primary, Community and Secondary Care.* Clinical guideline 28. Downloadable from http://www.nice.org.uk/nicemedia/pdf/word/CG028NICEguideline.doc

National Institute for Health and Clinical Excellence (2006) *Methylphenidate, Atomoxetine and Dexamfetamine for Attention Deficit Hyperactivity Disorder (ADHD) in Children and Adolescents.* Review of technology appraisal 13. Downloadable from http://www.nice.org.uk/nicemedia/pdf/TA098guidance.pdf

National Institute for Health and Clinical Excellence (2006) *Parent-Training/Education Programmes in the Management of Children with Conduct Disorders.* NICE technology appraisal guidance 102. Downloadable from http://www.nice.org.uk/nicemedia/pdf/TA102guidance.pdf

National Institute for Health and Clinical Excellence (2007) *Community-Based Interventions to Reduce Substance Misuse Among Vulnerable and Disadvantaged Children and Young People.* Public health intervention guideline 4. Downloadable from http://www.nice.org.uk/nicemedia/pdf/word/PHI004guidanceword.doc

Royal College of Psychiatrists, information leaflets for parents, children and young people (including information on growing up, common stressors, as well as specific disorders). Downloadable from http://www.rcpsych.ac.uk/mentalhealthinformation/childrenandyoungpeople.aspx

# References

Angold, A., Costello, E. J., Pickles, A., *et al* (1987) *The Development of a Questionnaire for Use In Epidemiological Studies of Depression in Children and Adolescents.* MRC Child Psychiatry Unit.

Asarnow, J. R., Jaycox, L. H., Duan, N., *et al* (2005) Depression and role impairment among adolescents in primary care clinics. *Journal of Adolescent Health*, **37**, 477–483.

Australian Health Ministers (2003) *National Mental Health Plan 2003–2008.* Australian Government.

Bailey, D. & Garralda, M. E. (1989) Referral to child psychiatry: parent and doctor motives and expectations. *Journal of Child Psychology and Psychiatry*, **30**, 449–458.

Bailey, V., Graham, P. & Boniface, D. (1978) How much child psychiatry does a general practitioner do? *Journal of the Royal College of General Practitioners*, **28**, 621–626.

Barnes, J. & Richman, N. (2003) *Early Years Behaviour Checklist Handbook.* nfer–Nelson.

Bernard, P., Garralda, E., Hughes, T., *et al* (1999) Evaluation of a teaching package in adolescent psychiatry for general practitioners. *Education for General Practice*, **10**, 21–28.

Blum, R. W. & Bearinger, L. H. (1990) Knowledge and attitudes of health professionals toward adolescent health care. *Journal of Adolescent Health Care*, **11**, 289–294.

Borowsky, I. W., Mozayeny, S. & Ireland, M. (2003) Brief psychosocial screening at health supervision and acute care visits. *Pediatrics*, **112**, 129–133.

Bower, P., Garralda, E., Kramer, T., *et al* (2001) The treatment of child and adolescent mental health problems in primary care: a systematic review. *Family Practice*, **18**, 373–382.

Briggs-Gowan, M. J., Horwitz, S. M., Schwab-Stone, M. E., *et al* (2000) Mental health in pediatric settings: distribution of disorders and factors related to service use. *Journal of the American Academy of Child and Adolescent Psychiatry*, **39**, 841–849.

Briggs-Gowan, M. J., Carter, A. S., Irwin, J. R., *et al* (2004) The Brief Infant–Toddler Social and Emotional Assessment: screening for social–emotional problems and delays in competence. *Journal of Pediatric Psychology*, **29**, 143–155.

Brugman, E., Reijneveld, S. A., Verhulst, F. C., *et al* (2001) Identification and management of psychosocial problems by preventive child health care. *Archives of Pediatrics and Adolescent Medicine*, **155**, 462–469.

Burns, B. J., Costello, E. J., Angold, A., *et al* (1995) Children's mental health service use across service sectors. *Health Affairs (Millwood)*, **14**, 147–159.

Campo, J. V., Jansen-McWilliams, L., Comer, D. M., *et al* (1999) Somatization in pediatric primary care: association with psychopathology, functional impairment, and use of services. *Journal of the American Academy of Child and Adolescent Psychiatry*, **38**, 1093–1101.

Campo, J. V., Bridge, J., Ehmann, M., *et al* (2004) Recurrent abdominal pain, anxiety, and depression in primary care. *Pediatrics*, **113**, 817–824.

Campo, J. V., Shafer, S., Strohm, J., *et al* (2005) Pediatric behavioral health in primary care: a collaborative approach. *Journal of the American Psychiatric Nurses Association*, **11**, 276–282.

Chang, G., Warner, V. & Weissman, M. M. (1988) Physicians' recognition of psychiatric disorders in children and adolescents. *American Journal of Disorders of Childhood*, **142**, 736–739.

Cheng, T. L. (2004) Primary care pediatrics: 2004 and beyond. *Pediatrics*, **113**, 1802–1809.

Cooper, P. & Murray, L. (1997) The impact of psychological treatments of postpartum depression on maternal mood and infant development. In *Post Partum Depression and Child Development* (eds L. Murray & P. Cooper), pp. 201–220. Guilford Press.

Costello, E. J. & Edelbrock, C. S. (1985) Detection of psychiatric disorders in pediatric primary care: a preliminary report. *Journal of the American Academy of Child and Adolescent Psychiatry*, **24**, 771–774.

Costello, E. J., Costello, A. J., Edelbrock, C., *et al* (1988) Psychiatric disorders in pediatric primary care. Prevalence and risk factors. *Archives of General Psychiatry*, **45**, 1107–1116.

Cullen, K. J. (1976) A six-year controlled trial of prevention of children's behavior disorders. *Journal of Pediatrics*, **88**, 662–667.

Cullen, K. J. & Cullen, A. M. (1996) Long-term follow-up of the Busselton six-year controlled trial of prevention of children's behavior disorders. *Journal of Pediatrics*, **129**, 136–139.

de Jong, J. T. (1996) A comprehensive public mental health programme in Guinea-Bissau: a useful model for African, Asian and Latin-American countries. *Psychological Medicine*, **26**, 97–108.

Department of Health (2004) *National Service Framework for Children, Young People and Maternity Services: The Mental Health and Psychological Well-being of Children and Young People*. Department of Health.

Dogra, N., Frake, C., Bretherton, K., *et al* (2005) Training CAMHS professionals in developing countries: an Indian case study. *Child and Adolescent Mental Health*, **10**, 74–79.

Dulcan, M. K., Costello, E. J., Costello, A. J., *et al* (1990) The pediatrician as gatekeeper to mental health care for children: do parents' concerns open the gate? *Journal of the American Academy of Child and Adolescent Psychiatry*, **29**, 453–458.

Ellingson, K. D., Briggs-Gowan, M. J., Carter, A. S. , *et al* (2004) Parent identification of early emerging child behavior problems: predictors of sharing parental concern with health providers. *Archives of Pediatrics and Adolescent Medicine*, **158**, 766–772.

Frankenfield, D. L., Keyl, P. M., Gielen, A., *et al* (2000) Adolescent patients – healthy or hurting? Missed opportunities to screen for suicide risk in the primary care setting. *Archives of Pediatrics and Adolescent Medicine*, **154**, 162–168.

Freed, G. L., Nahra, T. A. & Wheeler, J. R. C. (2004) Which physicians are providing health care to America's children? Trends and changes during the past 20 years. *Archives of Pediatrics and Adolescent Medicine*, **158**, 22–26.

Garralda, M. E. & Bailey, D. (1986) Children with psychiatric disorders in primary care. *Journal of Child Psychology and Psychiatry*, **27**, 611–624.

Garralda, M. E. & Bailey, D. (1987) Psychosomatic aspects of children's consultations in primary care. *European Archives of Psychiatry and Neurological Science*, **236**, 319–322.

Garralda, M. E. & Bailey, D. (1988) Child and family factors associated with referral to child psychiatrists. *British Journal of Psychiatry*, **153**, 81–89.

Garralda, M. E. & Bailey, D. (1989) Psychiatric disorders in general paediatric referrals. *Archives of Disease in Childhood*, **64**, 1727–1733.

Garralda, M. E. & Bailey, D. (1990) Paediatrician identification of psychological factors associated with general paediatric consultations. *Journal of Psychosomatic Research*, **34**, 303–312.

Gask, L., Sibbald, B. & Creed, F. (1997) Evaluating models of working at the interface between mental health services and primary care. *British Journal of Psychiatry*, **170**, 6–11.

Giel, R., de Arango, M. V., Climent, C. E., *et al* (1981) Childhood mental disorders in primary health care: results of observations in four developing countries. A report from the WHO collaborative study on strategies for extending mental health care. *Pediatrics*, **68**, 677–683.

Gilbody, S., Whitty, P., Grimshaw, J., *et al* (2003) Educational and organizational interventions to improve the management of depression in primary care: a systematic review. *JAMA*, **289**, 3145–3151.

Glazebrook, C., Hollis, C., Heussler, H., *et al* (2003) Detecting emotional and behavioural problems in paediatric clinics. *Child: Care, Health and Development*, **29**, 141–149.

Gledhill, J., Kramer, T., Iliffe, S., *et al* (2003) Training general practitioners in the identification and management of adolescent depression within the consultation: a feasibility study. *Journal of Adolescence*, **26**, 245–250.

Goldberg, I. D., Roghmann, K. J., McInerny, T. K., *et al* (1984) Mental health problems among children seen in pediatric practice: prevalence and management. *Pediatrics*, **73**, 278–293.

Goodman, R. (1997) The Strengths and Difficulties Questionnaire: a research note. *Journal of Child Psychology and Psychiatry*, **38**, 581–586.

Gureje, O., Omigbodun, O. O., Gater, R., *et al* (1994) Psychiatric disorders in a paediatric primary care clinic. *British Journal of Psychiatry*, **165**, 527–530.

Health Advisory Service (1995) *Child and Adolescent Mental Health Services: Together We Stand*. HMSO.

Horwitz, S. M., Leaf, P. J., Leventhal, J. M., *et al* (1992) Identification and management of psychosocial and developmental problems in community-based, primary care pediatric practices. *Pediatrics*, **89**, 480–485.

Horwitz, S. M., Leaf, P. J. & Leventhal, J. M. (1998) Identification of psychosocial problems in pediatric primary care: do family attitudes make a difference? *Archives of Pediatric and Adolescent Medicine*, **152**, 367–371.

Hughes, T., Garralda, E. & Tylee, A. (1995) *Child Mental Health Problems*. St Mary's Hospital Medical School.

Iliffe, S., Gledhill, J., da Cunha, F., *et al* (2004) The recognition of adolescent depression in general practice: issues in the acquisition of new skills. *Primary Care Psychiatry*, **9**, 51–56.

Jacobson, A. M., Goldberg, I. D., Burns, B. J., *et al* (1980) Diagnosed mental disorder in children and use of health services in four organized health care settings. *American Journal of Psychiatry*, **137**, 559–565.

Jacobson, L., Churchill, R., Donovan, C., *et al* (2002) Tackling teenage turmoil: primary care recognition and management of mental ill health during adolescence. *Family Practice*, **19**, 401–409.

Kang, M., Bernard, D., Booth, M., *et al* (2003) Access to primary health care for Australian young people: service provider perspectives. *British Journal of General Practice*, **53**, 947–952.

Katon, W., Von, K. M., Lin, E., *et al* (1999) Stepped collaborative care for primary care patients with persistent symptoms of depression: a randomized trial. *Archives of General Psychiatry*, **56**, 1109–1115.

Katz, M., Rubino, A., Collier, J., et al (2002) Demography of pediatric primary care in Europe: delivery of care and training. *Pediatrics*, **109**, 788–796.

Klasen, H. & Goodman, R. (2000) Parents and GPs at cross-purposes over hyperactivity: a qualitative study of possible barriers to treatment. *British Journal of General Practice*, **50**, 199–202.

Kovacs, M. (1992) *Children's Depression Inventory*. Multi-Health Systems.

Kramer, T. & Garralda, M. E. (1998) Psychiatric disorders in adolescents in primary care. *British Journal of Psychiatry*, **173**, 508–513.

Kramer, T., Iliffe, S., Murray, E., et al (1997) Which adolescents attend the GP? *British Journal of General Practice*, **47**, 327.

Laclave, L. J. & Campbell, J. L. (2006) Psychiatric intervention in children: sex differences in referral rates. *Journal of the American Academy of Child and Adolescent Psychiatry*, **24**, 430–432.

Lavigne, J. V., Arend, R., Rosenbaum, D., et al (1998) Mental health service use among young children receiving pediatric primary care. *Journal of the American Academy of Child and Adolescent Psychiatry*, **37**, 1175–1183.

Leaf, P. J., Owens, P. L., Leventhal, J. M., et al (2004) Pediatricians' training and identification and management of psychosocial problems. *Clinical Pediatrics*, **43**, 355–365.

Levav, I., Jacobsson, L., Tsiantis, J., et al (2004) Psychiatric services and training for children and adolescents in Europe: results of a country survey. *European Child and Adolescent Psychiatry*, **13**, 395–401.

Luby, J. L., Heffelfinger, A., Koenig-McNaught, A. L., et al (2004) The Preschool Feelings Checklist: a brief and sensitive screening measure for depression in young children. *Journal of the American Academy of Child and Adolescent Psychiatry*, **43**, 708–717.

Luk, E. S. L., Brann, P., Sutherland, S., et al (2002) Training general practitioners in the assessment of childhood mental health problems. *Clinical Child Psychology and Psychiatry*, **7**, 571–579.

Macdonald, W., Bradley, S., Bower, P., et al (2004) Primary mental health workers in child and adolescent mental health services. *Journal of Advanced Nursing*, **46**, 78–87.

March, J., Silva, S., Petrycki, S., et al (2004) Fluoxetine, cognitive–behavioral therapy, and their combination for adolescents with depression: Treatment for Adolescents With Depression Study (TADS) randomized controlled trial. *JAMA*, **292**, 807–820.

Martinez, R. (2006) Factors that influence the detection of psychological problems in adolescents attending general practices. *British Journal of General Practice*, **56**, 594–599.

Monck, E., Graham, P., Richman, N., et al (1994) Adolescent girls. I. Self-reported mood disturbance in a community population. *British Journal of Psychiatry*, **165**, 760–769.

Nicol, R., Stretch, D. & Fundudis, T. (1993) *Preschool Children in Troubled Families*. Wiley.

Office of Population Censuses and Surveys (1995) *Morbidity Statistics From General Practice*. HMSO.

Offord, D. R., Boyle, M. H., Szatmari, P., et al (1987) Ontario Child Health Study. II. Six-month prevalence of disorder and rates of service utilization. *Archives of General Psychiatry*, **44**, 832–836.

Olds, D. L. (2002) Prenatal and infancy home visiting by nurses: from randomized trials to community replication. *Preventive Science*, **3**, 153–172.

Olds, D. L., Eckenrode, J., Henderson, C. R., et al (1997) Long-term effects of home visitation on maternal life course and child abuse and neglect. Fifteen-year follow-up of a randomized trial. *JAMA*, **278**, 637–643.

Olds, D. L., Henderson, C. R., Cole, R., et al (1998) Long-term effects of nurse home visitation on children's criminal and antisocial behavior: 15-year follow-up of a randomized trial. *JAMA*, **280**, 1238–1244.

Olds, D. L., Kitzman, H., Cole, R., et al (2004) Effects of nurse home-visiting on maternal life course and child development: age 6 follow-up results of a randomized trial. *Pediatrics*, **114**, 1550–1559.

Olson, A. L., Kelleher, K. J., Kemper, K. J., et al (2001) Primary care pediatricians' roles and perceived responsibilities in the identification and management of depression in children and adolescents. *Ambulatory Pediatrics*, **1**, 91–98.

Omigbodun, O., Bella, T., Dogra, N., *et al* (2007) Training health professionals for child and adolescent mental health care in Nigeria: a qualitative analysis. *Child and Adolescent Mental Health*, **12**, 132–137.

Patel, V., Flisher, A. J., Hetrick, S., *et al* (2007) Mental health of young people: a global public-health challenge. *Lancet*, **369**, 1302–1313.

Patterson, J., Barlow, J., Mockford, C., *et al* (2002) Improving mental health through parenting programmes: block randomised controlled trial. *Archives of Disease in Childhood*, **87**, 472–477.

Pfaff, J. J., Acres, J. G. & McKelvey, R. S. (2001) Training general practitioners to recognise and respond to psychological distress and suicidal ideation in young people. *Medical Journal of Australia*, **174**, 222–226.

Pignone, M. P., Gaynes, B. N., Rushton, J. L., *et al* (2002). Screening for depression in adults: a summary of the evidence for the U.S. Preventive Services Task Force. *Annals of Internal Medicine*, **136**, 765–776.

Puura, K., Davis, H., Papadopoulou,K., *et al* (2002) The European Early Promotion Project: a new primary health care service to promote children's mental health. *Infant Mental Health Journal*, **23**, 606–624.

Rahman, A., Mubbashar, M., Harrington, R., *et al* (2000) Developing child mental health services in developing countries. *Journal of Child Psychology and Psychiatry*, **41**, 539–546.

Ramchandani, P. G., Stein, A., Hotopf, M., *et al* (2006) Early parental and child predictors of recurrent abdominal pain at school age: results of a large population-based study. *Journal of the American Academy of Child and Adolescent Psychiatry*, **45**, 729–736.

Rushton, J., Bruckman, D. & Kelleher, K. (2002) Primary care referral of children with psychosocial problems. *Archives of Pediatric and Adolescent Medicine*, **156**, 592–598.

Sanci, L., Coffey, C., Patton, G., *et al* (2005) Sustainability of change with quality general practitioner education in adolescent health: a 5-year follow-up. *Medical Education*, **39**, 557–560.

Sayal, K. & Taylor, E. (2004) Detection of child mental health disorders by general practitioners. *British Journal of General Practice*, **54**, 348–352.

Sayal, K., Taylor, E., Beecham, J., *et al* (2002) Pathways to care in children at risk of attention-deficit hyperactivity disorder. *British Journal of Psychiatry*, **181**, 43–48.

Scott, S., Spender, Q., Doolan, M., *et al* (2001) Multicentre controlled trial of parenting groups for childhood antisocial behaviour in clinical practice. Commentary: nipping conduct problems in the bud. *BMJ*, **323**, 194.

Shatkin, J. & Belfer, M. (2004) The global absence of child and adolescent mental health policy. *Child and Adolescent Mental Health*, **9**, 104.

Shaw, K. A., Mitchell, G. K., Wagner, I. J., *et al* (2002) Attitudes and practices of general practitioners in the diagnosis and management of attention-deficit/hyperactivity disorder. *Journal of Paediatrics and Child Health*, **38**, 481–486.

Sonuga-Barke E. J., Daley, D., Thompson, M. J. J., *et al* (2001) Parent based therapies for ADHD. A randomised trial with a community sample. *Journal of the American Academy of Child and Adolescent Psychiatry*, **40**, 402–408.

Starfield, B., Gross, E., Wood, M., *et al* (1980) Psychosocial and psychosomatic diagnoses in primary care of children. *Pediatrics*, **66**, 159–167.

Stiffman, A. R., Chen, Y. W., Elze, D., *et al* (1997) Adolescents' and providers' perspectives on the need for and use of mental health services. *Journal of Adolescent Health*, **21**, 335–342.

Turner, K. M. & Sanders, M. R. (2006) Help when it's needed first: a controlled evaluation of brief, preventive behavioral family intervention in a primary care setting. *Behavior Therapy*, **37**, 131–142.

US Public Health Service (2000) *Report of the Surgeon General's Conference on Children's Mental Health. A National Action Agenda*. Department of Health and Human Services.

Veit, F. C., Sanci, L. A., Young, D. Y., *et al* (1995) Adolescent health care: perspectives of Victorian general practitioners. *Medical Journal of Australia*, **163**, 16–18.

Verhulst, F. C. & van der Ende, J. (1997) Factors associated with child mental health service use in the community. *Journal of the American Academy of Child and Adolescent Psychiatry*, **36**, 901–909.

Webster-Stratton, C., Hollinsworth, T. & Kolpacoff, M. (1989) The long-term effectiveness and clinical significance of three cost-effective training programs for families with conduct-problem children. *Journal of Consulting and Clinical Psychology*, **57**, 550–553.

Webster-Stratton, C., Reid, M. J. & Hammond, M. (2001) Preventing conduct problems, promoting social competence: a parent and teacher training partnership in head start. *Journal of Clinical Child Psychology*, **30**, 283–302.

White, D., Leach, C., Atkinson, M., *et al* (1999) Validation of the Hospital Anxiety and Depression Scale for use with adolescents. *British Journal of Psychiatry*, **175**, 452–454.

World Health Organization (2004) *What Is the Evidence of Capacity Building of Primary Health Care Professionals in the Detection, Management and Outcome of Depression?* WHO.

Wren, F. J., Scholle, S. H., Heo, J., *et al* (2005) How do primary care clinicians manage childhood mood and anxiety syndromes? *International Journal of Psychiatry in Medicine*, **35**, 1–12.

# CHAPTER 15

# Psychosis

Helen Lester

Summary

This chapter explores the potential roles and responsibilities of the primary care team in providing care and advice for people with psychosis. It starts with a challenge to all primary care practitioners, regardless of the health system in which they work, describing the issues that face people living with psychosis. After a brief overview of the definition and epidemiology of psychosis, the chapter then focuses on the role that primary care currently plays both at diagnosis and in the longer term. It also encompasses service users' views of services and ideas for promoting a culture of recovery. The chapter concludes with some reflections on international work at the 'cutting edge' in this field. Above all, this chapter shows how the contribution of generalism and family practice are essential and valued aspects of effective healthcare for people with psychosis.

## The challenges

People who develop a psychosis can find themselves strangers in their own land (Box 15.1). The health and social effects create spirals of decline and a loss of autonomy which can quickly become entrenched and difficult to address. This situation would be unacceptable in almost any other area of healthcare. It is time, therefore, to re-examine not only how primary care practitioners think about people with psychosis, but also how health services can be better organised to provide 21st-century care for patients.

## What do we mean by the term 'psychosis'?

Terminology in this area can be fraught with difficulty and 'psychosis' is not, of itself, a diagnosis. The primary care version of ICD–10 (World Health Organization, 2004) offers a condensed ICD–10 classification, with 23 diagnostic categories for use by generalists in primary care settings.

---

**Box 15.1** The reality of living with a serious mental illness

- In 2003, while 83% of people in the UK agreed that a more tolerant attitude towards people with mental illness was needed, this still meant that nearly one in five believed there was no need to do so (Department of Health, 2003).
- Someone with psychosis is four times more likely than an 'average' person to have no close friends (Huxley & Thornicroft, 2003).
- In England, only 24% of people with mental health problems are currently in work (Office for National Statistics, 2003).
- Deaths from infectious diseases and endocrine, circulatory, respiratory, digestive and genito-urinary system disorders are significantly more likely for adults with psychosis (Harris & Barraclough, 1998).
- A person with schizophrenia can expect to live for 10 years less than someone without a mental health problem (Allebeck, 1989).
- Ninety-five per cent of carers are members of service users' families (Rethink, 2003).
- Twenty-nine per cent of carers provide support and care in excess of 50 hours per week (Rethink, 2003).
- Ninety per cent of carers are adversely affected by the caring role in terms of leisure activities, career progress, financial circumstances and family relationships (Rethink, 2003).

---

However, since psychoses have, historically, been regarded as disorders of adulthood, ICD–10 has yet to classify adolescent psychosis.

The most commonly used categories are probably:

- F23, acute psychotic disorder
- F20, chronic psychotic disorder
- F31, bipolar affective disorder.

The British Psychological Society (2000) estimated that around 10–15% of the general population experience what could be described as psychotic phenomena (i.e. hearing voices or hallucinations). Most are neither distressed nor seek help. Research shows that such people in the general population will not have received a diagnosis or have needed treatment for such experiences (van Os *et al*, 2000; Johns *et al*, 2004). There is also growing evidence that some people can have psychotic experiences following extremely stressful or traumatic life experiences such as solitary confinement, social isolation, sleep deprivation, abuse and assault. This chapter, however, is focused on the majority of people who are distressed and do seek help for their symptoms.

# Epidemiology

If all individuals with schizophrenia, bipolar disorder and chronic psychosis are included, psychosis affects approximately 3% of the population in the

UK (Bird, 1999). This means a diagnosis of psychosis is about as common as one of insulin-dependent diabetes.

Much work has focused on the risk factors for psychosis, although it is also important to remember that a risk factor only indicates a link and is not necessarily causal. Although studies about the effects of urban life extend back to Faris and Dunham in the 1930s in Chicago (Owen *et al*, 1941), recent data from the UK suggest that the incidence of psychosis may also be linked to socio-economic deprivation. The Aetiology and Ethnicity in Schizophrenia and Other Psychoses (AESOP) study (Kirkbride *et al*, 2006) examined the incidence of first-episode psychosis (FEP) in three English cities (it recruited 568 participants) and found that significant variation existed in the incidence of schizophrenia and other psychoses in terms of:

- gender (schizophrenia was significantly more common in men and affective disorders occurred equally in men and women)
- age (80% of first episodes occur in young people between 16 and 30 years of age)
- ethnicity (there were increased rates of diagnosis among Black and minority ethnic groups for all psychoses).

This and other studies suggest that the incidence is not uniform and that environmental effects, perhaps at the neighbourhood level, may interact together and with genetic factors to cause psychosis. A recent systematic review also underlined decades of debate over whether prolonged cannabis use increases an individual's risk of developing a psychosis (Moore *et al*, 2007).

## How do people with a psychosis present in primary care?

Most general practitioners (GPs) in the UK see only one or two new people with FEP each year. However, despite this low incidence, the role of primary care is important for a number of reasons. GPs are frequently consulted at some point during a developing FEP and are the most common final referral agent to mental health services in the patient pathway (Skeate *et al*, 2002). GP involvement is also associated with a reduced use of the Mental Health Act in the UK (Burnett *et al*, 1999).

Studies across the world of FEP have consistently found an average duration of untreated psychosis (DUP), the time interval between onset of psychotic symptoms and the start of antipsychotic treatment, of 1–2 years (McGlashen, 1999). It is highly likely that an association exists between long DUP and a poorer outcome of FEP, particularly functional and symptomatic outcome at 12 months and symptom reduction once treatment begins (Harrigan *et al*, 2003). Long-term follow-up studies have also shown that outcome at 2 years strongly predicts outcomes 15 years later. Birchwood *et al* (1998) argue that such observations support the concept that the early phase of psychosis represents a 'critical period' in treatment, with major implications for secondary prevention of impairments and disabilities, and provide a further rationale for intervening intensively and early.

In summary, while FEP is relatively rare from an individual GP's perspective, it is a life-changing event for the person and family. High-quality care at the outset offers the possibility of a less traumatic and shorter pathway into mental health services, and the hope of improved longer-term outcomes.

## Making a diagnosis

Early detection is a challenge for primary care practitioners. Psychosis can take several months to emerge from a prodrome of non-specific psychological and social disturbances of varying intensity without clear-cut psychotic symptoms. These disturbances can include poor sleep, panic and mood changes and social withdrawal and isolation. It is also important to look for evidence of poor personal hygiene, delusional or bewildered mood, abstract or vague speech and outbursts of anger or irritation. Positive symptoms (e.g. hallucinations and delusions) and negative symptoms (e.g. social withdrawal and depression) are rarely volunteered spontaneously and may need to be actively sought (Box 15.2).

If the GP or other primary professional suspects the person may be developing a psychosis, it is advisable also to ask about changes in:

- social functioning (e.g. problems in relationships with friends and family)
- cognition (e.g. poor concentration and memory)
- mood (e.g. feeling depressed, anxious or irritable)
- drug use
- ideas of suicide.

---

**Box 15.2** Seeking positive symptoms of psychosis

Questions a primary care practitioner may want to ask include:

- Have you felt that something odd might be going on that you cannot explain?
- Have you been feeling that people are talking about you, watching you or giving you a hard time for no reason?
- Have you been feeling, seeing or hearing things that others cannot?
- Have you felt especially important in some way, or that you have powers that let you do things that others cannot?

---

There may be a temptation to label some of the earlier and more vague symptoms as 'normal teenage behaviour' or as a consequence of cannabis use. However, it is important to keep an active watching brief, to follow up missed appointments and to take family concerns seriously. A better GP–patient/family relationship may well have been built up by the time a referral is needed. In summary, GP recognition of early changes, clinical intuition and acting on family worries are key to earlier detection.

## Management issues

### At diagnosis

Once a diagnosis is suspected or made, the young person needs to be referred to an appropriate mental health service, ideally a service that specialises in early intervention.

Early intervention in psychosis is a relatively new concept in policy terms, although claims for its benefits are not. In 1828, the British Metropolitan Commissioners of Lunacy cited statistical tables 'exhibiting the large proportion of cures effected in cases where patients are admitted within three months of their attacks' and the *Westminster Review* endorsed 'the very great probability of cure in the early stages of insanity' (Scull, 1979, p. 112). However, during the past two decades, effective, early intervention has become a priority in a number of countries, including England, Canada, New Zealand and Australia, and parts of the USA and Scandinavia.

In the UK, the IRIS (Initiative to Reduce the Impact of Schizophrenia) lobby group and charity Rethink have been at the forefront of early intervention activism and they have generated consistent pressure grounded in user and carer dissatisfaction with services (Rethink, 2002). Evidence has also demonstrated that community mental health teams (CMHTs) are less able than specialist mental health teams to engage young people effectively or provide specific treatments needed during the critical early period of the illness (Yung *et al*, 2003). Randomised controlled trials have shown that integrated intensive services at an early state in the illness can lead to improved clinical outcomes in relation to both positive and negative psychotic symptoms (Peterson *et al*, 2005) and lower relapse rates (Craig *et al*, 2004). This confluence of activism and evidence led to an 'Early Psychosis Declaration' endorsed by the World Health Organization that identified a set of expected standards of care for people with FEP (see e-resources at the end of the chapter).

In the UK, in 2000 the National Health Service (NHS) underwent a major policy reform with *The NHS Plan*, which stated that:

> fifty early intervention teams will therefore be established over the next three years … [so that] by 2004 all young people who experience a first episode of psychosis, such as schizophrenia, will receive the early and intensive support they need. (Department of Health, 2000, p. 119)

This was supported by a number of policy implementation guides (Department of Health, 2001, 2002) that provided technical detail and practical strategies for newly funded services to follow, and a National Early Intervention Programme to oversee the roll-out of new services.

By March 2005, an audit by the National Early Intervention Programme found that 86 new 'functionalised' early intervention services (EIS) had been implemented and were able to deliver services to approximately one-third of the population in England (Pinfold *et al*, 2007). For primary care practitioners in the UK, however, this means that the most common pathway into services when they suspect a young person has a FEP is still a referral to existing CMHTs.

## In the longer term

Internationally, access to healthcare in the longer term is inevitably influenced by whether primary care practitioners have a gatekeeper role and the social or insurance-based nature of the wider health system within the country. In the UK, up to 30% of people with established (chronic) psychosis are seen only in the primary care setting and have no regular mental health follow-up (Kendrick *et al*, 1994, 2000; Jeffreys *et al*, 1997; Rodgers *et al*, 2003). There are a number of reasons for this, including resolution of acute symptoms, secondary care service capacity, and service user choice. We also know that people with a chronic psychosis consult primary care practitioners in the UK more frequently than do the general population (Nazareth *et al*, 1993) and are in contact with primary care services for a longer cumulative time than patients without mental health problems (Kai *et al*, 2000). In the USA, where a quarter of inhabitants are without health insurance, and serious illness is a common cause of bankruptcy, the national mental health system for adults with psychosis has been frequently criticised as 'a system in shambles'. Access to practitioners and treatments is variable; 'many people [are] not provided with the essential treatment they need ... and [are] allowed to falter to the point of crisis' (National Alliance on Mental Illness, 2006, p. 2) (see e-resources at the end of the chapter for further details).

There are commonalities across countries in terms of both poorer health outcomes for people with psychosis compared with the general population, and health professionals' attitudes towards people with mental illness. As Chapter 20 shows, across health systems, patients with psychosis have higher morbidity and mortality rates from physical conditions than the general population. A systematic review that included 37 articles drawn from 25 nations concluded that not only does a substantial gap exist between the health of people with schizophrenia and the general community, but the differential mortality has in fact worsened in recent decades (Saha *et al*, 2007).

These statistics reflect a complex web of factors beyond health systems. Even if access were equal, lifestyle, diet, physical activity, smoking, obesity and drug side-effects all contribute to poor health outcomes for people with psychosis. Some 90% of people with schizophrenia and about 30% of people with bipolar disorder smoke (Brown *et al*, 1999). A number of psychotropic drugs, including clozapine, risperidone and olanzapine, also have a high risk of harmful side-effects. A 5-year follow-up of people starting clozapine found that 37% developed diabetes and most showed significant weight gain, particularly in the first 12 months (Henderson *et al*, 2000).

In terms of the stigma attached to the diagnosis within primary care, UK studies comparing patients with and without a diagnosis of schizophrenia found that the patients with schizophrenia were more likely to encounter reluctance by GPs to participate in their care (Lawrie *et al*, 1996, 1998). A survey of Norwegian GPs found that psychosis was ranked 34 of 38 in a 'disease prestige' list (Album & Westin, 2007), perhaps reflecting a dislike of working with people with mental illness.

It is important also to examine the other side of the relationship, that is, the views on primary care of patients with psychosis. Bindman *et al* (1997) found generally high satisfaction scores for primary care services in the UK but mixed patient views on greater primary care involvement in shared care. Longitudinal and interpersonal continuity of care, relative ease of access and the option of a home visit were valued features of primary care (Lester *et al*, 2003) and primary care was often contrasted with secondary care mental health services, in particular the difficulty presented by seeing a constant stream of new faces. A study that involved GPs and people with severe and enduring mental illness talking together about how to configure good-quality care found that primary care was seen as the 'cornerstone' of care (Lester *et al*, 2005). Patients prioritised continuity of care, attitudes and willingness to listen and learn over a GP with specialised mental health knowledge. This challenges some health professionals' assumptions that focused mental health expertise is vital in providing care for patients with psychosis (Box 15.3).

## Can people recover from psychosis?

Kraepelin's original description (1896) of 'dementia praecox' (literally 'dementia of young mind') as a single disease entity (now termed 'schizophrenia') with a universally poor outcome has dominated a whole century of treatment approaches. This concept of a relentless, downward, deteriorating course survived, virtually unchallenged, until Manfred Bleuler's classic observations of the course of schizophrenia over 20 years in 208 patients and families. Bleuler (1977) discovered that even the most severely affected person could achieve a partial or even complete recovery. Subsequent long-term follow-up studies have suggested that approximately half the people diagnosed with a psychotic illness have a favourable outcome (Harrison *et al*, 2001). Recent work on service users' views of primary care has also emphasised the importance of therapeutic optimism from health professionals, and reflects the importance of underpinning

**Box 15.3** Providing 'good enough' primary care

Lester *et al*'s (2005) study involved GPs and people with severe and enduring mental illness talking together about how to configure good-quality care. Some of the key findings are presented here.

- Most patients viewed primary care as the 'cornerstone' of their physical and mental healthcare.
- Patients and GPs agreed that the latter had a responsibility to continue prescribing drugs started in secondary care, monitor side-effects and tackle physical health issues.
- Both groups recognised, however, that it was sometimes difficult to present with or diagnose physical complaints once a mental health disorder had been diagnosed. Some GPs suggested this was related to difficulties in communicating effectively with people with serious mental illness.
- Most health professionals perceived the mental healthcare of people with serious mental illness as too specialised for routine primary care and felt they lacked sufficient skills and knowledge.
- All participants felt that interpersonal and longitudinal continuity was vital for good-quality care. However, most health professionals felt continuity was threatened by other national primary care policies.
- Patients felt that continuity: helped to ensure accurate diagnosis, particularly at times of mental health crisis; prevented the retelling of painful stories; enabled trust to develop, which in turn facilitated discussions of treatment options; and, above all, allowed patients and health professionals to understand each other as people.
- Most patients favoured seeing the same GP for their physical and mental health needs, preferring a continuous doctor–patient relationship and a positive attitude and willingness to learn, rather than the opportunity to consult a different GP with special expertise in mental health.
- Most patients knew that their GP had little formal training in mental health and did not expect expert advice from primary care professionals.

recovery principles (Warner, 2003). Although many health professionals associate a diagnosis of psychosis with notions of chronicity, service users do not necessarily identify themselves as people living with a *chronic* illness. Many prefer a social model of illness, one that emphasises recovery, at least in terms of quality-of-life issues, such as returning to work and regaining family ties (Lester *et al*, 2005).

In summary, there are a number of relatively simple issues that all health practitioners, regardless of the system they work in, can think about in terms of reducing levels of stigma and improving the care of people with psychosis (Lester & Gask, 2006) (Box 15.4). Although primary care health professionals may feel that lack of knowledge inhibits greater involvement in care, patients with a chronic psychosis appear to value continuity of care, listening skills, advocacy and willingness to learn more than specific

---

**Box 15.4** How can primary care practitioners improve care for people with psychosis?

- It is all too easy to be pessimistic and underrate the patient's capacity to respond to treatment – health professionals should remember that therapeutic optimism is important.
- All health professionals need to admit to any stigmatising attitudes, and to check their thoughts and behaviour repeatedly – just as they do with other areas of discrimination.
- All health practitioners should possess sufficient understanding of mental health issues to help patients with psychiatric illness, but this does not mean they have to have specialist-level skills.

---

knowledge about mental health. A primary care practitioner who knows the patient, listens, can access help for mental health problems when required and approaches individuals with therapeutic optimism would be viewed by almost all patients as 'good enough'.

## Where next?

There are a number of cutting-edge issues in terms of primary healthcare and psychosis nationally and internationally, including the role of primary care in detecting young people with 'at risk' mental states' and the role of primary care in improving physical healthcare through pay-for-performance initiatives.

As the markers for those individuals at highest risk become more refined, there is hope that very early detection and intervention could reduce the progression to psychosis. Several studies are currently testing whether cognitive–behavioural therapy (CBT) and/or low-dose antipsychotic medication offered to individuals at ultra-high risk of psychosis can reduce the risk of subsequent psychosis, as well as ameliorate prodromal symptoms. Two such trials have already reported promising results. The PACE study in Melbourne (McGorry *et al*, 2002) has shown a reduction in the risk of FEP from 35% to 10% when patients were treated with low-dose atypical antipsychotics and CBT, but the benefits disappeared when the treatment was withdrawn. Morrison *et al* (2004) demonstrated almost the same lowered conversion rate to psychosis (i.e. 12%) with CBT alone in a similar group of patients. So far, however, these studies have been conducted in relatively small samples of people at high risk of psychosis, willing to seek help and in a research setting. It remains to be seen if the findings can be translated into a real-world intervention that is widely available to individuals with 'at risk' mental states. Nevertheless, for primary care, the implications of these studies are considerable. They could, for example, shift the focus towards primary care recognition and flagging up of individuals with key 'at risk' indicators and a different access route to a youth-oriented specialist assessment and psychological treatment service.

Perhaps the biggest sea change in terms of the delivery of primary care for people with psychosis in the UK was precipitated by the introduction of a pay-for-performance scheme in April 2004 (British Medical Association & NHS Confederation, 2003). The Quality and Outcomes Framework (QOF) is a voluntary scheme focused on achieving health-related targets across a variety of chronic disease, organisational, patient experience and additional service areas. Despite the voluntary nature of QOF and the independent contractor status of most GPs, it has been taken up by 99.6% of practices across the UK. Mental health indicators encourage: the development of a register of people with psychosis; monitoring of patients on lithium therapy; an annual review of physical health medication and coordination arrangements with secondary care; an indicator encouraging GPs to document a 'comprehensive care plan' in the primary care record, including a list of the patient's early-warning signs; and an indicator encouraging practices to follow up people who do not attend their annual review. The health check was included in response to evidence of minimal health promotion and prevention activity for primary care patients with psychosis, despite their risk factors (Kendrick, 1996; Burns & Cohen, 1998; Disability Rights Commission, 2005) (see also Box 15.1).

It is still too soon to see if these largely process measures will have a positive effect on patient health outcomes but, in implementation terms, it is encouraging to see that practices across England achieved an average of 89% of the points in the mental health domain in year 1 (2004–2005), 95% in year 2 (2005–2006), 92% in year 3 (2006–2007) and 93% in year 4 (2007–2008). There is now every reason to expect positive changes in the morbidity and mortality of people with psychosis in the UK over the next decade. (See Chapter 8 for information on QOF and depression in the UK.)

## Conclusion

Primary care is a key pathway player at the point of diagnosis and has an ongoing role in providing good-quality, proactive physical and mental healthcare. The primary care team also need to remember that they are supporting not just an individual, but their wider family, as they come to terms with the diagnosis and seek to make sense of the illness.

The biggest hurdle for primary care is the self-realisation that the contributions of generalism and family practice are essential and valued aspects of effective healthcare. A key clinical tool in this respect is an ethical, respectful, optimistic and trusting doctor–patient relationship.

Key points

- Primary care is an important partner in providing good-quality holistic care for patients with psychosis both at the point of diagnosis and in the longer term.
- General Practitioner (GP) recognition of early changes, clinical intuition and acting on family worries are key to earlier detection.
- High-quality care at the outset offers the possibility of a less traumatic and shorter pathway into mental health services, and the hope of improved longer-term outcomes. Primary care is uniquely placed by the nature of its long-term view of the clinical pathway, allowing it to make the connections between early detection of emerging illness and relapse, health promotion, physical illness and support for patients and families with longer-term difficulties.
- Primary care practitioners who know their patient, listen and can access help for mental health problems when required, are viewed by almost all patients as 'good enough'.
- The primary care team needs to remember that they are supporting not just an individual, but also their wider family, as they come to terms with the diagnosis and seek to make sense of the illness.

# Further reading and e-resources

Burns, T. & Kendrick, T. (1997) The primary care of patients with schizophrenia: a search for good practice. *British Journal of General Practice*, **47**, 515–520.

Thornicroft, G. (2006) *Shunned: Discrimination Against People with Mental Illness*. Oxford University Press. This book presents a fascinating and humane portrayal of the problem of stigma and discrimination, and shows how we can work to reduce it.

Warner, R. (2003) *Recovery from Schizophrenia: Psychiatry and Political Economy* (3rd edn). Brunner-Routledge. This book argues convincingly, but controversially, how political, economic and labour market forces shape social responses to people with mental illness, mould psychiatric treatment philosophy, and influence the onset and course of schizophrenia. It provides a guide on how to combat the stigma of mental illness at a local and national levels.

NHS West Midlands Regional Development Centre, http://www.westmidlands.csip.org.uk/mental-health/mental-health/early-intervention/early-intervention-resources.html. This page is a useful resource for health professionals, service users and carers, and includes links to pages such as the Early Psychosis Declaration jointly issued by the World Health Organization and International Early Psychosis Association in Newcastle, UK, in 2002.

Royal College of Psychiatrists, 'Changing Minds', http://www.rcpsych.ac.uk/campaigns/changingminds.aspx. This page on the UK Royal College of Psychiatrists' website is dedicated to the campaign to increase the understanding of mental health problems and to reduce stigma and discrimination.

US National Alliance on Mental Illness, http://www.nami.org/content/navigationmenu/grading_the_states/NAMIs_Grading_the_States_2006_Report.htm. This website contains information about a recent detailed report on the US health system for people with serious mental illness. The National Alliance on Mental Illness (NAMI) is the largest grass-roots mental health organisation in the USA dedicated to improving the lives of persons with serious mental illness and their families.

It is also worth noting that the National Institute for Health and Clinical Excellence (NICE) is revising the 2002 guidance on the treatment and management of schizophrenia in adults in primary and secondary care. This should be in the public domain from late 2009. See http://www.nice.org.uk/guidance/index.jsp?action=byId&o=11657

# References

Album, D. & Westin, S. (2007) Do diseases have a prestige hierarchy? A survey among physicians and medical students. *Social Science and Medicine*, **66**, 182–188.

Allebeck, P. (1989) Schizophrenia: a life-shortening disease. *Psychiatric Bulletin*, **15**, 81–89.

Bindman, J., Johnson, S., Wright S., *et al* (1997) Integration between primary and secondary services in the care of the severely mentally ill: patients' and general practitioners' views. *British Journal of Psychiatry*, **171**, 169–174.

Birchwood, M., Todd, P. & Jackson, C. (1998) Early intervention in psychosis, the critical period hypothesis. *British Journal of Psychiatry*, **172** (Suppl. 33), 53–59.

Bird, L. (1999) *The Fundamental Facts About Mental Illness*. Mental Health Foundation.

Bleuler, M. (1977) *The Schizophrenic Disorders* (trans. S. M. Clemens). Yale University Press.

British Medical Association & NHS Confederation (2003) *Investing in General Practice: The New General Medical Services Contract*. BMA.

British Psychological Society Report (2000) *Recent Advances in Understanding Mental Illness and Psychotic Experiences*. British Psychological Society.

Brown, S., Birtwhistle, J., Roe, L., *et al* (1999) The unhealthy lifestyle of people with schizophrenia. *Psychological Medicine*, **29**, 697–701.

Burnett, R., Mallett, R., Bhugra, G., *et al* (1999) The first contact of patients with schizophrenia with psychiatric services: social factors and pathways to care in multi-ethnic population. *Psychological Medicine*, **29**, 475–483.

Burns, T. & Cohen, A. (1998) Item of service payments for general practitioner care of severely mentally ill persons: does the money matter? *British Journal of General Practice*, **48**, 1415–1416.

Craig, T., Garety, P., Power, P., *et al* (2004) The Lambeth Early Onset (LEO) Team: randomised controlled trial of the effectiveness of specialised care for early psychosis. *BMJ*, **329**, 1067–71.

Department of Health (2000) *The NHS Plan. A Plan for Investment. A Plan for Reform.* Cm 4818-I. The Stationery Office.

Department of Health (2001) *The Mental Health Policy Implementation Guide.* Department of Health.

Department of Health (2002) *Improvement, Expansion and Reform – The Next 3 Years: Priorities and Planning Framework 2003–2006.* Department of Health.

Department of Health (2003) *National Statistics on Adults' Attitudes to Mental Illness in Great Britain.* Department of Health.

Disability Rights Commission (2005) *Equal Treatment: Closing the Gap.* DRC.

Harrigan, S. M., McGorry, P. D. & Krstev, H. (2003) Does treatment delay in first episode psychosis really matter? *Psychological Medicine*, **33**, 97–110.

Harris, E. C. & Barraclough, B. (1998) Excess mortality of mental disorder. *British Journal of Psychiatry*, **173**, 11–53.

Harrison, G., Hopper, K., Craig, T., *et al* (2001) Recovery from psychotic illness: a 15- and 25-year international follow-up study. *British Journal of Psychiatry*, **178**, 506–517.

Henderson, D., Cagliero, E., Gray, C., *et al* (2000) Clozapine, diabetes mellitus, weight gain, and lipid abnormalities: a five-year naturalistic study. *American Journal of Psychiatry*, **157**, 975–81.

Huxley, P. & Thornicroft, G. (2003) Social inclusion, social quality and mental illness. *British Journal of Psychiatry*, **182**, 298–290.

Jeffreys, S., Harvey, C., McNaught, A., *et al* (1997) The Hampstead schizophrenia survey 1991. 1: Prevalence and service use comparisons in an inner London health authority, 1986–91. *British Journal of Psychiatry*, **170**, 301–306.

Johns, L. C., Cannon, M., Singleton, N., *et al* (2004) Prevalence and correlates of self-reported psychotic symptoms in the British population. *British Journal of Psychiatry*, **185**, 298–305.

Kai, J., Crossland, A. & Drinkwater, C. (2000) Prevalence of enduring and disabling mental illness in the inner city. *British Journal of General Practice*, **50**, 922–924.

Kendrick, T. (1996) Cardiovascular and respiratory risk factors and symptoms among general practice patients with long-term mental illness. *British Journal of Psychiatry*, **169**, 733–739.

Kendrick, T., Burns, T., Freeling, P., *et al* (1994) Provision of care to general practice patients with disabling long-term mental illness: a survey in 16 practices. *British Journal of General Practice*, **44**, 301–305.

Kendrick, T., Burns, T., Garland, C., *et al* (2000) Are specialist mental health services being targeted on the most needy patients? The effects of setting up specialist services in general practice. *British Journal of General Practice*, **50**, 121–126.

Kirkbride, J. B., Fearon, P., Morgan, C., *et al* (2006) Heterogeneity in incidence rates of schizophrenia and other psychotic syndromes: findings from the 3-center AeSOP study. *Archives of General Psychiatry*, **63**, 250–258.

Lawrie, S. M., Parsons, C., Patrick, J., *et al* (1996) A controlled trial of general practitioners' attitudes to patients with schizophrenia. *Health Bulletin (Edinburgh)*, **54**, 210–213.

Lawrie, S. M., Martin, K., McNeill, G., *et al* (1998) General practitioners' attitudes to psychiatric and medical illness. *Psychological Medicine*, **28**, 1463–1467.

Lester, H. E. & Gask, L. (2006) Delivering medical care for patients with serious mental illness or promoting a collaborative model of recovery? *British Journal of Psychiatry*, **188**, 510–512.

Lester, H. E., Tritter, J. & England, E. (2003) Satisfaction with primary care: the perspectives of people with schizophrenia. *Family Practice*, **20**, 508–513.

Lester, H. E., Tritter, J. Q. & Sorohan, H. (2005) Providing primary care for people with serious mental illness: a focus group study. *BMJ*, **330**, 1122–1128.

McGlashan, T. M. (1999) Duration of untreated psychosis in first episode schizophrenia: marker or determinant of course? *Biological Psychiatry*, **46**, 899–907.

McGorry, P., Yung, A. R., Phillips, L. J., *et al* (2002) Randomized controlled trial of interventions designed to reduce the risk of progression to first-episode psychosis in a clinical sample with subthreshold symptoms. *Archives of General Psychiatry*, **59**, 921–928.

Moore, T., Zammit, S., Lingford-Hughes, A., *et al* (2007) Cannabis use and risk of psychosis or affective mental health outcomes: a systematic review. *Lancet*, **370**, 319–328.

Morrison, A. P., French, P., Walford, L., *et al* (2004) Cognitive therapy for the prevention of psychosis in people at ultra-high risk: randomized controlled trial. *British Journal of Psychiatry*, **185**, 291–297.

National Alliance on Mental Illness (2006) *Grading the States. A Report on America's Health Care System for Serious Mental Illness*. NAMI.

Nazareth, I., King, M. & Haines, A. (1993) Care of schizophrenia in general practice. *BMJ*, **307**, 910.

Office for National Statistics (2003) *Labour Force Survey, Autumn 2003*. ONS.

Owen, M. G., Faris, R. E. L. & Dunham, W. (1941) Alternative hypotheses for the explanation of some of Faris' and Dunham's results. *American Journal of Sociology*, **47**, 48–52.

Peterson, L., Jeppesen, P., Thorup, A., *et al* (2005) A randomised multicentre trial of integrated versus standard treatment for patients with a first episode of psychotic illness. *BMJ*, **331**, 602–606.

Pinfold, V., Smith, J. & Shiers, D. (2007) Audit of early intervention in psychosis service development in England in 2005. *Psychiatric Bulletin*, **31**, 7–10.

Rethink (2002) *Reaching People Early*. RETHINK.

Rethink (2003) *Under Pressure*. RETHINK.

Rodgers, J., Black, G., Stobbart, A., *et al* (2003) Audit of primary care of people with schizophrenia in general practice in Lothian. *Quality in Primary Care*, **11**, 133–140.

Saha, S., Chant , D. & McGrath, J. (2007) A systematic review of mortality in schizophrenia. *Archives of General Psychiatry*, **64**, 1123–1131.

Scull, A. T. (1979) *Museums Of Madness: The Social Organization of Insanity in Nineteenth Century England*. St Martin's Press.

Skeate, A., Jackson, C., Birchwood, M., *et al* (2002) Duration of untreated psychosis and pathways to care in first-episode psychosis. *British Journal of Psychiatry*, **181**, s73–s77.

van Os, J., Hanssen, M., Bijl, R. V., *et al* (2000) Strauss (1969) revisited: a psychosis continuum in the normal population? *Schizophrenia Research*, **45**, 11–20.

Warner, R. (2003) *Recovery from Schizophrenia: Psychiatry and Political Economy* (3rd edn). Brunner-Routledge.

World Health Organization (2004) *Guide to Mental and Neurological Health in Primary Care*. Royal Society of Medicine Press.

Yung, A. R., Organ, B. A. & Harris, M. G. (2003) Management of early psychosis in a generic adult mental health service. *Australian and New Zealand Journal of Psychiatry*, **37**, 429–436.

# CHAPTER 16

# Emergencies in primary care

Tony Kendrick and Helen Lester

### Summary

This chapter discusses what primary care professionals need to do when they are called upon to help people with acutely disturbed behaviour, and people at risk of suicide. It covers diagnosis, the management of the acute situation, including drug treatment and referral, and issues to consider when compulsory admission to hospital seems to be required. The Mental Health Act (applicable to England and Wales) is summarised and brief reference is made to the legal framework for compulsory admission in other countries.

## Acutely disturbed behaviour

General practitioners (GPs) are not regularly called to attend people with acutely disturbed behaviour, but when they do it is often as an emergency, and assessment may be quite challenging. It is usually necessary to see the person at home, in a public place, or a police station, and family, friends, or the police are expecting urgent action to help defuse a tense situation, as well as advice and help for the person in acute distress.

First and foremost, it is crucial to determine whether an episode of acute disturbance in a person's behaviour is due to physical illness (especially in elderly patients), the effects of drugs (whether prescribed or recreational), or an acute mental health problem, because the management of these different types of problem is quite different.

It is important therefore to obtain a history wherever possible from a family member or other carer who can describe the person's behaviour before the acute disturbance and any drugs they may have taken, as this is key to making a correct diagnosis.

### Acute confusional state (or delirium)

This usually occurs in elderly patients, and more often among those with pre-existing dementia. The onset is quick, over a few hours, and typically there is fluctuation in the level of consciousness, with periods of drowsiness between bouts of disturbed behaviour or mood swings, which distinguishes acute confusion from psychiatric disorders. Patients may have visual and tactile hallucinations and disorientation in time and place, and sometimes an altered level of consciousness. They may also present as being either overaroused (e.g. restlessness, overactivity, psychotic symptoms), or underaroused (e.g. slowness, reduced speech, inactivity).

As well as chest or urinary infections, less common causes include drug side-effects (opiate analgesics, sedatives, anti-Parkinson drugs, hypoglycaemics, etc.), renal failure, heart failure, liver failure and subdural haematoma (Box 16.1). Immediate investigations for physical problems should be instigated (blood count, electrolytes, chest X-ray, urine testing, etc.) and the cause treated as appropriate. Often patients with acute confusion need to be admitted to hospital if they cannot be nursed at home satisfactorily by family or home nursing teams. If admission is necessary, this should be under the care of the *medical* team rather than to a psychiatric ward. Very rarely sedation is required to help the person calm down enough to admit him or her to hospital or to allow nursing care. Usually it should be avoided, as it will only add to the confusion. Where it is unavoidable, a fast-acting and short-lived benzodiazepine such as lorazepam (0.5–1 mg orally) may be used.

---

**Box 16.1** Causes of acute behavioural disturbance

**Physical causes**

- Acute infections in the elderly (consider urinary infection if there is no history to suggest chest or other infection) causing an *acute confusional state*, or delirium
- Hypoglycaemia in patients on treatment for diabetes
- Hypoxia due to heart or lung disorders
- Acute head injury, or a chronic subdural haematoma following previous head injury in an older person
- Post-ictal confusion after an epileptic convulsion

**Drug and substance misuse**

- Acute alcohol intoxication, or delirium tremens due to alcohol withdrawal
- Steroid 'psychosis'
- Amphetamine 'psychosis'

**Acute mental health problems**

- Acute schizophrenia or psychotic depression
- Hypomanic episode of bipolar disorder
- Personality disorder
- Severe anxiety disorder, panic disorder

# Acute mental health problems

## Non-psychotic

Non-psychotic acute mental health problems include acute anxiety states, agitated depression and impulsive behaviours arising from fear or from poor anger control. The person may have received a previous diagnosis of anxiety disorder (particularly panic disorder) or agitated depression, or the label of 'personality disorder' if a pattern of repeated disturbed behaviour has been established in the absence of diagnosable anxiety, depressive or psychotic disorder. Such a pattern may be exacerbated by drug or alcohol misuse.

It is important to get relevant information from the patient, from the medical record and where possible from a family member or friend, and to obtain any past history of mental health problems or any use of prescribed or recreational drugs, and a description of the circumstances leading up to the acute disturbance in behaviour.

## Psychotic

A history of changes in mood, sleep pattern, fatigue, irritability, loss of appetite and heightened sensitivity to pain is common to both non-psychotic and psychotic mental health problems. However, auditory hallucinations and delusions suggest a psychotic problem, which is likely to take longer to settle and to pose more challenges in management (see also Chapter 15). Amphetamine misuse is a possible cause of acute psychotic symptoms, and the use of recreational drugs should be enquired after, from the patient and, if there is any doubt, from immediate family or friends (see also Chapter 17).

## Approach to the consultation

If the person has a history of violent behaviour, it is crucial to ask for support from the police before seeing him or her. As much information as possible should be gathered beforehand from the medical records, and the patient's family or friends, especially about possible drug or alcohol misuse. If the person is at home, visiting health professionals should inform someone else at 'base' that they are visiting, arrange to let them know when they have seen the patient, and that they should call the police if they do not call them back at the end of the visit as expected.

When seeing the patient, it is advisable to talk slowly and move slowly. Health professionals should position themselves between the patient and the exit to avoid getting trapped, and be prepared to leave quickly if they feel at all threatened or acutely uncomfortable. The patient should not be made to feel trapped either, and a health professional should not try to restrain them.

## Management

Management at home is advisable only where the cause of the behavioural disturbance is clear, the behaviour is already settling or likely to settle quickly, and the person is well supported by family or friends. Sedation at home should usually be avoided. Occasionally sedation may help defuse the situation and avoid referral to hospital, if the patient will accept it. If so, suitable drugs include a single dose of an oral benzodiazepine such as diazepam(5–10 mg) or lorazepam (0.5–1 mg).

Referral to specialist mental health services is often indicated for psychotic behavioural disturbance, if not immediately then within hours or a few days at most. In the UK, functionalised teams such as assertive outreach and home treatment teams are often used as alternatives to a hospital admission. These teams are staffed by individuals with experience of working with people who are acutely unwell, and provide support in the community 24 hours a day, 7 days a week. If patients decline to go to hospital voluntarily, then compulsory admission under mental health law may be necessary. Occasionally, sedation with an antipsychotic medication (i.e. a neuroleptic or major tranquilliser) may help calm the situation pending referral to hospital, but this should usually be avoided unless absolutely necessary. Suitable medications include oral chlorpromazine (50–100 mg) or, very unusually, intramuscular chlorpromazine (50 mg) or haloperidol (1–3 mg). However, sedation should be avoided if the patient has any respiratory problems, or is thought to have taken any sedatives or alcohol.

## Iatrogenic states

### Acute dystonias

Torticollis of the neck or oculogyric crisis (distortion of the face and frozen eye movements) may occur within hours (after an oral dose) or minutes (if given intramuscularly) of giving chlorpromazine or haloperidol, but can be quickly relieved with intramuscular procyclidine (5–10 mg).

### Neuroleptic malignant syndrome (NMS)

This is a potentially fatal condition caused by psychotropic drugs (usually antipsychotics). Patients usually present with sweating/pyrexia, rigidity and confusion, and their level of consciousness may fluctuate. Sometimes they have tachycardia and a fluctuating blood pressure. The symptoms may develop rapidly, over 24–72 hours. In people with intellectual disability, the syndrome may present as an increase in challenging behaviour. If NMS is suspected, the antipsychotic drug should be stopped and the patient immediately referred to the medical team.

Patients at greater risk of developing NMS include:

* males
* agitated or dehydrated individuals
* those who recently started taking a neuroleptic drug or an increased dose
* people on intramuscular or high-dose neuroleptic drugs
* people with a history of organic brain disease (including intellectual disability and dementia).

## Lithium toxicity

Symptoms usually occur at a serum-lithium level over 1.5 mmol/litre. The patient may present with confusion and ataxia associated with diarrhoea, vomiting, drowsiness and a coarse tremor.

- If symptoms are mild, urgent testing of kidney function and lithium levels is requried. If levels are high (over 1.2 mmol/l), then the lithium should be stopped and further management discussed with the responsible psychiatrist.
- If the patient is unwell and lithium toxicity is suspected, an immediate referral should be made to the medical team for hydration.

## Serotonin syndrome

Rarely, serotonergic drugs, usually in combination, can cause a syndrome of diarrhoea, shivering, myoclonus, hyper-reflexia and/or agitation. Treatment generally involves withdrawing the medication and supportive measures. Symptoms usually resolve within 24 hours. In rare, more severe cases, autonomic instability can occur and if this is the case the patient should be referred urgently to the medical team.

## Antidepressant withdrawal

All antidepressants can cause withdrawal symptoms on stopping. These symptoms are usually mild and self-limiting but can occasionally be severe, particularly if the drug is stopped abruptly. Of the selective serotonin reuptake inhibitors, paroxetine and venlafaxine seem to be associated with a greater frequency of withdrawal reactions. The most commonly experienced reactions include dizziness, numbness and tingling, gastrointestinal disturbances (particularly nausea and vomiting), headache, sweating, anxiety, agitation and sleep disturbances.

These usually occur in the first days of discontinuing but may occur after a 'missed' dose. If the withdrawal symptoms are mild, reassurance that they will resolve is usually all that is needed. If the symptoms are severe, the antidepressant should be restarted at the dose that was effective (or changed to a drug with a longer half-life, e.g. fluoxetine) and the dose gradually reduced while the symptoms are monitored.

## Benzodiazepine withdrawal

Symptoms of benzodiazepine withdrawal include agitation, restlessness, poor concentration, hypersensitivity to light and sound, depression and flu-like symptoms. Rarely, abrupt withdrawal can precipitate fits or psychosis. Patients who have had a fit should immediately be referred to the emergency department. Patients managed in primary care should have their benzodiazepines restarted, but changed to diazepam, which has a longer half-life, which is then withdrawn gradually. Patients presenting complicated cases should be referred to a community drug team.

# Patients at risk of suicide

The important issue of suicide is discussed in detail in Chapter 9. However, the key issues are also highlighted in this section.

The average GP in the UK, with 1800 registered patients, is likely to have a patient commit suicide only once every 5 years (which means that there will be one every year on average in a group practice of 10 000 patients). However, many more patients will be seen who are at an increased risk of suicide, including those who present with depression or psychotic illness, and those who have made suicide attempts in the past. Health professionals working in areas of higher prevalence of mental disorders, particularly in inner cities, will see more suicides. Data for the three years 2003–05 show a rate of 8.5 deaths per 100 000 population – a reduction of 7.4% from 1995–97 (Care Services Improvement Partnership, 2006).

It is difficult to predict suicide in any individual case. Known risk factors are listed in Box 16.2, in ascending order of predictive utility (Crowley et al, 2004). Most of the socio-demographic risk factors, which are derived from epidemiological studies of completed suicides, are not very strong predictors by themselves or even in combination. The most significant predictor is a history of attempted suicide in the past.

## Assessment of risk

Many patients visit their GP or other member of the primary care team in the weeks or days leading up to a suicide attempt, which provides an opportunity for assessment (Houston et al, 2003). In assessing risk, it is important for the practitioner to ask specific questions about suicidal ideas and plans (such questioning is not in itself likely to put the thought of suicide into the minds of patients not already considering it). It is crucial to identify any specific plans for suicide, especially where preparatory steps have already been taken. Useful questions include (in order of intrusiveness):

- How does the future look to you? What are your hopes?
- Do you wish you could just not wake up in the morning?
- Have you considered doing anything to harm yourself, or to take your own life?
- Have you made actual plans to kill yourself? What are they?
- What has stopped you from doing anything so far?

A systematic review concluded that it is possible to identify people at higher risk of suicide (Hider, 1998). Suicide is (thankfully) a rare outcome, and it is not possible to mount randomised controlled trials large enough to demonstrate that suicide can be prevented by good primary care. Intuitively, however, a systematic assessment of risk factors and subsequent positive action when risk is high is the best way for primary care professionals to respond when faced with a person with depression or other mental health problem.

---

**Box 16.2** Risk factors for suicide

**Socio-demographic**

- Females more likely to attempt suicide
- Males more likely to die by suicide
- Younger people and older people more likely to kill themselves than middle-aged adults
- Lower socio-economic status; leaving education earlier; unemployment
- Same-sex sexual orientation
- Prisoners

**Family and childhood**

- Certain ethnic groups – in the UK young women from the Indian subcontinent
- Parental depression, substance misuse, or suicide
- Parental divorce, difficult family circumstances
- Bullying

**Mental health problems**

- Impulsive, aggressive, or socially withdrawn
- Poor problem-solving ability
- Mood disorders, especially bipolar disorder
- Substance misuse
- Schizophrenia
- Recent discharge from mental hospital

**Suicidal behaviour**

- Access to means (guns, drugs, tablets)
- History of suicide attempts
- Specific plans of suicide

---

## Interventions known to reduce suicide risk

### Limiting access to the means of suicide

There is evidence that limiting access to the means of suicide reduces the population risk (e.g. changing from coal gas to natural gas; restricting the amount of paracetamol sold per packet; Gunnell *et al*, 2004). Suicide attempts are often impulsive; patients who fail to kill themselves usually regret it and in the main do not repeat their attempt. Patients at risk of suicide should not be prescribed medication in large amounts, to reduce the risk of impulsive overdose. The selective serotonin reuptake inhibitors are safer in overdose than the tricyclics and related antidepressants, as they are less likely to cause ventricular tachycardia going on to ventricular fibrillation.

### Follow-up of patients discharged from hospital

The risk of suicide is high in the first 4 weeks after discharge from psychiatric hospital, especially if the patient is not actively followed up by the mental health team (King *et al*, 2001). Primary care teams should therefore ensure their discharged patients are enrolled in a care plan after discharge. *Avoidable Deaths*, a report from the National Confidential Inquiry into Suicide and Homicide by People with Mental Illness (2006), estimated that 56 mental health patients discharged from hospital died following non-compliance with medication or loss of contact with services. Supervised community treatment (SCT), a measure to improve clinical risk management that the government is introducing into the Mental Health Act 2007 (Box 16.3), has the potential to help prevent those deaths.

Patients who have attempted suicide need active follow-up. Nine out of 10 patients who attempt suicide do so with an overdose, and so may be admitted to an accident and emergency department for gastric lavage and observation overnight. Many leave the next day without waiting for a psychiatric assessment, and so it is important for the GP or other member of the primary care team to follow up patients who have taken overdoses, whether they seem to have been genuine attempts at suicide or seem more likely to have been attempts to communicate distress or change a painful life situation. A history of suicide attempts is the biggest single predictor of subsequent suicide, even though the large majority of those who take overdoses will not go on to kill themselves (Isometsa & Lonqvist, 1998).

## Emergency referral of patients at high risk

Where patients indicate their intent to kill themselves, and express hopelessness for the future, they should be referred for an immediate psychiatric assessment, especially in the presence of significant depression or other mental health problem, or drug or alcohol misuse. If patients decline to be assessed voluntarily, it may be necessary to admit them compulsorily under the Mental Health Act.

## Compulsory admission under the Mental Health Act (England & Wales) 1983

It is best for the patient, the family, and the health professionals to try to obtain voluntary admission. However, if that is impossible, for patients with a mental disorder who pose a risk to themselves or others, compulsion may be necessary. Mental illness is not defined by the Mental Health Act and is left to clinical judgement but does not include alcohol or drug misuse alone. More information can be found at http://www.hyperguide.co.uk/mha

Section 2, admission for assessment, is the most commonly used section of the Act in the community. It provides for compulsory admission and detention at a hospital for 28 days for assessment. The application must be made by an approved social worker (ASW) or the nearest relative. The ASW should make the application rather than the nearest relative wherever possible, to avoid adversely affecting family relationships. Following that, the recommendations of two independent doctors are needed, one of whom

**Box 16.3** Summary of the amendments to the 1983 Mental Health Act introduced by the Mental Health Act 2007

- *Definition of mental disorder*. It changes the way the 1983 Act defines mental disorder, so that a single definition applies throughout the Act, and abolishes references to categories of disorder. These amendments complement the changes to the criteria for detention.
- *Criteria for detention*. It introduces a new 'appropriate medical treatment' test, which will apply to all the longer-term powers of detention. As a result, it will not be possible for patients to be compulsorily detained or for their detention to be continued unless medical treatment that is appropriate to the patient's mental disorder and all other circumstances of the case is available to that patient. At the same time, the so-called 'treatability test' will be abolished.
- *Professional roles*. It is broadening the groups of practitioners who can take on the functions currently performed by the approved social worker (ASW) and responsible medical officer (RMO).
- *Nearest relative* (NR). It gives to patients the right to make an application to displace their NR and enables county courts to displace an NR where there are reasonable grounds for doing so. The provisions for determining the NR will be amended to include civil partners.
- *Supervised community treatment* (SCT). It introduces SCT for patients following a period of detention in hospital. It is expected that this will allow a small number of patients with a mental disorder to live in the community while subject to certain conditions under the 1983 Act, to ensure they continue with the medical treatment that they need. Currently, some patients leave hospital and do not continue with their treatment, their health deteriorates and they require detention again – the so-called 'revolving door'.
- *Mental health review tribunal* (MHRT). It introduces an order-making power to reduce the time before a case has to be referred to the MHRT by the hospital managers. It also introduces a single tribunal for England; the one in Wales remains in being.
- *Age-appropriate services*. It requires hospital managers to ensure that patients aged under 18 admitted to hospital for mental disorder are accommodated in an environment that is suitable for their age (subject to their needs).
- *Advocacy*. It places a duty on the appropriate national authority to make arrangements for help to be provided by independent mental health advocates.
- *Electroconvulsive therapy*. It introduces new safeguards for patients.

must be 'approved' under the Act and one, if practicable, must have prior knowledge of the patient. Ideally, therefore, a GP who knows the patient should attend wherever possible.

Section 4, emergency admission for assessment, can be used in situations where admission is urgent and compliance with section 2 would cause undesirable delay. It provides for 72 hours of admission for urgent assessment. In extreme urgency, the doctor can ask the nearest relative to make the application and apply the section alone. However, it should still ideally involve an ASW rather than the nearest relative.

In the UK, mental health practitioners across the country are now faced with the task of implementing the Mental Health Act 2007. The main changes to the 1983 Act are shown in Box 16.3.

---

Key points

- Patients experiencing a psychiatric emergency can feel overwhelmed and vulnerable and it is important to understand how distressing this can be for patients and those around them. Most patients with mental health problems pose no physical risk to either themselves or others.
- It is crucial to determine whether an episode of acute disturbance in a person's behaviour is due to physical illness, the effects of drugs, or an acute mental health problem, because the management of these different types of problem is quite different.
- Many patients visit their GP or other member of the primary care team in the weeks or days leading up to a suicide attempt, which provides an opportunity for assessment.

---

# Further reading and e-resources

National Institute for Health and Clinical Excellence (2004) *Self-Harm: The Short-Term Physical and Psychological Management and Secondary Prevention of Self-Harm in Primary and Secondary Care*. NICE. Downloadable from http://www.nice.org.uk

http://www.mhact.csip.org.uk/silo/files/national-suicide-prevention-strategy-for-england-annual-report-on-progress-2006.pdf. This report describes how measures to reduce the suicide rate have been implemented as part of the national suicide prevention strategy for England.

## *Legislation*

The Mental Health (Care and Treatment) (Scotland) Act 2003 was passed by the Scottish Parliament in March 2003 and came into effect in April 2005. See both:
http://www.scotland.gov.uk/Publications/2004/01/18753/31686
http://www.opsi.gov.uk/legislation/scotland/acts2003/asp_20030013_en_1.htm

The Mental Health Act 1983 applies only to people in England and Wales. See http://www.dh.gov.uk/en/Healthcare/NationalServiceFrameworks/Mentalhealth/DH_4001816
For a summary of the amendments to the 1983 Act see http://www.dh.gov.uk/en/Healthcare/NationalServiceFrameworks/Mentalhealth/DH_078743

# References

Care Services Improvement Partnership (2006) *National Suicide Prevention Strategy for England. Annual Report on Progress*. CSIP.

Crowley, P., Kilroe, J. & Burke, S. (2004) *Youth Suicide Prevention*. Health Development Agency.

Gunnell, D., Bennewith, O., Peters, T. J., *et al* (2004) The epidemiology and management of self-harm amongst adults in England. *Journal of Public Health*, **27**, 67–73.

Hider, P. (1998) Youth suicide prevention by primary healthcare professionals: a critical appraisal of the literature. New Zealand health technology assessment (NZHTA) 4. New Zealand Health Technology Assessment Clearing House.

Houston, K., Haw, C., Townsend E., *et al* (2003) General practitioner contacts with patients before and after deliberate self-harm. *British Journal of General Practice*, **53**, 365–370.

Isometsa, E. T. & Lonqvist, J. K. (1998) Suicide attempts preceding completed suicide. *British Journal of Psychiatry*, **173**, 531–535.

King, E. A., Baldwin, D. S., Sinclair, J. M., *et al* (2001) The Wessex Recent In-Patient Suicide Study, 1: case–control study of 234 recently discharged psychiatric patient suicides. *British Journal of Psychiatry*, **178**, 531–536.

National Confidential Inquiry into Suicide and Homicide by People with Mental Illness (2006) *Avoidable Deaths – Five Year Report of the National Confidential Inquiry into Suicide and Homicide by People with Mental Illness*. University of Manchester.

# CHAPTER 17

# Substance misuse

Clare Gerada

Summary

Primary care is a significant point of contact for drug users who require treatment. Managing drug users is a rewarding part of general practice work and can bring about significant and long-lasting positive changes in the patient.

Primary care is a significant point of contact for drug users who require treatment and many patients see this route of care as being readily accessible and less stigmatising than traditional specialist addiction services. Research shows that patients prefer care from a competent general practitioner (GP) rather than from other professionals.

In the UK, government policy has promoted GPs as an important facet of modern healthcare for these patients and, indeed, the past two decades are littered with policy documents, health service circulars and government strategies laying the foundations for effective primary care involvement in a primary-care-led National Health Service (NHS). To a large degree, GPs have responded to the challenge and collectively are undoubtedly the backbone of drug misuse treatment services, including the provision of substitute medication.

## Who uses drugs and why

The use of illicit drugs, such as cocaine, heroin, ecstasy and cannabis, is prevalent in every part of society and across all socio-economic groups. Use of illicit substances is, in the most part, transient and part of the adolescent stage of development. The factors that predict why an individual goes from experimental to problematic use are complex and are the result of the interplay between social, environmental and individual factors (Box 17.1).

Box 17.1 Predictive factors for problematic drug use

- Age (peaks among people in their mid-20s)
- Gender (use is much higher among men than among women)
- School failure (high rates of truancy or exclusion among drug users)
- History of inconsistent parenting
- Poverty
- Drug use

Adapted from Bry (1996).

Drug misuse or drug use is not the same as dependence. Dependence is a specific psychological state in which drug use takes an overriding importance in people's lives and when they do not have the drug, they crave it. Dependence is characterised by (World Health Organization, 1992):

- compulsion to use
- difficulty in controlling use (e.g. alcohol dependence is characterised by an inability to moderate drinking)
- a withdrawal state on cessation of use
- evidence of tolerance (i.e. requiring increasing amounts of the drug to produce the same effect)
- progressive neglect of other activity because of substance use
- persisting with use despite evidence that use is becoming or has become harmful.

Problem drug use is defined as injecting drug use or long duration/regular use of opiates, cocaine and/or amphetamines. Although small in terms of overall numbers, problem drug users are responsible for a disproportionate share of the health and social problems resulting from drug consumption. In the UK, problem drug use is characterised by the use of heroin, often in combination with other drugs.

## Impact of drug users on health and social care

### Case 1

Mary is a 39-year-old user of heroin and crack cocaine. She has three children, two of whom are in local-authority care. She currently has an 8-year-old child living with her and her partner. She is hepatitis C positive. Despite many treatment episodes, she continues to inject and has recently been admitted to the local hospital with septicaemia. During her in-patient stay, her child was cared for by foster parents.

Drug users are involved in all areas of the health and social care services. Some of the harmful effects of drug use are summarised below.

- *Accident and emergency*. Drug users utilise accident and emergency departments to a great extent. Gossop *et al* (2003) found that half of all drug users surveyed reported attending an accident and emergency department in the 2 years before treatment, most often because of a drug overdose.

- *Obstetrics, women's health and maternity services.* Around one in three drug users attending treatment services are women and most of these are of childbearing age. Babies born to women who use drugs are at greater risk of being born prematurely or small for dates, and if the exposed to opiates the infants risk neonatal addiction and withdrawal.
- *Primary care.* A national survey of English GPs estimated that at least half of all GPs have seen a drug user in the previous 4 weeks and half of these GPs had prescribed substitution medication to an average of four patients. Each GP is likely to have at least two patients per 1800 list with a drug use problem, and this increases to around 4–8/1800 in areas of high prevalence (Gerada & Harris, 2005).
- *Mental health (adult, child and adolescent) services.* It is estimated that 30% of patients attending community mental health services have substance misuse problems and drug misuse coexisting with mental health problems *and* are more likely to have prolonged in-patient stays. There are increasing concerns about adolescent mental health and drug use. Rates of drug use among young people are reported to be on the increase.
- *General medicine.* It is estimated that 25% of admissions to general hospital are alcohol-related and a significant proportion of these are likely to be a combination of drug and alcohol misuse. The National Treatment Outcome Research Study (NTORS) reported that 25% of patients entering drug treatment services had received treatment involving admission to a general hospital in the previous 2 years (Gossop *et al*, 2003). If this were reflected in the population as a whole, it would amount to approximately 50000 admissions per annum.
- *Child protection.* An estimated 200000–300000 children in England and Wales live in households where one or both parents have serious drug problems, and only 37% of fathers and 64% of mothers with drug problems live with their children. Although serious drug use does not automatically diminish the capacity to parent, it increases the potential for negative family processes and for disruptive lives (Advisory Council of the Misuse of Drugs, 2003).
- *Genito-urinary medicine.* It is well recognised that individuals attending sexual health services have high rates of alcohol and drug misuse.
- *Homelessness services.* Over half of homeless individuals have substance misuse problems (Wright, 2002).

## Physical complications of drug use

The complications of drug use are related to:

- the drug(s) used (e.g. opiates, amphetamines and benzodiazepines all have different effects and side-effects)

259

- the route of drug use (injecting is associated with more complications than smoking or oral route)
- the lifestyle associated with the drug-using habit (e.g. poor housing, unemployment, involvement in crime).

Injecting is a key factor in the transmission of blood-borne viruses (principally hepatitis B and C, and HIV) and in many overdose deaths. Tackling risky injecting behaviour lies at the heart of combating blood-borne viruses and overdose deaths among drug users (Health Protection Agency *et al*, 2006).

## Blood-borne viruses

Over a third (34%) of all cases of hepatitis B in England are associated with injecting drug use. The prevalence rate of hepatitis B among injecting drug users in the UK is estimated to be around 20%, with wide variation between countries and regions.

Over 90% of hepatitis C diagnoses are associated with injecting drug use in England, with current prevalence rates of hepatitis C among injecting drug users in England estimated to be 44% and in the UK almost 50% (meaning that one in two injecting drug users are infected).

Injecting drugs accounted for 5.6% of HIV diagnosis reported in England and 6.7% in Scotland. The overall prevalence of HIV among injecting drug misusers in England and Wales remains relatively low, at 2% (1 in 50) infected, but the prevalence in London is much higher, at 4% (1 in 25) infected.

## Drug-related overdose

Recorded rates of drug-related death due to overdose in the UK are among the highest in Europe. In the UK, acute drug-related deaths accounted for more than 7% of all deaths among those aged 15–39 years in 2004. Following steep increases in the rate of drug-related overdose deaths in the 1990s, just over 1500 drug-related overdose deaths were recorded in England alone in 2005. The vast majority of these were associated with injecting heroin misuse in combination with use of alcohol, benzodiazepines or other depressants. A significant proportion of drug-related overdose deaths occur among drug misusers who have just left prison. Deaths associated with methadone have significantly reduced over the past 5 years, probably partly reflecting implementation of supervised consumption of methadone prescriptions in the initial stages of drug treatment (European Monitoring Centre for Drugs and Drug Addiction, 2006).

# Treatment pathways

## Presentation

### Case 2
Charles, a 27-year-old man who is new to the surgery, comes late one evening complaining of skin infections. He looks unwell, seems gaunt and

generally unkempt. The GP examines him and finds that he has multiple small skin abscesses mainly around his forearms. On further questioning he admits that they are the result of injecting heroin under the skin (skin popping).

### Case 3

Philip is a 23-year-old patient of the practice. He has been registered for many years and the GP remembers him as a rather troubled young man. He attends accompanied by his mother. She begins to cry and says she has just found out that Philip has been using heroin for 2 years. She found some tin foil in his room and he admitted that he was smoking heroin. She begs the GP to help him.

As already discussed in this chapter, drug users, and especially injecting drug users, have high rates of ill health and therefore are high users of health services. A long-term follow-up of heroin addicts showed they had a mortality risk nearly 12 times greater than that of the general population (Oppenheimer *et al*, 1994). Another study of injecting drug misusers showed that they were 22 times more likely to die during the study period than their non-injecting peers (Frischer *et al*, 1997). Drug users may present to general practice either as a direct result of complications of their drug use (e.g. abscesses, infections) or they, or their families, may present requesting help for their drug problem. However the patient presents, it is important for the doctor, nurse or pharmacist to realise the importance of their role in helping to engage the user in treatment and hopefully beginning a treatment relationship that will succeed. All GPs should be able to:

- to take a drug history (what, what route, how much, how often, how long and why?)
- to take a treatment history (where, what, longest period of abstinence?)
- to assess for complications of drug taking (risk of hepatitis C, B, HIV, presence of abscesses, cellulitis)
- to develop treatment plans (what does the patient want?).

The level of involvement beyond this depends on the model of treatment provision in the particular area. Again, a GP should be able to provide, at the very least:

- advice about safer injecting (do not share!)
- testing for blood-borne viruses (hepatitis B, C and HIV)
- immunisation against hepatitis B
- advice about where to seek further help.

## Treatment

Treatment encompasses a range of interventions, which includes the provision of harm-minimisation advice and managing general health problems. Details are given in Table 17.1 for opiate users.

GPs with additional training and expertise may be in a position to offer specific interventions, such as:

- management of withdrawal
- maintenance treatment
- treatment aimed at relapse prevention.

Drug users are a heterogeneous group of individuals and treatments need to be flexible enough to meet their multiple needs. Abstinence is the overall treatment goal but to achieve this may take many years and will involve many treatment episodes.

Drug treatment in the UK has largely been focused on:

- engaging and attracting the patient into treatment by providing easily accessible 'walk-in' community-based services

**Table 17.1** Summary of different treatments for opiate users

| Intervention | Nature and objective of intervention |
|---|---|
| *Detoxification* | Term use used to describe withdrawal from drugs, with or without adjunctive medication, that lasts less than 12 weeks in a community setting or 4 weeks in a residential setting |
| Self-detoxification (reducing illicit heroin use over time) | Usually involves the patient withdrawing from opiates over a number of days or weeks |
| Non-opiate-based symptomatic treatments, such as clonidine, lofexidine, loperamide, diclofenac, temazepam | The patient may be placed on naltrexone after the detoxification process is complete – usually at least 5 days from last opiate use |
| Gradually tapering doses of methadone | |
| Gradually tapering doses of buprenorphine | |
| *Maintenance* | Usually implies stable prescribing for 6 months or more |
| Methadone (Farrell *et al*, 1994) | Considered to be the 'gold standard' for opiate substitution. There is a great deal of evidence, much derived from randomised controlled trails, to show that maintenance treatment works in reducing the harm associated with drug taking and in improving the physical, social and mental functioning of the individual. There is also evidence of a reduction in the rate of involvement in criminal activity |
| Buprenorphine | Newer treatment in the UK and potentially very useful. Trials are showing that it is as effective as methadone in improving outcomes for opiate users |
| *Relapse prevention* Naltrexone | Usually taken orally and blocks the effects of opiates for up to 72 hours |

- offering substitute medication for opiate addiction
- providing access to community-based or residential rehabilitation
- ensuring that out-of-treatment and hard-to-reach drug users are able to access harm-reduction interventions, for example needle-exchange programmes.

The general aims of treatment are for the patient:

- to reduce the physical, psychological and social problems associated with drug taking
- to reduce the harmful or risky behaviours associated with using drugs (e.g. sharing equipment, injecting drug use)
- to attain controlled, non-dependent or non-problematic drug use (e.g. intermittent and appropriate use of benzodiazepines)
- to abstain from illicit drug use
- to abstain from all drug use (prescribed, as well as drugs illicitly obtained).

Treatment works! A number of large-scale studies have shown the efficacy of evidence-based interventions. UK and international evidence consistently shows that different treatment interventions, in different treatment settings, and covering different types of drug problem, can reduce levels of drug use, offending, overdose risk and the spread of blood-borne viruses. The National Institute for Health and Clinical Excellence (NICE) has published two guidelines on a range of drug treatment interventions (National Institute for Health and Clinical Excellence, 2007a,b), and these endorse much of the mainstream drug treatment provided in the UK as evidence-based and cost-effective.

## Primary care involvement

Primary care is at the heart of the provision of healthcare (and increasingly social care) services to patients. Collectively there are around 1 million consultations per day in primary care in the UK and almost all patients will consult with their family doctor over a 3-year period. For drug users, primary care provides an accessible avenue to treatment and for the families and carers of drug users the GP or practice nurse is often the first port of call for help. The level of involvement of GPs will be determined by a number of factors, such as the local arrangements for the management of substance use and the level of training/competence and expertise of the different clinicians. Over the years, there has been a major expansion of GP management of drug users with demonstration of the feasibility and the value of such primary care provision. A national survey looking at community-dispensed prescriptions in England showed that GP involvement rose by 50% over the 10-year period 1995–2005 (Strang *et al*, 2007).

## Models of drug treatment

There are many different models of treatment and as more care is devolved into the community so the options for treatment increase (National Treatment Agency for Substance Misuse, 2006). A single 'shared care' model, as described in the 1999 clinical guidelines (Department of Health *et al*, 1999), as partnerships between primary and secondary/specialist providers, has, in practice, developed into a range of different models, often driven by local circumstances and including a wider range of providers. Moreover, primary care has moved on since the clinical guidelines were last published in 1999. There are new organisational arrangements and a new GP contract, introduced in 2003. GPs can now opt out of many 'non-core' aspects of work, which are then commissioned directly from other providers. GPs can develop areas of special clinical interest and many clinicians have done so, leading services within primary, secondary and custodial care settings. There are also new opportunities for non-medical prescribers, where nurses and pharmacists can acquire training to prescribe for their patients.

Whatever the local treatment model, the following principles are key (Department of Health *et al*, 2007).

### Joint working

As drug users have a myriad of health and social problems, treatment interventions must involve a range providers. Joint working – for example, between the GP and the pharmacist or the GP and the shared care or key worker – is the key to effective treatment. It is seldom the case that one clinician in isolation will be able to meet all the needs of a drug user. One of the special features and strengths of drug treatment in the UK is the valuable partnership between statutory NHS drug treatment services and non-statutory or voluntary sector drug treatment providers, which comprise up to half of service provision in some local areas.

### Doctors with a range of competencies

Each local health system will need to have a cohort of doctors providing treatment for drug misusers, ranging from those able to provide general medical services to those with specialist competencies in treating drug dependence.

### Involving patients

Involving patients as active partners in their drug treatment is essential and is associated with good outcomes. Patients should be fully involved in the development of their care or treatment plan, in setting appropriate treatment goals and in reviewing progress. It is also good practice to involve patients in the design, planning, development and evaluation of services, and in advocacy and support groups linked to local drug treatment systems. Patients may also be involved in peer education schemes to reduce the risk of overdose and blood-borne viruses.

---

**Key points**

- All doctors will come across patients whose present complaint is related to their use of illicit drugs.
- All health professionals should develop skills in managing patients who present with problems related to illicit drug use.
- Treating patients who use illicit drugs is effective and results in reductions in drug use, better health, social functioning and less involvement in criminal behaviour.
- Methadone or buprenorphine maintenance treatment is the mainstay of treatment for opiate addiction.

# Further reading and e-resources

Department of Health (England) & the Devolved Administrations (2007) *Drug Misuse and Dependence. UK Guidelines on Clinical Management*. Department of Health (England), the Scottish Government, Welsh Assembly Government and Northern Ireland Executive. Downloadable from http://www.dh.gov.uk/publications

Gerada, C. (2005) *The Management of Substance Misuse in Primary Care*. Royal College of General Practitioners.

National Institute for Health and Clinical Excellence (2007a) *Drug Misuse – Opioid Detoxification*. NICE.

Royal College of General Practitioners (2004) *Guidance for the Use of Buprenorphine for the Treatment of Opioid Dependence in Primary Care*. Royal College of General Practitioners.

Royal College of Psychiatrists & Royal College of Physicians (2000) *Drugs: Dilemmas and Choices*. Gaskell.

National Treatment Agency for Substance Misuse, http://www.nta.nhs.uk. The Agency is a special health authority that oversees treatment services across England. The organisation publishes a number of useful documents, including guidance documents and reviews.

Royal College of General Practitioners' Certificate in Substance Misuse (see also Gerada & Murnane, 2003). This course was established in 2000 and has now become the qualification for those who wish to become GPs with a special interest in substance misuse. The course is in two parts: part I involves free e-learning modules and a 1-day face-to-face course); part II is much more comprehensive and comprises 5 days of training spread over 5–6 months and written work and fieldwork as well as attendance at master classes.

Substance Misuse Management in General Practice (SMMGP), http://www.smmgp.org.uk. The SMMGP is a network that supports GPs and other members of the primary care team who work with substance misuse in the UK. The project team produces the SMMGP newsletter (*Network*) and organises the annual conference, 'Managing Drug Users in General Practice'. The site also contains all the material and information about the Royal College of General Practitioners' Certificate in Substance Misuse.

# References

Advisory Council on the Misuse of Drugs (2003) *Hidden Harm: Responding to the Needs of Children of Problem Drug Users*. Advisory Council on the Misuse of Drugs.

Bry, B. N. (1996) Psychological approaches to prevention. In *Drug Policy and Human Nature. Psychological Perspectives on the Prevention, Management, and Treatment of Illicit Drug Abuse* (eds W. K. Bickel & R. J. DeGrandpre), pp. 55–76. Plenum Press.

Department of Health (England) & the Devolved Administrations (2007) *Drug Misuse and Dependence. UK Guidelines on Clinical Management.* Department of Health (England), the Scottish Government, Welsh Assembly Government and Northern Ireland Executive. Downloadable from http://www.dh.gov.uk/publications

Department of Health, Scottish Office Department of Health, Welsh Office, Department of Health and Social Services, Northern Ireland (1999) *Drug Misuse and Dependence – Guidelines on Clinical Management.* The Stationery Office. Downloadable from http://drugs.homeoffice.gov.uk/

European Monitoring Centre for Drugs and Drug Addiction (2006) *Drug-Related Infectious Diseases and Drug-Related Deaths. Annual Report: The State of the Drug Problem in Europe.* EMCDDA.

Farrell, M., Ward, J., Mattick, R., *et al* (1994) Methadone maintenance treatment in opiate dependence: a review. *BMJ*, **309**, 997–1001.

Frischer, M., Goldberg, D., Rahman, M., *et al* (1997) Mortality and survival amongst a cohort of drug injectors in Glasgow 1982–1994. *Addiction*, **92**, 419–427.

Gerada, C. & Harris, L. (2005) General practitioners and the care of drug users: past, present and future. In *RCGP Guide to the Management of Substance Misuse in Primary Care* (ed. C. Gerada), pp. 55–70. Royal College of General Practitioners.

Gerada, C. & Murnane, M. (2003) Royal College of General Practitioners Certificate in Drug Misuse. *Drugs: Education, Prevention and Policy*, **10**, 369–379.

Gossop, M., Marsden, J., Stewart, D., *et al* (2003) The National Treatment Outcome Research Study (NTORS): 4–5 year follow-up results. *Addiction*, **98**, 291–303.

Health Protection Agency, Health Protection Scotland, National Public Health Service for Wales, CDSC Northern Ireland, CRDHB & UASSG (2006) *Shooting Up: Infections Among Injecting Drug Users in the United Kingdom 2005.* Health Protection Agency

National Institute for Health and Clinical Excellence (2007a) *Drug Misuse – Opioid Detoxification.* NICE.

National Institute for Health and Clinical Excellence (2007b) *Methadone and Buprenorphine for the Management of Opioid Dependence.* NICE.

National Treatment Agency for Substance Misuse (2006) *Models of Care for the Treatment of Adult Drug Misusers.* National Treatment Agency for Substance Misuse.

Oppenheimer, E., Tobutt C., Taylor, C., *et al* (1994) Death and survival in a cohort of heroin addicts from London clinics: a 22-year follow-up study. *Addiction*, **89**, 1299–1308.

Strang, J., Manning, V., Mayet, S., *et al* (2007) Does prescribing for opiate addiction change after national guidelines? Methadone and buprenorphine prescribing to opiate addicts by general practitioners and hospital doctors in England, 1995–2005. *Addiction*, **102**, 761–770.

World Health Organization (1992) *Classification of Mental and Behavioural Disorders. Clinical Descriptions and Diagnostic Guidelines* (10th revision) (ICD–10). WHO.

Wright, N. (2002) Common clinical problems. In *Homelessness: A Primary Care Response* (ed. N. Wright), pp. 45–67. RCGP.

# CHAPTER 18

# Management of alcohol problems

Helen Lester and Linda Gask

Summary

This chapter summarises current international evidence on the management of people with alcohol problems in primary care. After a brief overview of the definitions of different levels of alcohol use, it focuses on the costs and consequences of alcohol use and suggests a series of management strategies for primary care practitioners. The value of screening and the role of screening tools are discussed, as are the basic principles of providing a brief intervention. Barriers to brief intervention in primary care and the possible role of nurses in delivering intervention are highlighted. The chapter concludes with strategies for helping people with alcohol dependence, including community-based detoxification programmes.

Alcohol plays an important role in many societies. Over 90% of adults in the UK – nearly 40 million people – consume alcohol, and it is widely associated with pleasure and relaxation. Drinking in moderation can also confer some health benefits (Cabinet Office Strategy Unit, 2003). Sensible drinking may:

- reduce the risk of developing heart disease and peripheral vascular disease
- reduce the risk of dying of a heart attack
- possibly reduce the risk of strokes, particularly ischaemic strokes
- lower the risk of gallstones
- possibly reduce the risk of diabetes.

Alcohol makes a substantial contribution to the UK economy, with the drinks market generating approximately one million jobs and excise duties on alcohol raising about £7 billion per year (Cabinet Office Strategy Unit, 2003).

However, alcohol contributes 4% to the total disease burden worldwide, as measured by disability-adjusted life years (DALYs) (Rehm *et al*, 2003).

This burden is greater in high-income countries (9% DALYs), where alcohol ranks third after smoking and hypertension among the leading causes of morbidity and premature death.

The costs of alcohol misuse in the UK are around £20 billion a year (Cabinet Office Strategy Unit, 2003), with £1.7 billion directly related to health costs. In the UK, alcohol-related disease accounts for 1 in 26 hospital bed days and up to 35% of all attendances at accident and emergency departments and ambulance costs. Up to 150 000 hospital admissions are related to alcohol misuse. It has also been estimated that 1 in 15 doctors may, at some time, experience problems with drugs or alcohol (British Medical Association, 1998) (see Chapter 32 for further discussion of this issue).

The World Health Organization (WHO) has been committed to reducing the burden of alcohol-related problems for over three decades (Brunn et al, 1975). The first WHO European Alcohol Action Plan was introduced in 1992. It aimed to reduce consumption by 25% and had a particular focus on reducing harmful use, although in fact only three countries (Italy, Poland and Spain) achieved this target (Institute of Alcohol Studies, 2003). The current WHO 'health for all' target (WHO, 1999) states that:

> by 2015, the adverse health effects from the consumption of addictive substances such as tobacco, alcohol and psychoactive drugs should have been significantly reduced in all Member States.... In all countries, per capita alcohol consumption should not increase or exceed 6 litres per annum, and should be close to zero in under 15 year olds.

The 25-year WHO Collaborative Project on Identification and Management of Alcohol-Related Problems in Primary Health Care (WHO, 2006) concluded that widespread and routine implementation of brief interventions in each country represented a set of different challenges requiring unique solutions.

# Definitions of alcohol use

A report from the Royal College of Physicians (2001) defined alcohol use in the following terms:

- *Sensible drinker* – a man who drinks 21 or fewer units per week,[1] or a woman who drinks 14 or fewer units per week. The Department of Health guidelines (1995) in the UK have recommended drinking limits on a daily rather than weekly basis, suggesting that, for men, drinking 3–4 unit a day or less and for women 2–3 units a day presents no significant risk to health. It is also recommended that people do not drink up to the recommended limits every day.

---

1 One unit of alcohol in the UK is defined as a drink containing 8 g of ethanol. This is equivalent to half a pint of average-strength beer, lager or cider (3–4% alcohol by volume). A small glass (125 ml) of average-strength wine (12% alcohol by volume) contains 1.5 units of alcohol. See e-resources for an internet calculator for units in relation to actual drinks consumed.

- *Hazardous drinker* (also called an at-risk drinker) – very heavy drinkers and binge-drinkers who have drinking patterns that pose a considerable risk to their own and others' health. Other sources define 'hazardous drinkers' in terms of the units of alcohol consumed: those drinking above the recommended weekly levels, i.e. men drinking above 21 units and women drinking above 14 units per week.
- *Harmful drinker* (also called a 'problem drinker') – drinkers for whom there is clear evidence that alcohol use is responsible for (or substantially contributes to) physical, social or psychological harm, including impaired judgement or dysfunctional behaviour, which may lead to disability or have adverse consequences for interpersonal relationships. Other sources define 'harmful drinkers' as men drinking above 50 units per week and women drinking above 35 units per week.
- *Binge drinker*, those who engage in what is sometimes referred to as 'risky single-occasion drinking' (RSOD) or 'heavy episodic drinking' – a man who regularly drinks 10 or more units in a single session, or a woman who regularly drinks 7 or more units in a single session. However, there is considerable diversity in the way binge drinking is defined and measured.
- *Alcohol dependence* is defined in ICD–10 (WHO, 1992) as a cluster of physiological, behavioural and cognitive phenomena in which the use of alcohol takes on a much higher priority for a given individual than other behaviours. A central characteristic is the desire to drink alcohol, and a return to drinking after a period of abstinence is often associated with a reappearance of the features of the syndrome. A definite diagnosis of dependence is usually made only if three (or more) of the ICD–10 criteria for alcohol dependence are satisfied (Scottish Intercollegiate Guidelines Network, 2003) (Box 18.1).

## Alcohol trends

In 2002, 27% of men and 17% of women aged 16 years and over drank on average more than 21 and 14 units, respectively (Office for National Statistics, 2001). Drinking at these levels had remained stable among men since 1992 but had risen for women, from 12% (Department of Health, 2004). Binge drinking in the UK accounts for 40% of all drinking occasions for men and 22% for women. Young people (aged 16–24 years) are more likely to binge drink (Cabinet Office Strategy Unit, 2003). Alcohol use among children (11–15 years) has been rising steadily in England, from 21% in 1992 to 27% in 2003, and has since fluctuated within this range (Department of Health, 2004).

## Costs and consequences of alcohol misuse

There is growing evidence of the individual and social harms associated with alcohol consumption and misuse (Cabinet Office Strategy Unit, 2003):

**269**

---

**Box 18.1** ICD–10 criteria for alcohol dependence

Dependence is diagnosed if three or more of the following have been present together during the previous year:

- a strong desire or sense of compulsion to drink alcohol
- difficulty in controlling drinking in terms of its onset, termination or level of use
- a physiological withdrawal state (e.g. tremor, sweating, rapid heart rate, anxiety, insomnia, or, less commonly, seizures, disorientation, hallucinations) when drinking has ceased or reduced, or drinking to relieve or avoid such a withdrawal state
- evidence of tolerance, such that increased doses of alcohol are required in order to achieve effects originally produced by lower doses
- progressive neglect of alternative pleasures or interests because of drinking, and increased amounts of time necessary to obtain or take alcohol, or to recover from its effects
- Persisting with alcohol use despite awareness of overtly harmful consequences

---

- *Crime and disorder*. In 1999, an estimated 1.2 million violent incidents (half of all violent crimes) were alcohol related, some 360 000 of which involved domestic violence. There were 85 000 cases of drink driving.
- *Workplace*. Up to 17 million days are lost annually due to alcohol-related absence.
- *Family/social networks*. Between 0.78 million and 1.3 million children are affected by alcohol misuse in the family. Around a third of incidents of domestic violence are linked to alcohol misuse.

# Health effects of hazardous and harmful drinking

There is an extensive epidemiological evidence base linking excessive drinking to a range of health problems. The WHO Global Burden of Disease project quantified the link between alcohol consumption and both mortality and morbidity across a number of disease conditions (Ezzati *et al*, 2002, 2003).

In the UK, between 15 000 and 22 000 deaths each year are associated with alcohol misuse, mainly resulting from stroke, cancer, liver disease, accidental injury or suicide. Rates of alcohol-related mortality from liver disease have increased by about 90% over the past decade. There has been a 466% increase in mortality from alcohol-related liver cirrhosis since 1970 (Academy of Medical Sciences, 2004), with a nine- to ten-fold increase among men and women aged 25–44 years.

Excessive drinking has particular implications for mental health. About a third of patients with serious mental illness in the UK have a substance misuse problem, mostly involving alcohol. Alcohol increases the risk of accidental death and may be associated with 15–30% of such deaths (1700 deaths per year in the UK). Alcohol has been linked to 38–45% of deaths in fires, 7–25% of deaths at work and 23–28% of deaths by drowning (Cabinet Office, 2004). Up to 65% of suicides are thought to be linked to alcohol; 50% of those who present to hospital after an act of deliberate self-harm are regular excessive drinkers and 23% are alcohol dependent.

# Role of primary care in managing alcohol disorders

## Identification

Alcohol problems are underdiagnosed in primary care, for a variety of reasons, including poor recognition by healthcare professionals, or people not disclosing their drinking because of shame or fear of stigmatisation (Enoch & Goldman, 2002). An active request for help is more likely in people with harmful drinking or alcohol dependence (either the person him- or herself, or via friends or relatives). People with hazardous drinking will not usually seek medical help, even though they may be aware that their drinking is putting them at risk. However, evidence suggests that approximately 20% of patients presenting to primary care are likely to be hazardous drinkers (Anderson, 1993).

## Screening for alcohol problems

There is still some uncertainty whether screening should be carried out with every patient or just those who give cause for concern. US guidance calls for screening of all patients (Whitlock *et al*, 2004). Guidance from the Scottish Intercollegiate Guidelines Network (2003), however, suggests that it is confined to people who present conditions where alcohol is a 'possible contributory factor' (p. 4). Indeed, that guidance goes further and suggests:

> primary care practitioners should rely on case detection based on clinical presentation, with judicious use of questionnaire tools where there is suspicion, rather than screening the whole population. (p. 9)

The English Alcohol harm reduction strategy also supports a policy of targeted screening (Cabinet Office, 2004, p. 37).

A Delphi group study that involved 53 UK experts also concluded that routine screening and brief interventions should be carried out in special circumstances, such as new patient registrations, general health check-ups and special clinics where excessive drinkers are likely to be found, rather than opportunistic screening for all patients (Heather *et al*, 2004) (Box 18.2).

### Screening tests

#### The AUDIT questionnaire

During the 1980s, the WHO commissioned a study (Saunders *et al*, 1993) to develop an international screening test that could be used in different

---

**Box 18.2** Screening opportunities in primary care

- Opportunistic detection of problem drinking or alcohol dependence when an individual presents with an unrelated condition or for a health check (e.g. new patient medical examination).
- An active request for help with problem drinking or alcohol dependence, either from the patient, or from friends or relatives.
- Presentation with medical, psychiatric or social problems/complications related to problem drinking or dependence, including alcohol-related driving ban.
- When a person frequently requests sick notes, or presents with conditions that could be related to heavy drinking (e.g. gastritis and hypertension).
- Presentation of physical signs linked to heavy drinking:
  - injuries (including those in the elderly).
  - tremor of the hands and tongue.
  - excessive capillarisation of the facial skin and conjunctivae.
- Return of abnormal blood test results suggestive of excessive alcohol consumption:
  - raised gamma-glutamyl transferase (GGT) – although GGT is not a particularly sensitive or specific indicator of hazardous drinking, a raised value should prompt further questions or use of the AUDIT tool
  - raised mean corpuscular volume (MCV)
  - raised fasting triglyceride levels.
- Dependency on other drugs of misuse (alcohol and drug misuse are commonly associated in young drug misusers).
- Presentation of symptoms of withdrawal. These may occur on sudden cessation of use, vary in severity, and include tremor, nausea, vomiting and sweating. Generalised convulsions may also occur. Onset is 3–6 hours after the last drink and symptoms usually last 5–7 days.

---

countries. The project was inspired by the notion that once a standardised screening test was developed for use in primary care, it would stimulate early intervention, thereby reducing the burden of alcohol problems in different societies, including those without a specialised treatment system. Working with alcohol researchers in Norway, Bulgaria, the UK, Mexico, Australia and the USA, the WHO sponsored a validation study of different screening procedures that led to the development of the Alcohol Use Disorders Identification Test (AUDIT). AUDIT focuses on the preliminary signs of hazardous and harmful drinking and identifying mild dependence. It contains ten questions on quantity and frequency of alcohol consumption, drinking behaviour and alcohol-related problems or reactions. AUDIT has 92% sensitivity and 94% specificity. It takes 5 minutes to complete.

Shorter variants, including the AUDIT-PC (Piccinelli *et al*, 1997), AUDIT-C (Bush *et al*, 1998) and the Fast Alcohol Screening Test (FAST; Hodgson *et al*, 2002), are increasingly being used as screening questionnaires in busy environments such as primary care. They allow detection of hazardous and harmful drinking with only slightly diminished diagnostic accuracy compared with the longer questionnaires. FAST, for example, detects 90% of those AUDIT detects. AUDIT-PC has five, FAST four and AUDIT-C three questions and each takes about 1 minute to complete.

The CAGE questionnaire (Mayfield *et al*, 1974) asks 'ever' questions, rather than focusing on the person's current alcohol consumption, which can be misleading. The score is the sum of the 'yes' responses to the following questions:

1   Have you ever felt you should **C**ut down on your drinking?
2   Have people **A**nnoyed you by criticising your drinking?
3   Have you ever felt bad or **G**uilty about your drinking?
4   Have you ever had a drink in the morning to get rid of a hangover (**E**ye opener)?

It is less sensitive than the AUDIT questionnaire in detecting hazardous drinking, unless it is supplemented by additional questions on maximum daily or weekly consumption (CAGE Plus Two).

## Taking a drinking history

The practitioner needs to establish what the patient's consumption has been over the previous week, taking each day at a time back over the previous 7 days, in order to estimate the *total number of units consumed per week*. It may be helpful to obtain a simple guide to the alcohol content of various types of beer, wine and spirits as an *aide-memoir* (see e-resources for an internet calculator). Some people may be at very high risk of alcohol-related harm due to bingeing on one or two nights of the week, so it is necessary to check not just a 'typical day' but consumption over the week. Patients should be asked whether that had been a typical week, as some people have a pattern of binge drinking followed by a period of abstinence.

Then the practitioner should establish:

- whether the first drink of the day is taken to combat withdrawal symptoms
- whether the patient drinks throughout the day without getting drunk, or in bouts – usually at lunchtime and the evening
- how much is drunk at each session
- whether a single drink always leads to many more, and whether the person generally becomes drunk (and if so, whether this has led to blackouts or falls)
- whether drinking takes place alone, and whether the person drinks only in response to certain moods or situations.

Having established the current drinking pattern, the practitioner should ascertain the *development of heavy drinking* over the years. There are often key points in the patient's life, such as working in the armed forces or in the wine trade, when a great increase in drinking occurred. It may be useful to ask what the longest period of abstinence has been. Contacts with the police may also be dated. In this way the practitioner can establish the duration of heavy drinking, which of the related disabilities have developed and the pattern of their development over time.

## Management

Once alcohol misuse has been identified and a pattern of consumption established, the primary care practitioner and patient have to decide on an appropriate course of action (Box 18.3).

---

**Box 18.3** Overview of management strategies

- Confirm the diagnosis and assess the extent of the problem using a screening tool (e.g. AUDIT) and ICD– 10 criteria if dependence is suspected.
- Assess whether there are any related physical, psychological or social problems associated with alcohol use.
- Determine the person's physical, psychological and social well-being.
- Determine the impact of the person's drinking on others (family members, friends, children, wider community).
- Determine the person's motivation and readiness to change the drinking habit. Prochaska & DiClemente's (1986) 'stages of change' model provides a helpful framework for understanding and staging the process of change for any behaviour, including alcohol or drug use. It suggests that there are six stages: pre-contemplation, contemplation, preparation, action, maintenance and relapse. See Chapter 26 for further information.
- For people who are drinking hazardous amounts of alcohol, discuss cutting down (see 'The value of brief interventions' below). For people who are experiencing harm from drinking, treat alcohol-related problems in primary care where possible, or refer to appropriate specialists, including agencies for advice on social and financial concerns.
- Ideally, refer people who are dependent on alcohol to a specialist service for detoxification, as they often have greater comorbidity, more complications and a worse prognosis than people without dependence. Also, studies of brief interventions have excluded people with alcohol dependence, so there is only limited evidence to support such approaches in this cohort.
- If the person refuses a referral and the healthcare professional has appropriate experience, then consider detoxification in primary care:
  - A tapered-dosing regimen of chlordiaxepoxide is recommended, ideally with the drug dispensed and symptoms reviewed on a daily basis. Advise the person about the expected adverse effects of alcohol withdrawal.
  - After detoxification, follow up quickly and offer help in maintaining abstinence or reduction. Acamprosate may help ease cravings. Counselling should be continued, and mutual-aid groups such as Alcoholics Anonymous may benefit some people.
  - The level of follow-up should be based on the degree of alcohol consumption, the presence of alcohol-related problems, and/or dependence.

Based on Raistrick *et al* (2006).

---

## The value of brief interventions

If the patient is a hazardous but not dependent drinker, then a brief intervention can be offered. There is no standard definition of a brief intervention but it often consists of a structured, 'talk-based' therapy of short duration, delivered usually in four or fewer sessions and often with a motivational component. The goal is usually 'moderate drinking' or a reduction in alcohol-related problems rather than abstinence (Bien *et al*, 1993). Brief interventions are not merely traditional treatment done in a shortened time frame; they have a basic structure on top of which may be added various additional components, such as self-help manuals, behavioural skills training and motivational interviewing.

A brief intervention has been defined as having six essential elements, summarised by the acromym FRAMES (Miller & Sanchez, 1993) (Box 18.4).

Practical advice on how to reduce alcohol intake could include:

- recognising and avoiding high-risk situations for drinking
- recognising personal cues for drinking (e.g. stress, being alone)
- drinking a soft drink for every alcoholic drink and eating before drinking
- trying alternative activities to drinking (coping strategies) – exercise, reading, exploring other interests
- keeping a drinking diary and asking close contacts for help (if acceptable).

Management should involve setting goals, with daily and weekly limits of alcohol consumption (moderation) or abstinence. People should be provided with written information on the consequences of hazardous and harmful drinking and given tips on cutting down. Follow-up should be organised after the initial appointment. If trained, the primary healthcare professional should consider giving an extended brief intervention, such as motivational interviewing (see Chapter 26).

There is a body of research evidence on the effectiveness of brief interventions for alcohol problems, including at least 56 controlled trials.

---

**Box 18.4** Essential elements of a brief intervention

A brief intervention has been defined as having six essential elements, summarised by the acromym FRAMES (Miller & Sanchez, 1993):

- Feedback – on the client's risk for alcohol problems
- Responsibility – the individual is responsible for change
- Advice – on alcohol reduction or explicit direction to change
- Menu – a variety of options for change
- Empathy – a warm, reflective and understanding approach
- Self-efficacy – optimism about changing behaviour

---

Moyer *et al* (2002), in a rigorous meta-analysis that included 34 opportunistic brief interventions in generalist settings among individuals not seeking treatment for alcohol (as well as 20 specialist brief interventions among those seeking treatment), reported that they were effective on a composite of various drinking-related outcomes, including measures of alcohol-related problems. The US Preventive Services Task Force (Whitlock *et al*, 2004) found good evidence that brief counselling interventions with follow-up produce small to moderate reductions in alcohol consumption that are sustained over 6–12 months or longer.

There have been a number of systematic reviews specifically focused on the effectiveness of brief interventions in primary care. A meta-analysis by Bertholet *et al* (2005) concluded that brief interventions were effective in reducing consumption among both men and women at 6 and 12 months. Fleming *et al* (1997) reported that brief interventions delivered in primary care were also effective among older adults (those over 65 years).

There is mixed evidence on longer-term effects of brief interventions. A trial based in family medicine in Wisconsin, USA, reported continuing benefits for alcohol use, binge-drinking episodes and frequency of excessive drinking compared with controls 4 years after a brief intervention (Fleming *et al*, 1997). An Australian study reported that the benefits of a brief intervention had disappeared after 10 years (Wutzke *et al*, 2001) and it was suggested that booster sessions would be necessary to maintain the effect over this period. The WHO (2006) estimated that the cost-effectiveness is approximately £1300 per year of ill health or premature death averted. This is similar to the cost-effectiveness of smoking cessation interventions in primary healthcare.

## Barriers to brief intervention in primary care

Research from a number of different countries, including a WHO survey of 1300 GPs in nine countries, has suggested that brief interventions have yet to be integrated into routine clinical primary care practice (Anderson *et al*, 2003). Common barriers to implementation include lack of time, lack of training, a belief that patients will not take advice to change drinking behaviour and a lack of suitable screening and counselling materials (Kaner *et al*, 1999).

General practitioners who have tried to include a screening and brief intervention programme in their practice found the extra workload onerous and had problems establishing rapport with hazardous and harmful drinkers identified through screening (Beich *et al*, 2002).

Other work has suggested that GPs and nurses can be trained to use 5- to 10-minute brief interventions in a 2.5-hour training session (Ockene *et al*, 1999). There is also evidence that, when GPs and nurses are adequately trained and supported for the work, their use of brief interventions increases (Anderson *et al*, 2004). Brief interventions can also be cost-effectively delivered by primary care nurses (Tomson *et al*, 1997; Kaner *et al*, 2003). Nurses are a relatively underexplored resource in this area, but work in the front line of healthcare in many countries, and would be in an excellent position, with training, to screen, advise and monitor patients, and to deliver brief interventions to hazardous and harmful drinkers (Sullivan & Handley, 1994).

However, there is still a lack of evidence on how to achieve routine implementation of screening and brief interventions in primary care (WHO, 2006). A number of structural changes would also need to occur, at least in the UK, to encourage implementation, including the provision of training, dissemination of information about the success of brief interventions, government support for alcohol prevention in primary care and funding for alcohol support agencies.

## Alcohol dependence

If the patient is identified as a dependent drinker or drinking at levels that have harmful health or social effects, referral to a local alcohol service and detoxification should be considered, ideally through a shared care scheme, if available. If the person refuses a referral and the healthcare professional feels confident (i.e. has previous experience with successful assisted withdrawal), knows the person and has the appropriate amount of time (including follow-up arrangements), an attempt at community-based withdrawal could be tried. This also requires that the social circumstances are in place to favour community withdrawal (particularly if the person lives alone) and there is no history of fits or delirium tremens, suicide risk, history of illicit drug misuse or existing dependence on benzodiazepines (Department of Health et al, 1999).

Chlordiazepoxide is the usual benzodiazepine of choice for the community-based detoxification of people who are dependent on alcohol (Raistrick et al, 2006). Chlordiazepoxide has a slower onset of action than diazepam or lorazepam, and has less potential for misuse (Mayo-Smith, 1997). Diazepam is an alternative. It has similar efficacy to chlordiazepoxide, but has a greater potential for misuse, as it has a faster onset of action.

A tapered fixed-dose regimen of a benzodiazepine is recommended for alcohol detoxification in primary care, with daily monitoring wherever possible. The dose of chlordiazepoxide should be gradually reduced over the course of a week (see Table 18.1 for an example of a typical regimen). The initial dose and the length of treatment will depend on the severity of alcohol dependence and on individual patient factors (e.g. weight, gender, liver function). A loading dose of chlordiazepoxide 100 mg can be used to prevent delirium if prodromal symptoms appear.

## Drugs that promote abstinence or attenuate drinking behaviour

The two drugs with the most promise in this area are acamprosate, a synthetic GABA analogue, and naltrexone, an opioid antagonist (Drummond

**Table 18.1** Reducing dose of chlordiazepoxide (mg) over 7 days for alcohol detoxification

|  | First thing | 12:00 | 18:00 | Bedtime |
|---|---|---|---|---|
| Day 1 | 20–30 | 20–30 | 20–30 | 20–30 |
| Day 2 | 20–30 | 20–30 | 20–30 | 20–30 |
| Day 3 | 15 | 15 | 15 | 15 |
| Day 4 | 15 | 15 | 15 | 15 |
| Day 5 | 10 | 10 | 10 | 10 |
| Day 6 | 10 | – | – | 10 |
| Day 7 | – | – | – | 10 |

Department of Health *et al* (1999).

*et al*, 2004). Treatment with acamprosate should be initiated immediately after detoxification. It will usually be initiated by a specialist service, which may review treatment at regular intervals (often under a shared care agreement). However, if detoxification has been carried out within primary care, acamprosate should be considered by the GP during the maintenance phase. The dose of acamprosate prescribed depends on the weight of the person, with people weighing less than 60 kg receiving a lower dose than heavier individuals (ABPI Medicines Compendium, 2003). Where effective, it should be continued for up to 12 months.

## Support groups

Alcoholics Anonymous (AA) is helpful for some patients. It advocates a strict abstinence policy and provides a social structure to replace drinking. Support is available at all times and often from ex-drinkers, with whom the patient can identify. Al-Anon and Al-Ateen are support groups for the partners and children of drinkers. Other people who are aiming to cut down their drinking but not to achieve abstinence may benefit from support groups run by a range of different alcohol- and drug-related voluntary agencies in the community.

## Prognosis

The majority of people who drink alcohol will go in and out of different drinking patterns, sometimes involving problem drinking, without engaging any professional services. A systematic review showed that approximately 21% of people with an untreated alcohol problem were abstinent after a 30-year follow-up (Moyer & Finney, 2002). The majority of people drinking at hazardous levels will recover without any professional or formal help (Klingemann & Schibli, 2004). Alcohol dependence, however, is thought to have a chronic and relapsing course.

# Conclusion

Despite a wealth of evidence on the individual social and health harms and the costs to society of alcohol misuse, screening and brief interventions in primary care are far from a reality in most countries. Routine screening and implementation of brief interventions in primary care require more evidence on the best way to roll out programmes that work in that setting, and on who is best placed to deliver them; they will also require greater support and financial backing from central government.

---

**Key points**

- Excessive drinking is a global health problem, responsible for a wide range of both chronic and acute illness.
- The challenge for governments is to balance the tension between the risks and benefits of alcohol, including the economic benefit to individual communities and the state, the social and health benefits from low levels of drinking and the significant harms caused by alcohol.
- Despite the fact that brief interventions in primary care can be effective in reducing alcohol consumption, there is little evidence that primary care practitioners are aware of them, let alone incorporate them into routine clinical practice.
- Implementation of screening and brief interventions in primary care requires high-level government support, funding for the provision of training and dissemination of information about their value and success.

---

# Further reading and e-resources

An internet calculator for number of units consumed is available at http://www.drinkaware.co.uk/how-many-units.html

Useful WHO websites include:
http://www.who.int/substance_abuse/publications/alcohol/en/index.html
http://www.who.int/topics/alcohol_drinking/en/

Screening tools for hazardous drinking, including AUDIT, AUDIT-PC, AUDIT-C, FAST and the Single Alcohol Screening Questionnaire (SASQ), can be downloaded from the website of the Institute of Health and Society, Newcastle University, http://www.ncl.ac.uk/ihs

General information is available on the Alcohol Concern website, http://www.alcoholconcern.org.uk

A primary care alcohol information services fact sheet can be downloaded from http://www.alcoholconcern.org.uk/files/20030910_143338_Screening%20factsheet%20final%20for%20web%202.pdf

Bandolier (2004) Brief interventions for alcohol problems. Downloadable from http://www.medicine.ox.ac.uk/bandolier/band126/b126-4.html

# References

ABPI Medicines Compendium (2003) Summary of product characteristics for Campral EC. *Electronic Medicines Compendium*. Datapharm Communications Ltd.

Academy of Medical Sciences (2004) *Calling Time: The Nation's Drinking as a Major Health Issue*. Academy of Medical Sciences.

Anderson, P. (1993) Effectiveness of general practice interventions for patients with harmful alcohol consumption. *British Journal of General Practice*, **43**, 386–389.

Anderson, P., Kaner, E., Wutzke, S., *et al* (2003) Attitudes and management of alcohol problems in general practice: descriptive analysis based on findings of a World Health Organization international collaborative study. *Alcohol and Alcoholism*, **38**, 597–601.

Anderson, P., Kaner, S., Wutzke, S., *et al* (2004) Attitudes and managing alcohol problems in general practice: an interaction based on findings from a WHO collaborative study. *Alcohol and Alcoholism*, **39**, 351–359.

Beich, A., Gannick, G. & Malterud, K. (2002) Screening and brief intervention for excessive alcohol use: qualitative interview study of the experiences of general practitioners. *BMJ*, **325**, 870–872.

Bertholet, N., Daeppen, J. B., Wietlisbach, V., *et al* (2005) Brief alcohol intervention in primary care: systematic review and meta-analysis. *Archives of Internal Medicine*, **165**, 986–995.

Bien, T. H., Miller, W. R. & Tonigan, J. S. (1993) Brief interventions for alcohol problems: a review. *Addiction*, **88**, 315–336.

British Medical Association (1998) *The Misuse of Alcohol and Other Drugs by Doctors*. BMA.

Brunn, K., Edwards, G., Lunio, M., *et al* (1975) *Alcohol Control Policies in Public Health Perspectives*. Finnish Foundation for Alcohol Studies.

Bush, K., Kivlahan, D. R., McDonell, M. B., *et al* (1998) The AUDIT alcohol consumption questions (AUDIT-C): an effective brief screening test for problem drinking. *Archives of Internal Medicine*, **158**, 1789–1795.

Cabinet Office (2004) *Alcohol Harm Reduction Strategy for England*. Strategy Unit.

Cabinet Office Strategy Unit (2003) Alcohol Misuse: Interim Analytical Report. *Cabinet Office*.

Department of Health (1995) *Sensible Drinking: The Report of an Interdepartmental Working Group*. Department of Health.

Department of Health (2004) *Statistics on Alcohol: England, 2004*. Statistical Bulletin. Department of Health.

Department of Health, Scottish Office Department of Health, Welsh Office & Department of Health and Social Services of Northern Ireland (1999) *Drug Misuse and Dependence: Guidelines on Clinical Management*. Department of Health.

Drummond, C., Oyefeso, A., Phillips, T., *et al* (2004) *Alcohol Needs Assessment Research Project (Anarp). The 2004 National Alcohol Needs Assessment for England*. Department of Health.

Enoch, M. A. & Goldman, D. (2002) Problem drinking and alcoholism: diagnosis and treatment. *American Family Physician*, **65**, 441–448.

Ezzati, M., Lopez, A., Rodgers, A., *et al* (2002) Selected major risk factors and global and regional burden of disease. *Lancet*, **360**, 1347–1360.

Ezzati, M., Vander Hoorn, S., Rodgers, A., *et al* (2003) Estimates of global and regional potential health gains from reducing multiple major risk factors. *Lancet*, **362**, 271–280.

Fleming, M. F., Barry, K. L., Manwell, L. B., *et al* (1997) Brief physician advice for problem alcohol drinkers: a randomized controlled trial in community-based primary care practices. *JAMA*, **277**, 1039–1045.

Heather, N., Dalloloio, E., Hutchings, D., *et al* (2004) Implementing routine screening and brief alcohol intervention in primary health care: a Delphi survey of expert opinion. *Journal of Substance Misuse*, **9**, 68–85.

Hodgson, R., Alwyn, T., John, B., *et al* (2002) The FAST Alcohol Screening Test. *Alcohol and Alcoholism*, **37**, 61–66.

Institute of Alcohol Studies (2003) *Counterbalancing the Drinks Industry. A Summary of the Eurocare Report on Alcohol Policy in the European Union.* Eurocare.

Kaner, E., Heather, N., McAvoy, B. R., *et al* (1999) Intervention for excessive alcohol consumption in primary health care: attitudes and practices of English general practitioners. *Alcohol and Alcoholism*, **24**, 559–566.

Kaner, E., Lock, C., Heather, N., *et al* (2003) Promoting brief alcohol intervention by nurses in primary care: a cluster randomised controlled trial. *Patient Education and Counselling*, **51**, 277–284.

Klingemann, H. & Schibli, D. (2004) Times for healing: towards a typology of time-frames in Swiss alcohol and drug clinics. *Addiction*, **99**, 1418–1429.

Mayfield, D. G., McLeod, G. & Hall, P. (1974) The CAGE questionnaire: validation of a new alcoholism screening instrument. *American Journal of Psychiatry*, **131**, 1121–1123.

Mayo-Smith, M. F. (1997) Pharmacological management of alcohol withdrawal: a meta-analysis and evidence-based practice guideline. *JAMA*, **278**, 144–151.

Miller, W. & Sanchez, V. (1993) *Motivating Young Adults for Treatment and Lifestyle Change.* University of Notre Dame Press.

Moyer, A. & Finney, J. W. (2002) Outcomes for untreated individuals involved in randomized trials of alcohol treatment. *Journal of Substance Abuse Treatment*, **23**, 247–252.

Moyer, A., Finney, J., Swearingen, C., *et al* (2002) Brief interventions for alcohol problems: a meta-analytic review of controlled investigations in treatment-seeking and non-treatment seeking populations. *Addiction*, **97**, 279–292.

Ockene, J., Adamms, A., Hurley, T., *et al* (1999) Brief physician and nurse practitioners delivered counselling for high risk drinkers. *Archives of Internal Medicine*, **159**, 2198–2205.

Office for National Statistics (2001) *General Household Survey.* The Stationary Office.

Piccinelli, M., Tessari, E., Bortolomasi, M., *et al* (1997) Efficacy of the Alcohol Use Disorders Identification Test as a screening tool for hazardous alcohol intake and related disorders in primary care: a validity study. *BMJ*, **314**, 420–424.

Prochaska, J. O. & DiClemente, C. C. (1986) Towards a comprehensive model of change. In *Treating Addictive Behaviours: Processes of Change* (eds W. R. Miller & N. Heather), pp. 3–27. Plenum Press.

Raistrick, D., Heather, N. & Godfrey, C. (2006) *Review of the Effectiveness of Treatment for Alcohol Problems.* National Treatment Agency for Substance Misuse.

Rehm, J., Room, R., Monteiro, M., *et al* (2003) Alcohol as a risk factor for global burden of disease. *European Addiction Research*, **9**, 157–164.

Royal College of Physicians (2001) *Alcohol – Can the NHS Afford It? A Report of a Working Party of the Royal College of Physicians.* Royal College of Physicians.

Saunders, J. B., Aasland, O. G., Babor, T. F., *et al* (1993) Development of the Alcohol Use Disorders Identification Test (AUDIT): WHO collaborative project on early detection of persons with harmful alcohol consumption II. *Addiction*, **88**, 791–804.

Scottish Intercollegiate Guidelines Network (2003) *The Management of Harmful Drinking and Alcohol Dependence in Primary Care.* National clinical guidelines. SIGN.

Sullivan, E. J. & Handley, S. M. (1994) The role of nurses in primary care: managing alcohol-abusing patients. *Alcohol Health and Research World*, **18**, 185–161.

Tomson, Y., Romelsjo, A. & Aberg, H. (1997) Excessive drinking – brief invention by a primary health care nurse: a randomised controlled trial. *Scandinavian Journal of Primary Care*, **15**, 188–192.

Whitlock, E. P., Polen, M. R., Green, C. A., *et al* (2004) Behavioral counselling interventions in primary care to reduce risky/harmful alcohol use by adults: a summary of the evidence for the US Preventive Services Task Force. *Annals of Internal Medicine*, **140**, 557–568.

WHO (1992) *Classification of Mental and Behavioural Disorders. Clinical Descriptions and Diagnostic Guidelines* (10th revision) (ICD–10). WHO.

WHO(1999) *The Health for All Policy Framework for the WHO European Region.* WHO.

WHO (2006) *WHO Collaborative Project on Identification and Management of Alcohol-Related Problems in Primary Health Care. Report on Phase IV: Development of Country-Wide Strategies for Implementing Early Identification and Brief Intervention in Primary Health Care.* WHO.

Wutzke, S. E., Shiell, A., Gomel, M. K., *et al* (2001) Cost effectiveness of brief interventions for reducing alcohol consumption. *Social Science and Medicine,* **52**, 863–870.

# CHAPTER 19

# Eating disorders

## Geoffrey Wolff

### Summary

Eating disorders are common and are associated with high rates of morbidity and mortality. However, they are under-recognised and often go untreated. Many health professionals feel ill-equipped to manage them and the availability of specialist provision is very variable. However, there are simple steps which can be taken in primary care to engage and support both patients and carers as well as monitor and manage medical risk. This may be sufficient for mild cases, and primary care protocols have been developed to guide both early management and the transition to specialist care.

Eating disorders are common and are associated with high rates of morbidity and mortality. However, sufferers are often ambivalent about seeking treatment. On average, they present only after several years and they commonly present with non-specific physical and psychological symptoms, which may not initially be attributed to the eating disorder. They are therefore under-recognised and often go untreated (Hoek, 1993). Furthermore, once they are diagnosed, many health professionals feel ill-equipped to manage them and the availability of specialist provision is very variable (Royal College of Psychiatrists, 2000). Mild cases may, though, be managed in primary care.

## Definitions

An eating disorder is a disturbance of eating habits or weight control behaviour that results in significant impairment of physical health or psychosocial functioning (which is not secondary to a medical condition or other psychiatric disorder). The two major categories are anorexia nervosa and bulimia nervosa (Box 19.1) but most eating disorders (more than half) do not satisfy criteria for these full syndromes (Fairburn & Harrison, 2003). Hence ICD–10 (World Health Organization, 1992) recognises partial syndromes of atypical anorexia nervosa and atypical bulimia nervosa as well as a number of minor categories: overeating associated with other psychological disturbances (excludes simple obesity); vomiting associated with other psychological disturbances; other eating disorders (including pica in adults and psychogenic loss of appetite); and eating disorder, unspecified. DSM–IV (American Psychiatric Association, 1994) also includes the category of 'eating disorder not otherwise specified' (EDNOS) and a further provisional category of binge eating disorder (where there is recurrent binge eating without the use of compensatory strategies such as purging).

# Epidemiology

The prevalence of anorexia nervosa in young females is of the order of 0.3%, that of bulimia nervosa around 1%, and that of EDNOS around 1–3% (Hoek *et al*, 2003). Eating disorders are much more common in females than in males (anorexia nervosa 12:1, bulimia nervosa 6:1, and binge eating disorder 4:1) (Fichter & Krenn, 2003). General practitioners (GPs) with a list of 2000 patients will have around 3 patients with anorexia nervosa and 11 patients with bulimia nervosa on their list (Hoek, 1993). In addition to this, they will be likely to have a further 15 or so with EDNOS.

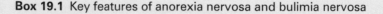

**Box 19.1** Key features of anorexia nervosa and bulimia nervosa

**Anorexia nervosa**

- Self-induced weight loss (to body mass index of 17.5 kg/m² or less or less than 85% of expected body weight) motivated by a fear of fatness
- Amenorrhoea.
- DSM–IV recognises two subtypes: restricting type (no binge eating or purging behaviour) and binge eating/purging type (self-induced vomiting or the misuse of laxatives, diuretics or enemas).

**Bulimia nervosa**

- Recurrent episodes of binge eating (at least twice a week for 3 months).
- Repeated use of compensatory strategies to counteract calorie intake, such as fasting, vomiting, purging or use of drugs.
- Preoccupation with weight and shape.
- DSM–IV recognises two subtypes: purging (self-induced vomiting, laxatives, diuretics or enemas); and non-purging (only fasting or exercise to counteract calorie intake).

# Physical and psychological morbidity

Eating disorders are associated with high levels of both physical and psychological morbidity. The physical morbidity can affect all body systems (Rome & Ammerman, 2003). Eating disorders in general are also associated with marked impairment of quality of life through lack of energy, emotional distress, social isolation and sleep disturbance (Keilen *et al*, 1994).

Anorexia nervosa in particular is also associated with high levels of chronic disability from, for example, reduced mobility and pain. The mortality from anorexia nervosa is ten times that of the general population, standardised for age and gender. Among patients ill enough to require specialist psychiatric in-patient care, the mortality rate is twice that of other psychiatric in-patients (Sullivan, 1995; Nielsen *et al*, 1998; Herzog *et al*, 2000). The main causes of death are infections, cardiovascular collapse and suicide. There are high levels of psychiatric comorbidity, including depression, obsessive–compulsive disorder and social phobia, and suicide rates are higher than for any other psychiatric disorder: 60 times that of the general population when standardised for age and gender (Herzog *et al*, 2000). Patients with anorexia nervosa tend to have anxious, obsessional and avoidant personality traits. Many complain that their illness causes them to feel out of control, taken over, preoccupied with thoughts about food and that it damages their personal relationships (Serpell *et al*, 1999).

Bulimia nervosa is also associated with high levels of psychological comorbidity, including depression and substance misuse. People with bulimia nervosa tend to have borderline and impulsive personality traits. Medical comorbidity is less than that for anorexia nervosa. Patients with bulimia nervosa complain that their illness causes them to feel shame or low self-esteem and leads to obsessive thoughts about weight and shape (Serpell & Treasure, 2002).

# Presentation and detection in primary care

Patients with eating disorder present more frequently than controls in the 5 years prior to diagnosis, with: gynaecological symptoms (e.g. amenorrhoea or irregular periods); gastrointestinal symptoms (constipation or diarrhoea, secondary to laxative abuse); and psychological complaints (depression, anxiety and emotional distress) (Ogg *et al*, 1997). Indeed, 90% of patients with eating disorder present to a GP with symptoms related to their eating disorder (Noordenbos, 1991), but the mean period between the start of their eating disorder and the first visit to the physician is nearly 4 years (Daaleman, 1991).

However, detection rates for eating disorders are low. Only 40% of cases of anorexia nervosa and 10% of cases of bulimia nervosa are detected in primary care. Often, anorexic patients hide their emaciation, and bulimic patients look well (Hoek, 1993).

In the UK, the National Institute for Health and Clinical Excellence (NICE) recommends screening for eating disorders in high-risk target groups (Box 19.2). In these groups, it recommends either two simple screening questions ('Do you think you have an eating disorder?', 'Do you worry excessively about your weight?') or the use of the SCOFF questionnaire (Box 19.3) (NICE, 2004).

# Assessment

## History

In taking the history (Box 19.4) it is important to ask about eating patterns and anorexic behaviour (including food restriction, bingeing and compensatory strategies); to elicit psychopathology both specific to the eating disorder (including the motivations and triggers for food restriction and bingeing) and general (including poor concentration, anxiety, depression, hopelessness and suicidality); and to explore physical symptoms (including

---

**Box 19.2** Target groups for screening for eating disorder in primary care

- Young women with low body mass index
- Patients consulting with weight concerns who are not overweight
- Women with menstrual disturbances or amenorrhoea
- Patients with gastrointestinal symptoms
- Patients with physical signs of starvation or repeated vomiting
- Children with poor growth

From NICE (2004).

---

**Box 19.3** The SCOFF questionnaire

- Do you make yourself **S**ick because you feel uncomfortably full?
- Do you worry you have lost **C**ontrol over how much you eat?
- Have you recently lost more than **O**ne stone in a 3-month period?
- Do you believe yourself to be **F**at when others say you are too thin?
- Would you say that **F**ood dominates your life?

One point is scored for every 'yes'; a score of 2 or more indicates a likely case of anorexia nervosa or bulimia.

Reproduced with permission from Morgan *et al* (1999): © BMJ Publishing Group Ltd.

**Box 19.4** Questions the primary care professional needs to ask

**Eating and anorexic behaviour**

- Can you tell me what you eat in a typical day?
- Which foods feel 'safe' and what do you avoid?
- Do you avoid eating with others?
- Do you ever vomit, exercise, abuse laxatives and/or diuretics? If so, how much and when?
- Do you ever lose control or binge? How often and what do you eat?

**Eliciting psychopathology**

- What do you think of your current weight?
- What do you see as your ideal weight?
- How would you feel if you were the normal weight for your height?
- How much of the day do you spend thinking of food and your weight?
- Do you ever get depressed or guilty? Do you ever feel suicidal?
- Has your life become more ritualised?
- Do you have compulsions (e.g. bingeing, over-exercise)?

**Physical symptoms**

- When was your last period?
- Have you noticed any weakness in your muscles? What about climbing stairs or brushing your hair?
- Are you more sensitive to the cold than others?
- What is your sleep like?
- Have you fainted or had dizzy spells?
- Have you problems with your teeth (hot/cold sensitivity, etc.)?
- Have you had any problems with your digestive system?

amenorrhoea and infertility, gastrointestinal disturbance, weakness and lack of energy, dizziness, sleep disturbance) as well as enquiring about possible infections. In shorter primary care consultations this can be done over several visits.

## Physical examination

It is essential to check the patient's weight and height and to calculate the body mass index (BMI) for adults and the percentage average body weight for children and adolescents using centile charts, and to relate the results to any previous measurements in the medical records. Box 19.5 gives further details. It is also essential to check the pulse and blood pressure (lying and standing) as there may be bradycardia and hypotension in low-weight patients and cardiac arrhythmias, especially in patients with bulimic symptoms. In low-weight patients it is also very helpful to chart weight over time, as rate of weight loss is an important indicator of risk. It is also important to assess the peripheries for poor circulation and oedema, muscle

---

**Box 19.5** Eating disorders minimum physical examination

**All**

- Weight, height, body mass index for adults (criterion for anorexia 17.5 kg/m$^2$ or below)
- Centile charts (criterion for anorexia below 2nd centile) or percentage average body weight (criterion for anorexia below 85%) for children and adolescents
- Pulse and blood pressure (lying and standing)
- Temperature
- Peripheries for poor circulation and oedema
- Ability to rise from a squat for proximal myopathy

**Binging and vomiting**

- Parotid enlargement
- Callus on hand
- Dental enamel erosion

---

strength and temperature. In patients with bulimic symptoms there may be parotid enlargement, dental erosion and a callous on the back of the hand.

The results of the physical examination can be a useful guide to risk assessment. A short medical risk assessment for anorexia nervosa based on this is presented in Table 19.1.

## Investigations

Laboratory investigations (Box 19.6) are necessary for a more extensive assessment of medical risk. A full blood count and biochemical profile (including thyroid function tests) should be obtained for all patients with an eating disorder. In addition it may sometimes be helpful to request a urinary drug screen for laxative abuse. In patients with low weight and amenorrhoea of more than one year a bone density scan is recommended.

**Table 19.1** Short medical risk assessment in anorexia nervosa

|  | Moderate risk | High risk |
|---|---|---|
| Body mass index | Less than 14 kg/m$^2$ | Less than 12 kg/m$^2$ |
| Rate of weight loss | Greater than 0.5 kg | Greater than 1.0 kg |
| Pulse | Less than 50 b.p.m. | Less than 40 b.p.m. |
| Blood pressure | Less than 90/70 mmHg | Less than 80/60 mmHg |
| Postural drop | Greater than 10 mmHg | Greater than 20 mmHg |
| Squat test | Use arms for balance | Use arms as levers |
| Temperature | Less than 35.0°C | Less than 34.50°C |
| Circulation (capillary refill) | Blanching greater than 2 s | |
| Oedema | Present | |

**Box 19.6** Eating disorders investigations

- Blood count (especially if low weight)
  - anaemia (usually normochromic, normocyctic)
  - leucopenia
- Urea and electrolytes (especially if bulimic):
  - potassium < 3.5 mmol/l – vomiting or laxative abuse
  - bicarbonate > 30 mmol/l – vomiting
  - bicarbonate < 18 mmol/l – laxative abuse
- Other blood chemistry (especially if low weight)
  - glucose – hypoglycaemia a marker for recovery
  - thyroid function tests (hyperthyroidism as differential diagnosis of weight loss or secondary hypothyroidism due to weight loss)
  - liver function tests – raised liver enzymes in severe malnutrition
- Urinary drug screen
  - laxative abuse
- Bone density scan (in low-weight patients with amenorrhoea)
  - Osteopenia or osteoporosis may develop after 6–12 months of amenorrhoea.

# Managing eating disorders

The NICE guidelines recommend that, for people with eating disorders presenting in primary care, GPs should take responsibility for the initial assessment and the initial coordination of care. This includes the determination of the need for emergency medical or psychiatric assessment (NICE, 2004). The assessment needs to take account of physical, psychological and social needs and there needs to be ongoing assessment of the level of risk, as this may change. The initial care required will be regular support and monitoring and may require the involvement of a counsellor, practice nurse and dietician (if available).

Patients who do not respond or those with more severe illness may require referral to specialist services. Indeed, 80% of cases of anorexia nervosa and 60% of cases of bulimia nervosa will eventually be referred to a specialist (Turnbull *et al*, 1996).

The first steps in managing patients in primary care are: establishing a therapeutic relationship; monitoring risk; establishing nutritional health and regular eating; and engaging and supporting the family (especially in younger patients and those with anorexia nervosa).

## Establishing a therapeutic relationship

Many patients initially presenting are not yet ready or willing to take decisive action to overcome their eating disorder. They are likely to be at the very least ambivalent about change and some may deny that they have a problem at all. Even if they are motivated to change, they may lack confidence in their ability to change. In establishing a therapeutic relationship, therefore, a motivational interviewing approach may be helpful (see Box 19.7 and also Rollnick *et al*, 1999).

The practitioner also needs to be an expert resource of information about eating disorders and nutrition, including the effects of starvation, bingeing and weight-control strategies such as vomiting and laxative misuse, as well as being able to direct patients to other resources such as websites and books (Box 19.8). In addition, counselling over wider psychosocial issues such as relationship problems or psychological trauma may be helpful. This may be provided by a practice counsellor, or by referral to specialist eating disorder services.

## Monitoring risk and establishing nutritional health and regular eating

The patient needs to be weighed regularly as part of the ongoing risk assessment and progress needs to be charted. The patient needs to be encouraged to establish an eating pattern that is regular (three meals and three snacks are recommended), sufficient and varied.

In bulimic patients (who are usually of normal weight), the main goal is regular eating, which will probably prevent most binges (self-monitoring with food diaries may be helpful to establish this). A further goal will be a reduction in weight-control strategies such as vomiting, laxative misuse and over-exercise (simple behavioural strategies may be helpful in this respect, such as delaying vomiting, planning activities incompatible with vomiting, graded reduction of laxative use and exercise). Self-help resources (see below) may be utilised in achieving these goals.

In low-weight patients, in addition to regular eating, the main goal is to eat sufficient to achieve a weight gain of around 0.5 kg per week.

---

**Box 19.7** Motivational interviewing

**Assumptions**

- People are naturally ambivalent about change
- If a practitioner advocates change, resistance to change increases
- Evoking a person's own change talk increases the likelihood of behaviour change

**Principles**

- Express empathy
- Develop discrepancy
- Avoid arguments
- Roll with resistance
- Support self-efficacy

---

---

**Box 19.8** Sources of information and support

**Self-help books**

- Janet Treasure (1997) *Anorexia Nervosa: A Survival Guide for Families, Friends and Sufferers*. Psychology Press.
- Ulrike Schmidt & Janet Treasure (1993) *Getting Better Bit(E) by Bit(E): A Survival Guide for Sufferers of Bulimia Nervosa and Binge Eating Disorders*. Lawrence Erlhaum.
- J. Treasure, G. Smith & A. Crane (2007) *Skills-Based Learning for Caring for a Loved One with an Eating Disorder: The New Maudsley Method*. Routledge.
- Chris Fairburn (1995) *Overcoming Binge Eating*. Guilford.

**Websites and helplines**

- Beat (beating eating disorders), http://www.b-eat.co.uk, helpline 0845 634 1414, youthline 0845 634 7650
- NHS Direct, http://www.nhsdirect.nhs.uk, telephone 0845 4647
- Institute of Psychiatry, http://www.eatingresearch.com
- Royal College of Psychiatrists, http://www.rcpsych.ac.uk/college/sections/eatingdisorders.aspx

---

This requires around an extra 500 kcal per day on top of normal daily requirements. A female patient of average height will probably need a total of around 2500 kcal per day.

In the majority of patients with eating disorders a secondary goal is to work on increasing variety and challenging avoidance of 'forbidden' foods.

## Engaging and supporting the family

Engaging carers is essential, especially with younger and low-weight patients. It is helpful to include the family in any treatment plan and to provide information about eating disorders. Carers need to be clear about treatment goals and they need to be calm, consistent and empathic. Teaching carers reflective listening and motivational interviewing skills can be helpful and there are resources available to facilitate this (Treasure *et al*, 2007; http://www.eatingresearch.com).

## Primary care protocols

The National Service Framework for Mental Health (Department of Health, 1999) specifies that primary care protocols for the management of eating disorders should be in place. An example of such a protocol (for adults with anorexia nervosa or bulimia nervosa), which was adapted by the Eating Disorders Section of the Royal College of Psychiatrists from one developed by Croydon Health Authority, is posted on the Royal College of Psychiatrists' website (Royal College of Psychiatrists, 2001). A simplified version of this protocol is presented in Tables 19.2 and 19.3.

The protocol does not mention specifically the needs of patients with the diagnosis of eating disorder not otherwise specified (EDNOS). However, it should be possible to make a clinical decision on whether an EDNOS case is more similar to anorexia nervosa or bulimia nervosa and to follow the paths outlined for either of these two disorders.

The protocol does not cover the management of children and adolescents with eating disorders. Anorexia nervosa in children often requires more rapid intervention than advocated here, as children are more vulnerable to rapid physical deterioration.

The protocol also assumes that access to an eating disorder unit is available to the referring GP. This is not the case in many areas and local protocols will vary accordingly, to fit local needs. Furthermore, clear local agreements need to be made around who will be responsible for physical monitoring of patients for whom care is shared between primary care and specialist services.

**Table 19.2** Primary care guidelines for anorexia nervosa

| Condition | Definition | Primary care management |
|---|---|---|
| Mild anorexia nervosa | BMI > 17 kg/m$^2$ No additional comorbidity (e.g. depression, diabetes, inflammatory bowel disease, gastrointestinal disorders) | Support and monitoring by GP Give information Explore problem, comorbidity, causes Monitor for 8 weeks and consider referral to eating disorders specialist if patient fails to respond |
| Moderate anorexia nervosa | BMI 15–17 kg/m$^2$ No evidence of system failure | Routine referral to eating disorder unit |
| Severe anorexia nervosa | BMI < 15 kg/m$^2$ Rapid weight loss Evidence of system failure | Urgent referral to eating disorder specialist (or medical unit if life threatening) |

**Table 19.3** Primary care guidelines for bulimia nervosa

| Condition | Characteristics | Primary care management |
|---|---|---|
| Mild to moderate bulimia nervosa | Less than daily purging No comorbidity (e.g. depression, diabetes) | Support and monitoring by GP Give information Explore problem, comorbidity, causes Monitor for 8 weeks and consider referral to eating disorders specialist if patient fails to respond |
| Severe bulimia nervosa | Daily purging with electrolyte imbalance Comorbidity (e.g. diabetes) | Urgent referral to eating disorder specialist |

Guidelines have also been produced by the American Academy of Eating Disorders for the treatment of children and adolescents with eating disorders (Rome & Ammerman, 2003). They advise that although it may be ideal to have a formal eating disorders team, a primary care professional in communication with a dietician and therapist can do much. An abbreviated summary is presented in Table 19.4.

In adolescents, because of the potentially irreversible effects of an eating disorder on physical, psychological and emotional growth and development, the high mortality and the evidence suggesting improved outcome with early treatment, the Society for Adolescent Medicine advises that the threshold for intervention should be lower than in adults (Golden *et al*, 2003). Indeed, guidelines from the UK National Library for Health (http://www.library.nhs.uk) advise liaison with the child and adolescent mental health service and that referral should be made for both anorexia nervosa (this should be done urgently if body mass index is low or there has been rapid weight loss) and bulimia nervosa if there is a lack of rapid improvement.

# Conclusion

Primary care services play a vital role in the recognition and management of eating disorders. Practitioners need to be aware that sufferers often present with non-specific symptoms and that the patient may not link these with the eating disorder or may be reluctant to reveal the eating disorder. Primary

**Table 19.4** Suggested guidelines for children and adolescents with eating disorder

| Condition | Characteristics | Primary care management |
|---|---|---|
| Mild or early eating disorder | 85–95% ideal body weight and vital signs stable | Begin food plan (3 meals, 3 snacks, at least 1200–1500 calories per day) Set weight gain goals See weekly Parental supervision of meals for continued failure to gain Refer to dietician and therapist |
| Moderate or established eating disorder | 75–85% ideal body weight may have downhill trend in vital signs and minor laboratory abnormalities | As above plus: Dietician and therapist should be mandatory Discuss possibility of hospitalisation if weight loss not reversed |
| Severe eating disorder | Less than 75% ideal body weight, medically unstable, pulse below 50 b.p.m., may be dehydrated | Admit to hospital |

care practitioners need to be aware of the possibility of eating disorders, especially in high-risk groups, and a few simple screening questions can help in detection. However, it is important to have protocols in place as a prerequisite for screening (Johnston *et al*, 2007).

Once the diagnosis has been made, an empathetic and motivational stance is helpful in establishing a therapeutic relationship and engaging the patient. Is important to monitor risk and focus on establishing nutritional health and/or regular eating as well as engaging and supporting the family.

Primary care protocols should be established to guide referral to specialist services where necessary.

---

### Key points

- Patients with eating disorders often present to their primary care physicians with symptoms related to their illness but the eating disorder may go undiagnosed.
- Screening of high-risk groups is recommended but protocols for management need to be in place.
- The initial assessment and the initial coordination of care include the determination of the need for emergency medical or psychiatric assessment. The threshold for intervention in adolescents should be lower than in adults.
- Is important to monitor risk and focus on establishing nutritional health and regular eating as well as engaging and supporting the family.

---

## Further reading and e-resources

See Box 19.8 for a list of useful self-help books, websites and helplines.

## References

American Psychiatric Association (1994) *Diagnostic and Statistical Manual of Mental Disorders* (4th edition) (DSM–IV). APA.

Daaleman, C. J. (1991) *More or Less: Research on the Prevalence of Anorexia Nervosa, Bulimia Nervosa and Obesity* [in Dutch]. RIGG Oost Gelderland.

Department of Health (1999) *A National Service Framework for Mental Health*. Department of Health.

Fairburn, C. G. & Harrison, P. F. (2003) Eating disorders. *Lancet*, **361**, 407–416.

Fichter, M. & Krenn, K. (2003) Eating disorders in males. In *Handbook of Eating Disorders* (2nd edn) (eds J. Treasure, U. Schmidt & E. van Furth), pp. 219–235. Wiley.

Golden, N. H., Katzman, D. K., Kreipe, R. E., *et al* (2003) Eating disorders in adolescents: position paper of the Society for Adolescent Medicine. *Journal of Adolescent Health*, **33**, 496–503.

Herzog, W., Greenwood, D. N., Dorer, D. J., *et al* (2000) Mortality in eating disorders: a descriptive study. *International Journal of Eating Disorders*, **28**, 20–26.

Hoek, H. W. (1993) Review of the epidemiological studies of eating disorders. *International Review of Psychiatry*, **5**, 61–74.

Hoek, H. W., van Hoeken, D. & Katzman, M. A. (2003) Epidemiology and cultural aspects of eating disorders: a review. In *Eating Disorders* (eds M. Maj, K. Halmi, J. J. Lopez-Ibor, *et al*), pp. 75–104. Wiley.

Johnston, O., Fornai, G., Cabrini, S., *et al* (2007) Feasibility and acceptability of screening for eating disorders in primary care. *Family Practice*, **24**, 511–517.

Keilen, M., Treasure, T., Schmidt, U., *et al* (1994) Quality of life measurements in eating disorders, angina and transplant candidates: are they comparable? *Journal of the Royal Society of Medicine*, **87**, 441–444.

Morgan, J. F., Reid, J. & Lacey, J. H. (1999) The SCOFF questionnaire: assessment of a new screening tool for eating disorders. *BMJ*, **319**, 1467–1468.

NICE (2004) *Eating Disorders: Core Interventions in the Treatment and Management of Anorexia Nervosa, Bulimia Nervosa and Related Eating Disorders*. British Psychological Society and Gaskell.

Nielsen, S., Møller-Madsen, S., Isager, T., *et al* (1998) Standardized mortality in eating disorders – a quantitative summary of previously published and new evidence. *Journal of Psychosomatic Research*, **44**, 413–434.

Noordenbos, G. (1991) Eating disorders: prevention and therapy [Dutch]. *De Psycholoog*, **3**, 122–129.

Ogg, E. C., Millar, H. R., Pusztai, E. E., *et al* (1997) General practice consultation patterns preceding diagnosis of eating disorders. *International Journal of Eating Disorders*, **22**, 89–93.

Rollnick, S., Mason, P. & Butler, C. (1999) *Health Behaviour Change: A Guide for Practitioners*. Churchill Livingstone.

Rome, E. S. & Ammerman, S. (2003) Medical complications of eating disorders: an update. *Journal of Adolescent Mental Health*, **33**, 418–426.

Royal College of Psychiatrists (2000) *Eating Disorders in the UK: Policies for Service Development and Training*. Council Report CR87. Royal College of Psychiatrists

Royal College of Psychiatrists (2001) *Primary Care Protocols for Common Mental Illnesses. Protocol III: Eating Disorders*. Royal College of Psychiatrists (http://www.rcpsych.ac.uk/pdf/pcProtocol.pdf).

Serpell, L. & Treasure, J. (2002) Bulimia nervosa: friend or foe? The pros and cons of bulimia nervosa. *International Journal of Eating Disorders*, **32**, 164–170.

Serpell, L., Treasure, J., Teasdale, J., *et al* (1999) Anorexia nervosa: friend or foe? *International Journal of Eating Disorders*, **25**, 177–186.

Sullivan, P. F. (1995) Mortality in anorexia nervosa. *American Journal of Psychiatry*, **152**, 1073–1074.

Treasure, J., Smith, G. & Crane, A. (2007) *Skills-Based Learning for Caring for a Loved One with an Eating Disorder: The New Maudsley Method*. Routledge.

Turnbull, S., Ward, A., Treasure, J., *et al* (1996) The demand for eating disorder care. An epidemiological study using the general practice research database. *British Journal of Psychiatry*, **169**, 705–712.

World Health Organization (1992) *Classification of Mental and Behavioural Disorders. Clinical Descriptions and Diagnostic Guidelines* (10th revision) (ICD–10). WHO.

# CHAPTER 20

# Physical health of people with mental illness

Richard Holt, Tony Kendrick and Robert Peveler

### Summary

This chapter explores the reasons why physical illness occurs more frequently among people with mental illness and the responsibilities of the primary care team in screening and treatment. The physical healthcare of people with severe mental illness is a frequently neglected component of their holistic care. Guidelines and policy documents have recommended that registers of people with severe mental illness and systems of regular review of their care should be set up in general practice to reduce the burden of physical illness.

The physical healthcare of people with severe mental illness has probably never been of the highest quality and is a frequently neglected yet essential component of the holistic care of the person with mental illness (Peveler *et al*, 2000). The standardised mortality ratio is increased threefold in those with schizophrenia and life expectancy is reduced by 10–20 years (Brown *et al*, 2000). While the risk of suicide and traumatic death is increased 12-fold in people with schizophrenia, mortality associated with physical illness is also doubled and accounts for around 75% of all deaths of people with schizophrenia (Fig. 20.1). Cardiovascular disease is the most common cause, accounting for 30–50% of all deaths (Osborn *et al*, 2007). Mortality rates are also higher in those with depression, which is as strong a risk factor for cardiovascular disease as smoking (Yusuf *et al*, 2004). The reasons for excess physical illness include both genetic and environmental factors as well as disease-specific factors and treatment effects (Holt *et al*, 2004).

The National Institute for Health and Clinical Excellence (NICE) has placed the responsibility for the management of physical health within primary care and so an understanding of the scale of the problem, of the underlying aetiology and of the management strategies is important for all professionals caring for people with mental illness (NICE, 2002).

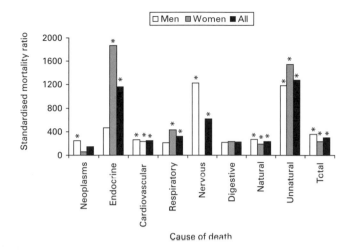

**Fig. 20.1** Standardised mortality ratio for causes of death in 79 people with schizophrenia. *Increase significantly different from the general population. Adapted from Brown *et al* (2000).

# Cardiovascular disease

The increased rates of cardiovascular disease in people with mental illness present an important clinical problem. Much of the increased risk is explained by an excess of traditional cardiovascular risk factors but a direct effect of the mental illness cannot be excluded (Osborn *et al*, 2007).

Smoking rates are high in people with severe mental illness (Brown *et al*, 1999). Although dyslipidaemia has been less well studied in people with mental illness (Bushe & Paton, 2005), in people with chronic schizophrenia treated with phenothiazines, levels of high-density lipoprotein (HDL) cholesterol are lower and those of serum triglycerides higher than in normal controls (Sasaki *et al*, 1984). Antipsychotic drugs have a modest adverse effect on lipid profile. Low-density lipoprotein (LDL) cholesterol is increased with treatment, while HDL cholesterol is decreased, with little difference between drugs (Bushe & Paton, 2005). In contrast, triglyceride concentrations may be markedly raised by antipsychotic treatment. The mechanism appears to be mediated at least partially by weight change and therefore drugs associated with the most weight gain are most consistently associated with hypertriglyceridaemia.

Diabetes and obesity are increased in people with mental illness and are covered separately within this chapter.

Studies of the prevalence of hypertension in severe mental illness have yielded inconsistent findings, with some finding it increased (Kendrick, 1996) and others not (Osborn *et al*, 2003). Antipsychotic drugs have multiple opposing effects on blood pressure; weight gain will tend to increase blood pressure, while α-adrenergic blockade may lower it (Markowitz *et al*, 1995).

In addition to atherosclerotic vascular disease, there is a small increase in arrhythmia, notably the potentially fatal *torsades de pointes*, in people with mental illness receiving certain antipsychotic or antidepressant drugs (Witchel *et al*, 2003).

## Clinical implications

It is important to assess cardiovascular risk factors in people with mental illness on an annual basis. It is likely that the Joint British Societies' risk factor tables (British Cardiac Society *et al*, 2005) underestimate the risk of cardiovascular disease, but without specific risk engines for people with mental illness more precise estimates are not possible.

Primary preventive treatment is recommended for those at high risk through systematic treatment of cardiovascular risk factors (Box 20.1). Advice about smoking cessation is needed. There is no evidence that statins or aspirin are any less effective in people with mental illness and therefore patients should not be denied these effective treatments because of their mental illness (Hanssens *et al*, 2007). It is important to treat the mental illness effectively to ensure that the patient is in the best position to understand the need for concordance with treatment.

# Diabetes

The link between diabetes and severe mental illness has been recognised for well over a century. Despite the difficulties in obtaining accurate

---

**Box 20.1** Interventions to reduce cardiovascular disease in people with severe mental illness

- Annual assessment of cardiovascular risk factors
  - age
  - gender
  - family history
  - lifestyle (smoking, alcohol, exercise)
  - body mass index
  - lipid profile
  - glucose
  - blood pressure
- Calculate cardiovascular risk using established risk engines
- Ensure mental illness is adequately treated
- Offer advice on lifestyle modification
- For those at high risk, consider pharmacological therapy –
  - lipid-lowering therapy (especially statins)
  - aspirin
  - agents to reduce blood pressure

---

epidemiological data, the rates of diabetes in people with schizophrenia and bipolar illness are increased two- to threefold, to around 10–15%, in US and European settings (Holt *et al*, 2004). It is well recognised that there is a high prevalence of undiagnosed diabetes within the general population; among those with severe mental illness, as many as 70% of all cases of diabetes are undiagnosed (Subramaniam *et al*, 2003). This may reflect not only the reluctance of patients to volunteer symptoms but also the difficulties they have in accessing physical health services.

Although familial and genetic studies suggest inheritance as a factor (Gough & O'Donovan, 2005), it seems likely that environmental factors are the most important reason for the increased prevalence of diabetes (Fig. 20.2) (Holt & Peveler, 2006*a*,*b*). Compared with the general population, people with severe mental illness are less physically active and have diets that are poor in fruit and vegetables, and high in saturated fat and refined sugars (Brown *et al*, 1999).

Much attention has been paid to the effect of antipsychotics on the risk of diabetes. The evidence concerning the antipsychotics remains inconclusive; while a small number of individuals have developed diabetes rapidly following treatment, overall the risk appears to be low and the vast majority of those receiving antipsychotics will not develop diabetes as a result of their treatment (Holt & Peveler, 2006*a*,*b*).

Depression is increased in people with diabetes but there is also evidence that depression increases the risk of subsequent diabetes (Engum, 2007). The reason for this link is unclear but may involve some of the same mechanisms that operate in severe mental illness.

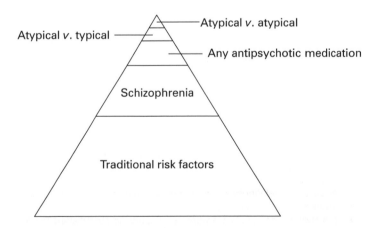

**Fig. 20.2** Factors influencing the risk of diabetes among patients with schizophrenia. The attributable risk for developing diabetes is greater for traditional risk factors such as family history, ethnicity, obesity and ageing than it is for receiving an antipsychotic. Adapted from Holt & Peveler (2006*b*).

## Clinical implications

The high prevalence of diabetes among those with severe mental illness has important clinical implications (Box 20.2). The first is the need to screen for diabetes and it is noteworthy that several national diabetes associations, including Diabetes UK, now recommend that those with severe mental illness should be routinely screened for diabetes, before treatment, 3–4 months after a treatment change and then annually. While the ideal test is a fasting blood glucose level, it is not always possible for those with severe mental illness to fast and under these circumstances a random blood glucose level is an acceptable alternative and certainly preferable to no test at all (Dinan *et al*, 2004).

Lifestyle modification is a highly effective intervention to reduce the incidence of new-onset diabetes and should be encouraged in people with severe mental illness (Fig. 20.3) (Pendlebury *et al*, 2007).

The complexity of the management of diabetes means that this should be undertaken by someone with suitable experience, although this would usually be within primary care in the first instance (Dinan *et al*, 2004). Adequate treatment of the psychosis is paramount in the successful management of diabetes and therefore antipsychotics should be stopped only after consultation with the mental health team if it is clear that they are the main cause of diabetes.

# Obesity

The rate of obesity among those with severe mental illness is increased (Dickerson *et al*, 2006). Obesity reduces self-esteem and is often associated with poor concordance with psychiatric treatment (Pendlebury *et al*, 2007).

All antipsychotics can lead to significant weight gain, although the risk is highest with clozapine and olanzapine (Allison *et al*, 1999). There is wide inter-individual variability regarding weight gain with second-generation antipsychotic treatment, making predictions about weight change difficult. The risk of weight gain seems to be highest for younger individuals (particularly first-episode patients), women, those with a family or personal

---

**Box 20.2** Clinical implications of the high prevalence rate of diabetes among those with mental illness

- People with mental illness should be screened for diabetes because of the high prevalence of undiagnosed diabetes
- Lifestyle modification programmes should be established to reduce the risk of diabetes
- A clear management plan involving psychiatric and physical health services is needed for those who develop diabetes

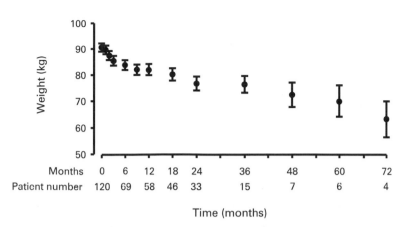

**Fig. 20.3** Change in weight of people with severe mental illness attending a weight management clinic in Salford run by Mr John Pendlebury. The points show the means, and the bars standard error. For further details of the programme, see Pendlebury *et al* (2007).

history of obesity, and those with a tendency to overeat at times of stress. Early weight gain in the first few weeks of treatment is probably the most reliable predictor of long-term weight change.

## Clinical implications

The prevention and management of obesity in people with severe mental illness is challenging but not insurmountable. Several studies have shown that weight loss or the prevention of weight gain is possible and lifestyle modification programmes, with advice about diet and physical activity, are at least as effective as they are in the general population (Pendlebury *et al*, 2007). Most of the studies report the effectiveness of group programmes and intuitively the benefits of peer support for the patient are appealing.

# Hyperprolactinaemia

Hyperprolactinaemia is a common problem among those taking antipsychotic medication, with both short-term and long-term clinical sequelae (Box 20.3) (Bushe & Shaw, 2007). For many years, this problem was ignored because it was believed to be an unavoidable consequence of antipsychotic medication through blockade with dopamine $D_2$ receptors. This is no longer the case, as several of the newer second-generation antipsychotics have a much lower propensity to cause hyperprolactinaemia.

## Clinical implications

It is important to ask the person with severe mental illness about symptoms of sexual dysfunction; in women this should also include enquiries about

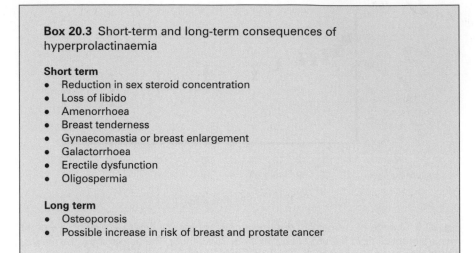

**Box 20.3** Short-term and long-term consequences of hyperprolactinaemia

**Short term**
- Reduction in sex steroid concentration
- Loss of libido
- Amenorrhoea
- Breast tenderness
- Gynaecomastia or breast enlargement
- Galactorrhoea
- Erectile dysfunction
- Oligospermia

**Long term**
- Osteoporosis
- Possible increase in risk of breast and prostate cancer

galactorrhoea and menstrual irregularities. It is important to monitor for changes in serum prolactin level following changes in antipsychotic medication (NICE, 2002). If there is evidence of hyperprolactinaemia, particularly if this is associated with sexual dysfunction or reduced sex steroid concentrations, it is important to consider dose reduction or switching to alternative antipsychotics with lower potential to raise prolactin, after discussion with the psychiatric team.

# Osteoporosis

The prevalence of osteoporosis is increased in people with severe mental illness and the consequences of osteoporotic fractures are more serious than in the general population (Yarden *et al*, 1989). In-patient stay and rehabilitation following fracture are often longer among those who are mentally ill and fracture may lead to a psychiatric relapse.

While hyperprolactinaemia leads to reduction in bone mineral density, predominantly through inhibition of the hypothalamic–pituitary–gonadal axis, there are other reasons for the increase in osteoporosis in mental illness, including diet and physical inactivity (Table 20.1).

## Clinical implications

The availability of dual X-ray absorptiometry (DEXA) varies according to health system and there is no systematic advice about the place of DEXA in screening people with severe mental illness for osteoporosis. It seems sensible to consider this investigation for any person with mental illness who has other risk factors (Table 20.1). It is also important to ensure that people with severe mental illness are given advice about the need for adequate

**Table 20.1** Risk factors for low bone mass in mental illness and within the general population

| People with mental illness | General population |
|---|---|
| Smoking | Advanced age |
| Alcoholism | Female |
| Reduced physical activity | White race |
| Extrapyramidal movement disorders | Previous fracture |
| Reduced calcium and vitamin D intake | Postmenopausal |
| Reduced caloric intake | Maternal history of hip fracture |
| Hyperprolactinaemia | Oral corticosteroid use |
| Hypogonadism | Low body mass index |
| Hypercortisolaemia | Falls |
| Polydipsia with obligatory hypercalcuria | |

calcium and vitamin D intake, as well as the importance of regular weight-bearing exercise. Where low bone mineral density is found, pharmacological therapy with bisphosphonates is appropriate, as in the general population.

As peak bone mineral density is often not reached until the early 20s, it is probably best to avoid prolactin-raising antipsychotics in younger patients, to reduce the risk of osteoporosis later in life. In amenorrhoeic premenopausal women, it is reasonable to use the oral contraceptive pill to maintain skeletal integrity where a change or dose reduction in antipsychotic medication is not possible.

# HIV and hepatitis

Patients with severe mental illness are at significantly increased risk for infection with human immunodeficiency virus (HIV), hepatitis C virus, or both (Cournos *et al*, 2005). Several factors underlie this increased risk, including substance misuse and high-risk sexual behaviour. Although overall sexual activity is lower in people with severe mental illness, those who are sexually active tend to engage in higher-risk behaviour than the general population. This probably reflects inadequate knowledge and understanding of the risks of HIV and hepatitis.

Infection with a life-threatening viral illness in people with severe mental illness worsens the prognosis for both conditions.

## Clinical implications

It is clearly important that the person who is mentally ill understands the risk of engaging in high-risk sexual activity. The delivery of factual information about this is often insufficient to bring about behavioural changes that reduce the risk of exposure and transmission, and so there is a responsibility to encourage the practice of safe sex.

For those who develop either HIV or hepatitis, effective pharmacotherapy exists, and antipsychotics and highly active antiretroviral treatments for

HIV can be used together successfully. Ensuring adherence to treatment is clinically challenging.

## Regular review in primary care

In the UK, in the 1990s, a number of randomised controlled trials of systems of regular review of patients with severe mental illness by their general practitioner or practice nurse showed that the process of care could be improved, in terms of the numbers of problems picked up, changes in treatment, and referrals to secondary care, for physical health as well as mental health problems (Kendrick *et al*, 1995; Nazareth *et al*, 1996; Burns *et al*, 1998). More recently, it has been shown that patients with schizophrenia are just as willing as other patients to attend their general practice for cardiovascular screening (Osborn *et al*, 2003).

Guidelines and policy documents in the UK (including the National Service Framework for Mental Health) have recommended that registers of people with severe mental illness, and systems of regular review of their care, be set up in general practice (Burns & Kendrick, 1997; Department of Health, 1999; NICE, 2002, 2006).

In 2003, the new GP contract introduced performance-related payments to reward the regular review of patients with a severe mental illness through the Quality and Outcomes Framework (QOF) (British Medical Association & NHS Employers, 2003). The aim was to ensure annual reviews of mental and physical health as well as drug treatment, and coordination of care with specialist services. In the 2006 version of the UK GP contract (British Medical Association & NHS Employers, 2006) more specific recommendations were made for the regular review of physical health (Box 20.4).

---

**Box 20.4** Recommendations for the annual review of patients with severe mental illness in general practice

- Cardiovascular
  - Smoking
  - Blood pressure
  - History suggestive of arrhythmias
  - Cholesterol where clinically indicated
  - Body mass index
- Alcohol or drug misuse
- Assessment of risk of diabetes
  - Especially patients on newer antipsychotics
- Preventive screening appropriate to age and gender
  - Cervical screening
  - Mammography

From the UK GP contract Quality and Outcomes Framework (British Medical Association & NHS Employers, 2006).

---

While the NICE guidance is clear that the responsibility for the physical health of people with mental illness lies with primary care, some patients never see their general practitioner and the responsibility for the physical health monitoring of these people lies with specialist psychiatric services (NICE, 2002). In theory, this should ensure that all people with mental illness are assessed in one clinical setting or another. In reality, however, many people are never screened and there is a high prevalence of undiagnosed disease (Taylor *et al*, 2005). It is therefore essential that there is excellent communication between primary care and specialist services at a local level to ensure that all people are screened and managed appropriately. The development of shared guidelines is important to delineate who has what responsibility within any given locality. In some settings, physical health nurses or dieticians are being employed by mental health trusts to promote physical health monitoring, management and promotion.

In conclusion, chronic physical ill health is common among people with mental illness and constitutes an important clinical problem. A coordinated approach is needed across primary and specialist care to ensure that this burden of disease is managed effectively.

---

Key points

- People with severe mental illness have a life expectancy which is shortened on average by 10–20 years; three-quarters of deaths are attributable to physical illness.
- Diabetes, cardiovascular disease and obesity are all more common among people with severe mental illness, as are hyperprolactinaemia, osteoporosis and sexual health problems.
- The causes of the increased risk of physical illness in people with severe mental illness are multiple, and include genetic and environmental risk factors as well as disease-specific and treatment-specific factors.
- The physical healthcare of people with severe mental illness is a frequently neglected component of the holistic care.
- Regular review of patients with severe mental illness in primary care improves both the diagnosis and the treatment of physical illness.

---

# Further reading and e-resources

NICE (2006) *Bipolar Disorder: The Management of Bipolar Disorder in Adults, Children and Adolescents, in Primary and Secondary Care*. NICE (http://www.nice.org.uk/nicemedia/pdf/CG38fullguideline.pdf).

NICE (2009) *Schizophrenia: Core Interventions in the Treatment and Management of Schizophrenia in Primary and Secondary Care*. NICE (http://www.nice.org.uk/nicemedia/pdf/CG82NICEGuideline.pdf).

# References

Allison, D. B., Mentore, J. L., Heo, M., *et al* (1999) Antipsychotic-induced weight gain: a comprehensive research synthesis. *American Journal of Psychiatry*, **156**, 1686–1696.

British Cardiac Society, British Hypertension Society, Diabetes UK, *et al* (2005) JBS 2: Joint British Societies' guidelines on prevention of cardiovascular disease in clinical practice. *Heart*, **91 (Suppl 5)**, v1–v52.

British Medical Association & NHS Employers (2003) *Investing in General Practice. The New General Medical Services Contract*. BMA & NHS Employers.

British Medical Association & NHS Employers (2006) *Revisions to the GMS Contract 2006/07. Delivering Investment in General Practice*. BMA & NHS Employers

Brown, S., Birtwistle, J., Roe, L., *et al* (1999) The unhealthy lifestyle of people with schizophrenia. *Psychological Medicine*, **29**, 697–701.

Brown, S., Inskip, H. & Barraclough, B. (2000) Causes of the excess mortality of schizophrenia. *British Journal of Psychiatry*, **177**, 212–217.

Burns, T. & Kendrick, T. (1997) The primary care of patients with schizophrenia: a search for good practice. *British Journal of General Practice*, **47**, 515–520.

Burns, T., Millar, E., Garland, C., *et al* (1998) Randomized controlled trial of teaching practice nurses to carry out structured assessments of patients receiving depot antipsychotic injections. British Journal of General Practice, 48, 1845–1848.

Bushe, C. & Paton, C. (2005) The potential impact of antipsychotics on lipids in schizophrenia: is there enough evidence to confirm a link? *Journal of Psychopharmacology*, **19**, 76–83.

Bushe, C. & Shaw, M. (2007) Prevalence of hyperprolactinaemia in a naturalistic cohort of schizophrenia and bipolar outpatients during treatment with typical and atypical antipsychotics. *Journal of Psychopharmacology*, **21**, 768–773.

Cournos, F., McKinnon, K. & Sullivan, G. (2005) Schizophrenia and comorbid human immunodeficiency virus or hepatitis C virus. *Journal of Clinical Psychiatry*, **66** (Suppl. 6), 27–33.

Department of Health (1999) *National Service Framework for Mental Health: Modern Standards and Service Models*. The Stationery Office.

Dickerson, F. B., Brown, C. H., Kreyenbuhl, J. A., *et al* (2006) Obesity among individuals with serious mental illness. *Acta Psychiatrica Scandinavica*, **113**, 306–313.

Dinan, T., Holt, R., Kohen, D., *et al* (2004) 'Schizophrenia and Diabetes 2003' Expert Consensus Meeting, Dublin, 3–4 October 2003: consensus summary. *British Journal of Psychiatry*, **47** (Suppl.), 112–114.

Engum, A. (2007) The role of depression and anxiety in onset of diabetes in a large population-based study. *Journal of Psychosomatic Research*, **62**, 31–38.

Gough, S. C. & O'Donovan, M. C. (2005) Clustering of metabolic comorbidity in schizophrenia: a genetic contribution? *Journal of Psychopharmacology*, **19**, 47–55.

Hanssens, L., De Hert, M., Kalnicka, D., *et al* (2007) Pharmacological treatment of severe dyslipidaemia in patients with schizophrenia. *International Clinical Psychopharmacology*, **22**, 43–49.

Holt, R. I. G. & Peveler, R. C. (2006a) Antipsychotic drugs and diabetes – an application of the Austin Bradford Hill criteria. *Diabetologia*, **49**, 1467–1476.

Holt, R. I. G. & Peveler, R. C. (2006b) Antipsychotic medication. *Diabetes, Obesity and Metabolism*, **8**, 125–135

Holt, R. I. G., Peveler, R. C. & Byrne, C. D. (2004) Schizophrenia, the metabolic syndrome and diabetes. *Diabetic Medicine*, **21**, 515–523.

Kendrick, T. (1996) Cardiovascular and respiratory risk factors and symptoms among general practice patients with long-term mental illness. *British Journal of Psychiatry*, **169**, 733–739.

Kendrick, T., Burns, T. & Freeling, P. (1995) Randomised controlled trial of teaching general practitioners to carry out structured assessments of their long term mentally ill patients. *BMJ*, **311**, 93–98.

Markowitz, J. S., Wells, B. G. & Carson, W. H. (1995) Interactions between antipsychotic and antihypertensive drugs. *Annals of Pharmacotherapy*, **29**, 603–609.

Nazareth, I., King, M. & See Tai, S. (1996) Monitoring psychosis in general practice: a controlled trial. *British Journal of Psychiatry*, **169**, 482.

NICE (2002) *Schizophrenia: Core Interventions in the Treatment and Management of Schizophrenia in Primary and Secondary Care*. NICE (http://www.nice.org.uk/nicemedia/pdf/ CG82NICEGuideline.pdf).

NICE (2006) *Bipolar Disorder: The Management of Bipolar Disorder in Adults, Children and Adolescents, in Primary and Secondary Care*. NICE (http://www.nice.org.uk/nicemedia/ pdf/CG38fullguideline.pdf).

Osborn, D. P., King, M. B. & Nazareth, I. (2003) Participation in screening for cardiovascular risk by people with schizophrenia or similar mental illnesses: cross sectional study in general practice. *BMJ*, **326**, 1122–1123.

Osborn, D. P., Levy, G., Nazareth, I., *et al* (2007) Relative risk of cardiovascular and cancer mortality in people with severe mental illness from the United Kingdom's General Practice Research Database. *Archives of General Psychiatry*, **64**, 242–249.

Pendlebury, J., Bushe, C. J., Wildgust, H. J., *et al* (2007) Long-term maintenance of weight loss in patients with severe mental illness through a behavioural treatment programme in the UK. *Acta Psychiatrica Scandinavica*, **115**, 286–294.

Peveler, R. C., Feldman, E. & Friedman, T. (2000) *Liaison Psychiatry: Planning Services for Specialist Settings*. Gaskell.

Sasaki, J., Kumagae, G., Sata, T., *et al* (1984) Decreased concentration of high density lipoprotein cholesterol in schizophrenic patients treated with phenothiazines. *Atherosclerosis*, **51**, 163–169.

Subramaniam, M., Chong, S. A. & Pek, E. (2003) Diabetes mellitus and impaired glucose tolerance in patients with schizophrenia. *Canadian Journal of Psychiatry*, **48**, 345–347.

Taylor, D., Young, C., Mohamed, R., *et al* (2005) Undiagnosed impaired fasting glucose and diabetes mellitus amongst inpatients receiving antipsychotic drugs. *Journal of Psychopharmacology*, **19**, 182–186.

Witchel, H. J., Hancox, J. C. & Nutt, D. J. (2003) Psychotropic drugs, cardiac arrhythmia, and sudden death. *Journal of Clinical Psychopharmacology*, **23**, 58–77.

Yarden, P. E., Finkel, M. G., Raps, C. S., *et al* (1989) Adverse outcome of hip fractures in older schizophrenic patients. *American Journal of Psychiatry*, **146**, 377–379.

Yusuf, S., Hawken, S., Ounpuu, S., *et al* (2004) Effect of potentially modifiable risk factors associated with myocardial infarction in 52 countries (the INTERHEART study): case–control study. *Lancet*, **364**, 937–952.

# CHAPTER 21

# Ethnic minorities

Waquas Waheed

Summary

The concept of ethnicity is multidimensional. The prevalence of psychiatric disorders is higher in ethnic minorities than in host populations. Ethnic minorities under-use mental health services and where services are accessed they may not adequately meet their cultural and religious needs. Non-detection and poor management of mental disorders in primary care increase the likelihood that patients in crisis will come into contact with non-health-related agencies, such as police or forensic services. There is a need to understand patients' own perspectives and experiences of their illness and healthcare systems. These observations need to be incorporated in management plans and service-delivery frameworks.

There has been a constant human migration over the centuries but this increased greatly after the middle of the 20th century. Geopolitical problems and economic disparities are cited as the major factors for this increase, which has been facilitated by improved means of travel. Countries in the West have been popular destinations, as they offer economic opportunities and safety from political strife. In European countries, ethnic minority groups are largely representative of historical colonial links, while in the USA and Canada migrants from South America and later generations of African slaves form the majority of minority ethnic groups.

## Defining ethnic minorities

The concept of ethnicity is multidimensional, and includes aspects such as race, origin or ancestry, identity, language and religion. It may also include more subtle dimensions, such as culture, the arts, customs and beliefs, and even practices such as dress and food preparation. It is also dynamic and in a constant state of flux. It will change as a result of new immigration flows, blending and intermarriage, and new identities may be formed (Statistics Canada, 2008).

# Rates of mental illness

Circumstances of migration and the status of being in a minority in the host country invariably put the individual under stress. The prevalence of psychiatric disorders is higher in ethnic minorities than in host populations. But this follows some peculiar trends, specific to certain ethnic groups. The incidence of schizophrenia has been found to be higher in African–Caribbean minority groups settled in the West (Selten & Sijben, 1994; Bhugra et al, 1997; Selten et al, 2007) but lower in Caribbean islands (Mahy et al, 1999). This higher prevalence persists in the second generations of African–Caribbean groups residing in the West (Bhugra & Bhui, 1998).

Ödegaard (1932) reported that migrant Norwegians in the USA had higher rates of schizophrenia than the host population, with a peak occurring 10–12 years after migration. Several later studies have similarly shown that rates of schizophrenia are higher among migrant groups than among native populations (Cooper, 2005). Cochrane & Bal (1989) observed that migrants had higher rates of admission than the native population. Similar high rates of schizophrenia have also been reported among migrant populations in The Netherlands (Selten & Sijben, 1994).

Epidemiological studies in the UK show that women of South Asian family origin, in particular from Pakistan, and Irish men show higher prevalence of depression and other common mental disorders (Husain et al, 1997; Bhui et al, 2001; Weich et al, 2004). Similarly, in the USA, Spanish-speaking migrants from Latin America, in particular women, have a higher prevalence of depression (Chung et al, 2003; Read & Gorman, 2007).

Research has demonstrated higher rates of self-harm and suicide among young ethnic minority women but not among men and older women (Husain et al, 2006; Fortuna et al, 2007; Walker, 2007). These women seek help at the point of desperation, and self-harm in the majority of cases is a consequence of interpersonal problems stemming from cultural conflicts (Chew-Graham et al, 2002).

# Factors associated with the increased prevalence of mental health problems

## Patient-related psychosocial risk factors

Some of the reasons cited for elevated rates are listed in Box 21.1.

Symptoms of illness in ethnic minority patients tend to persist and follow a chronic course to a greater extent than in the White population (Husain et al, 1997; Bhui et al, 2001; Chung et al, 2003; Weich et al, 2004; Read & Gorman, 2007). The main reasons for this chronic course appear

---

**Box 21.1** Reasons for elevated rates of mental ill health in ethnic minorities

- Poor housing
- Unemployment or low-paid work
- Racism, discrimination and abuse
- Low literacy levels and lack of English language skills
- Lack of social support
- Marital and family relationships (different traditional or religious expectations, including beliefs concerning marriage, divorce, widowhood and family honour)

---

to be lack of treatment seeking, lack of treatment provision and poorer adherence to treatment regimens in this group. This leads to non-resolution of symptoms and hence higher prevalence.

## Factors related to the health service

South Asian patients living in the UK visit their general practitioner (GP) more frequently than comparison White groups but are less likely to have their psychological difficulties identified (Gillam *et al*, 1989). It has also been reported that ethnic minorities under-use mental health services and where services are accessed they may not adequately meet their cultural and religious needs (Wilson & MacCarthy, 1994). This lack of help seeking from the patients, along with lower referral rates to secondary mental health services, is a barrier to the management of such patients (Bhui *et al*, 2002).

Access to psychological therapies is the key to effective management, particularly of mild to moderate illness. However, ethnic minorities in the UK are less likely to receive talking therapies than the host population (Bhui & Bhugra, 1998). Also, among Asian patients who had not used counselling services, the awareness of such services was found to be low (Netto *et al*, 2006). Data collected between 1993 and 2004 revealed that, in the USA, psychotherapy visits significantly decreased, from 2.4% to 1.3% in Hispanics, whereas they remained constant (2.5%) in non-Hispanics (Blanco *et al*, 2007).

Bhugra *et al* (1997), in a study examining the incidence and outcome of schizophrenia, found that only one in 36 African–Caribbean patients with schizophrenia presented via the GP. Healthcare systems that are not organised in accordance with the preferred pattern of help seeking do not readily lend themselves to early intervention. A systematic review of pathways to care in first-episode psychosis deduced that, compared with that for White British patients, GP referral was less frequent for both African–Caribbean and Black African patients and referral by a criminal justice agency was more common. Detention was also associated with lack of help seeking and lack of GP referral, while cases with GP referral were associated with lower detention rates (Singh & Grange, 2006).

## Factors related to primary care staff

The knowledge, skills and attitudes of staff working in primary care are crucially important in addressing the quality of treatment provided to ethnic minorities. The diagnostic and treatment practices of clinicians may vary according to the minority status of the patient they are seeing and there are considerable variations in the competence of health professionals to manage mental health problems presented by minority groups. The ability of primary care physicians to diagnose depression, for instance, was found to be poorer for African and Hispanic Americans in the Medical Outcomes Study database (Borowsky et al, 2000) and for Punjabi-speaking, South Asian minorities in London, UK (Bhui et al, 2002). Poor detection rates of mental health problems among South Asian patients have been attributed to linguistic and cultural barriers between patients and doctors (Jacob et al, 1998). It is suggested that the diverse culture-specific expressions of psychological distress, such as 'sinking heart', a Punjabi idiom of distress (Krause, 1989), and *ataque de nervios* in south American migrants (Guarnaccia et al, 2003), can mislead the general practitioner and make accurate diagnosis of depression more difficult.

Contrary to the claim that non-Westerners are prone to somatise their distress, recent research confirms that somatisation is ubiquitous. Somatic symptoms serve as cultural idioms of distress in many ethno-cultural groups and, if misinterpreted by the clinician, may lead to unnecessary diagnostic procedures or inappropriate treatment. Clinicians must learn to decode the meaning of somatic and dissociative symptoms, which are not simply indices of disease or disorder but part of a language of distress, with interpersonal and wider social meanings (Kirmayer, 2001). In Manchester, UK, 42% of a sample were assessed as depressed in a diagnostic interview in a primary care survey of Pakistani immigrants, and out of these not a single respondent was in receipt of any treatment for their depression (Husain et al, 1997).

The problem does not end with low rates of diagnosis: the quality of treatment provided to ethnic minorities is relatively poor. Hull et al (2001) found that the lowest prescription rates for antidepressants were found in areas of London where Asian immigrants were residing in higher proportions. A further analysis of the prescriptions revealed that Asians were given lower doses of medication, and for a shorter period (Cornwell & Hull, 1998).

Similarly, in the USA, African Americans among 13 065 Medicaid patients in a nationally representative survey in primary care who presented with depression were provided antidepressant prescriptions at a lower rate than Caucasians (27% versus 44%). In addition, Caucasians were significantly more likely to receive the newer, safer and better-tolerated antidepressants, whereas African Americans were more likely to be prescribed the older, less well-tolerated and less safe tricyclic antidepressants (Melfi *et al*, 2000). Such poor prescription choices may contribute to the lower adherence rates to psychotropic medication among people from an ethnic minority than among Caucasians (Diaz *et al*, 2005).

Non-detection and poor management of mental disorders in primary care increase the likelihood that patients in crisis will come into contact with non-health-related agencies, such as police or forensic services. This may lead to dissatisfaction with services, poor engagement and repeated relapses, leading in turn to a delay in diagnosis or treatment and to multiple involuntary hospital admissions. Lack of training in cross-cultural issues, stereotyping and poor communication skills are other contributing factors.

## Patient-related treatment factors

In addition to patient-related psychosocial factors, discussed above, which can lead to a delay in seeking care, other key factors that require further examination include acceptance, preferences and engagement with treatment. All these factors are determined not only by patients' own cultural beliefs, literacy and acculturation levels but also those of their immediate family and friends.

This area of research remains largely unexplored, particularly in the UK. What is available mainly originates in the USA, where it was found that African Americans and Hispanic Americans found antidepressants less acceptable as compared to other treatments (Cooper *et al*, 2003) and preferred counselling (Hazlett-Stevens *et al*, 2002). African Americans had a lower medication adherence rate than Caucasians (35% versus 61%) (Brown *et al*, 1999). A study in New Mexico at various university-affiliated clinics found that Hispanic patients were significantly less likely to adhere to their antidepressants than their Caucasian counterparts (Sleath *et al*, 2003).

Once individuals have been diagnosed with a mental illness, their problems become more obvious and they may feel stigmatised by the diagnosis and treatment. Through qualitative research it has been determined that stigma-related concerns are more common among immigrant women and may partly account for their under-use of mental healthcare services (Nadeem *et al*, 2007).

# How can we improve the outcome of treatment?

It is recognised that ethnic minorities are significantly less likely to obtain high-quality care than the general population. This has been highlighted in two key policy publications in the UK and the USA. *Inside Outside* (Department of Health, 2001) and the Surgeon General's report *Mental*

*Health: Culture, Race and Ethnicity* (Department of Health and Human Services, 2001) not only touch upon the disparities but also highlight the barriers. Both documents also make evidence-based suggestions on overcoming these barriers, particularly the role primary care can play in bridging these gaps (Box 21.2).

It is imperative that a paradigm shift in health policy is made to accommodate sensitivity towards the needs specific to ethnic minorities and that these are incorporated into established guidelines. Even small innovations can yield dividends and can be cost-effective as well. A multidimensional approach to tackling all the main factors can help to remove some of the disparities. As these factors are interrelated, a solution based on addressing individual factors will fail to achieve the desired results.

Perhaps the best level at which to incorporate these changes is in primary care (Ayalon *et al*, 2007), particularly in health systems that are modelled on the UK, where, unlike in the USA, socialised medicine is free to all citizens at the point of access. Primary care is the first point of contact and provides the majority of treatments, particularly for minor psychiatric morbidity. Even in the case of major illnesses, early detection will be in

---

**Box 21.2** Summary of official US and UK recommendations on overcoming barriers to primary care mental health experienced by ethnic minorities

- Establish consultation and discussion locally between various mental health agencies and other key stakeholders.
- Work collaboratively with the local voluntary sector in developing and sustaining a variety of service models for minority ethnic groups and promote mental health.
- Provide services that are congruent rather than conflicting with cultural norms.
- Establish accountability and ensure change through clinical governance.
- Provide language access for non-English speakers.
- Give all general practitioners training in cultural awareness.
- Incorporate culture and mental health into training for general practitioners.
- Improve geographical availability of culturally sensitive mental health services.
- Coordinate care to vulnerable, high-need ethnic groups.
- Regularly audit variations in consultation rates, referral rates to specialist mental health services and use of psychotropic drugs in different ethnic groups.
- Fund culturally sensitive research to find new evidence to dictate policy, service innovation and guideline development.

Derived from: *Inside Outside* (Department of Health, 2001) and the Surgeon General's report *Mental Health: Culture, Race and Ethnicity* (Department of Health and Human Services, 2001).

primary care, and referral to specialist services and subsequent follow-up are arranged through primary care. From a user perspective, this may also be more acceptable, as primary care is generally seen as less stigmatising than secondary care and more able to respond to the patient's own health beliefs. From a commissioning perspective, a focus on primary care means that more patients can be seen and treated, in a more cost-efficient way.

A multilevel approach that enhances the cultural competence of clinicians and healthcare systems is suggested as one solution to reducing racial/ethnic disparities in healthcare. Enhancing provider and clinic cultural competence may be synergistic strategies for reducing healthcare disparities (Paez et al, 2008). While training in cultural competency for physicians is increasingly promoted, few studies have evaluated the impact of such training. The available evidence suggests that whenever such interventions have been implemented, the result has been improved patient outcomes, particularly user satisfaction (Smith-Campbell, 2005; Thom et al, 2006; Dogra et al, 2007).

All pharmacological, psychological and social interventions are likely to be effective among ethnic minorities (Ward, 2007), but they need to be tailored to the needs of the minority population (Miranda et al, 2005). In particular, there is a need to understand patients' own perspectives and experiences of their illness and healthcare systems. These observations need to be incorporated in management plans and service delivery frameworks. Patients may prefer to be seen by a therapist of their own ethnic background, which may in turn increase adherence and satisfaction. If such options are not available, then formally trained interpreters rather than a family member should be used (Phelan & Parkman, 1995). Multilingual health information and self-report symptom measures can also aid diagnosis and help track progress.

The content and format of the psychological and social interventions need cultural adaptations to make them relevant and acceptable. Use of non-traditional delivery methods like guided self-help and multimedia should be explored, as traditional, face-to-face delivery of services is dependent on culturally trained therapists being available, which makes them costly and less widely available. Even in the case of pharmacological interventions, communication must include patient education about the medication, particularly side-effects, dose, duration and time lag before improvement, which should be repeatedly emphasised throughout the course of therapy. The therapeutic response to medication, along with the nature and degree of side-effects, may vary according to ethnic background (Burroughs et al, 2002), so physicians should be more vigilant and be ready to advise the patients and carers beforehand.

Assistance with child care, transportation, interpretation and multimedia information may help overcome barriers to services. Incorporating these measures into a stepped-care, enhanced and case management framework has shown promising outcomes (Miranda et al, 2006; Schraufnagel et al, 2006) (see also Chapter 27).

Persistent states of distress in the absence of timely intervention can culminate in presentation both in crisis and only when disorders are severe and patients' social networks and housing conditions are already compromised. Recovery times will then be longer and a greater intensity of input will be required to establish the necessary conditions for recovery and relapse prevention. If primary care could become involved at an earlier stage, identifying symptoms of relapse and keeping contact with non-statutory agencies with which ethnic minorities have regular contact, then this might enable earlier intervention. Finally, working through places of worship, leisure clubs, entertainment venues and the ethnic voluntary sector may also increase the engagement of minority ethnic communities, not only by extending services but also by providing education and advocacy (Gray, 1999). Such partnership would also facilitate recruitment and retention in research, which is of paramount importance when developing new interventions and evaluating targeted service delivery innovations (Wells *et al*, 2006).

---

**Key points**

- Ethnic minority populations are on the increase in high-income countries.
- There is huge diversity within these groups.
- Prevalence of mental illness is comparatively higher, and there is more unmet healthcare need in these groups.
- Currently there is lack of treatment evidence specific to ethnic minorities.
- As the risk factors are different, adaptations to the content and delivery of healthcare interventions are warranted.

---

## Further reading and e-resources

Bhugra, D. & Bhui, K. (2001) *Cross-cultural Psychiatry: A Practical Guide*. Arnold.

Online resources devoted to cultural competence:
http://www.culturalcompetence2.com/asian.html
US Department of Health and Human Services, Office of Minority Health, http://www.thinkculturalhealth.org

## References

Ayalon, L., Areán, P. A., Linkins, K., *et al* (2007) Integration of mental health services into primary care overcomes ethnic disparities in access to mental health services between black and white elderly. *American Journal of Geriatric Psychiatry*, **15**, 906–912.

Bhugra, D. & Bhui, K. (1998) Transcultural psychiatry: do problems persist in the second generation? *Hospital Medicine*, **59**, 126–129.

Bhugra, D., Leff, J., Mallett, R., *et al* (1997) Incidence and outcome of schizophrenia in whites, African-Caribbeans and Asians in London. *Psychological Medicine*, **27**, 791–798.

Bhui, K. & Bhugra, D. (1998) Psychotherapy for ethnic minorities: issues, context and practice. *British Journal of Psychotherapy*, **143**, 310–326.

Bhui, K., Bhugra, D., Goldberg, D., *et al* (2001) Cultural influences on the prevalence of common mental disorder, general practitioners' assessments and help-seeking among Punjabi and English people visiting their general practitioner. *Psychological Medicine*, **31**, 815–825.

Bhui, K., Bhugra, D. & Goldberg, D. (2002) Causal explanations of distress and general practitioners' assessments of common mental disorder among Punjabi and English attendees. *Social Psychiatry and Psychiatric Epidemiology*, **37**, 38–45.

Blanco, C., Patel, S. R., Liu, L., *et al* (2007) National trends in ethnic disparities in mental health care. *Medical Care*, **45**, 1012–1019.

Borowsky, S. J., Rubenstein, L. V., Meredith, L. S., *et al* (2000) Who is at risk of nondetection of mental health problems in primary care? *Journal of General Internal Medicine*, **15**, 381–388.

Brown, C., Schulberg, H. C., Sacco, D., *et al* (1999) Effectiveness of treatments for major depression in primary medical care practice: a post hoc analysis of outcomes for African American and white patients. *Journal of Affective Disorders*, **53**, 85–92.

Burroughs, V. J., Maxey, R. W. & Levy, R. A. (2002) Racial and ethnic differences in response to medicines: towards individualised pharmaceutical treatment. *Journal of the National Medical Association*, **94** (Suppl 10), 1–26.

Chew-Graham, C., Bashir, C., Chantler, K., *et al* (2002) South Asian women, psychological distress and self-harm: lessons for primary care trusts. *Health and Social Care in the Community*, **10**, 339–347.

Chung, H., Teresi, J., Guarnaccia, P., *et al* (2003) Depressive symptoms and psychiatric distress in low income Asian and Latino primary care patients: prevalence and recognition. *Community Mental Health Journal*, **39**, 33–46.

Cochrane, R. & Bal, S. S. (1989) Mental hospital admission rates of immigrants to England: a comparison of 1971 and 1981. *Social Psychiatry and Psychiatric Epidemiology*, **24**, 2–11.

Cooper, B. (2005) Schizophrenia, social class and immigrant status: the epidemiological evidence. *Epidemiolgica e Psichiatria Sociale*, **14**, 137–144.

Cooper, L. A., Gonzales, J. J., Gallo, J. J., *et al* (2003) The acceptability of treatment for depression among African-American, Hispanic, and white primary care patients. *Medical Care*, **41**, 479–489.

Cornwell, J. & Hull, S. (1998) Do GPs prescribe antidepressants differently for South Asian patients? *Family Practice*, **15** (Suppl. 1), S16–S18. Erratum in *Family Practice* (1998), **15**, 288.

Department of Health (2001) *Inside Outside: Improving Mental Health Services for Black and Minority Ethnic Communities in England*. Department of Health.

Department of Health and Human Services (2001) *Mental Health: Culture, Race and Ethnicity*. Supplement to *Mental Health*, a Surgeon General Report. DHSS.

Diaz, E., Woods, S. W. & Rosenheck, R. A. (2005) Effects of ethnicity on psychotropic medications adherence. *Community Mental Health Journal*, **41**, 521–537.

Dogra, N., Vostanis, P. & Frake, C. (2007) Child mental health services: cultural diversity training and its impact on practice. *Clinical Child Psychology and Psychiatry*, **12**, 137–142.

Fortuna, L. R., Perez, D. J., Canino, G., *et al* (2007) Prevalence and correlates of lifetime suicidal ideation and suicide attempts among Latino subgroups in the United States. *Journal of Clinical Psychiatry*, **68**, 572–581.

Gillam, S. J., Jarman, B., White, P., *et al* (1989) Ethnic differences in consultation rates in urban general practice. *BMJ*, **299**, 953–957.

Gray, P. (1999) Voluntary organisations. In *Ethnicity: An Agenda for Mental Health* (eds D. Bhugra & V. Bahl), pp. 202–210. Gaskell.

Guarnaccia, P. J., Lewis-Fernández, R. & Marano, M. R. (2003) Toward a Puerto Rican popular nosology: nervios and ataque de nervios. *Culture Medicine and Psychiatry*, **27**, 339–366.

Hazlett-Stevens, H., Craske, M. G., Roy-Byrne, P. P., et al (2002) Predictors of willingness to consider medication and psychosocial treatment for panic disorder in primary care patients. General Hospital Psychiatry, **24**, 316–321.

Hull, S. A., Cornwell, J., Harvey, C., et al (2001) Prescribing rates for psychotropic medication amongst east London general practices: low rates where Asian populations are greatest. Family Practice, **18**, 167–173.

Husain, M. I., Waheed, W. & Husain, N. (2006) Self-harm in British South Asian women: psychosocial correlates and strategies for prevention. Annals of General Psychiatry, **22**, 5–7.

Husain, N., Creed, F. & Tomenson, B. (1997) Adverse social circumstances and depression in UK persons of Pakistani origin. British Journal of Psychiatry, **171**, 434–437.

Jacob, K. S., Bhugra, D., Lloyd, K. R., et al (1998) Common mental disorders, explanatory models and consultation behaviour among Indian women living in the UK. Journal of the Royal Society of Medicine, **91**, 66–71.

Kirmayer, L. J. (2001) Cultural variations in the clinical presentation of depression and anxiety: implications for diagnosis and treatment. Journal of Clinical Psychiatry, **62 (Suppl 13)**, 22–28.

Krause, I. B. (1989) Sinking heart: a Punjabi communication of distress. Social Science and Medicine, **29**, 563–575.

Mahy, G. E., Mallett, R., Leff, J., et al (1999) First-contact incidence rate of schizophrenia on Barbados. British Journal of Psychiatry, **175**, 28–33.

Melfi, C. A., Croghan, T. W., Hanna, M. P., et al (2000) Racial variation in antidepressant treatment in a Medicaid population. Journal of Clinical Psychiatry, **61**, 16–21.

Miranda, J., Bernal, G., Lau, A., et al (2005) State of the science on psychosocial interventions for ethnic minorities. Annual Review of Clinical Psychology, **1**, 113–142.

Miranda, J., Green, B. L., Krupnick, J. L., et al (2006) One-year outcomes of a randomised clinical trial treating depression in low-income minority women. Journal of Consulting and Clinical Psychology, **74**, 99–111.

Nadeem, E., Lange, J. M., Edge, D., et al (2007) Does stigma keep poor young immigrant and U.S.-born Black and Latina women from seeking mental health care? Psychiatric Services, **58**, 1547–1554.

Netto, G., Gaag, S. & Thanki, M. (2006) Increasing access to appropriate counselling services for Asian people: the role of primary care services. Downloadable from http://priory.com/psych/counselling.htm

Ödegaard, O. (1932) Emigration and insanity. Acta Psychiatrica Scandinavica, **Suppl. 4**, 1–206.

Paez, K. A., Allen, J. K., Carson, J. A., et al (2008) Provider and clinic cultural competence in a primary care setting. Social Science and Medicine, **66**, 1204–1216.

Phelan, M. & Parkman, S. (1995) How to work with an interpreter. BMJ, **311**, 555–557.

Read, J. G. & Gorman, B. K. (2007) Racial/ethnic differences in hypertension and depression among US adult women. Ethnicity and Disease, **17**, 389–396.

Schraufnagel, T. J., Wagner, A. W., Miranda, J., et al (2006) Treating minority patients with depression and anxiety: what does the evidence tell us? General Hospital Psychiatry, **28**, 27–36.

Selten, J. P. & Sijben, N. (1994) First admission rates for schizophrenia in immigrants to The Netherlands. The Dutch National Register. Social Psychiatry and Psychiatric Epidemiology, **29**, 71–77.

Selten, J. P., Cantor-Graae, E. & Kahn, R. S. (2007) Migration and schizophrenia. Current Opinion in Psychiatry, **20**, 111–115.

Singh, S. P. & Grange, T. (2006) Measuring pathways to care in first-episode psychosis: a systematic review. Schizophrenia Research, **81**, 75–82.

Sleath, B., Rubin, R. H. & Huston, S. A. (2003) Hispanic ethnicity, physician–patient communication, and antidepressant adherence. Comprehensive Psychiatry, **44**, 198–204.

Smith-Campbell, B. (2005) A health professional students' cultural competence and attitudes toward the poor: the influence of a clinical practicum supported by the National Health Service Corps. Journal of Allied Health, **34**, 56–62.

Statistics Canada (2008) http://www.statcan.ca/english/concepts/definitions/ethnicity. htm

Thom, D. H., Tirado, M. D., Woon, T. L., *et al* (2006) Development and evaluation of a cultural competency training curriculum. *BMC Medical Education*, **26**, 38.

Walker, R. L. (2007) Acculturation and acculturative stress as indicators for suicide risk among African Americans. *American Journal of Orthopsychiatry*, **77**, 386–391.

Ward, E. C. (2007) Examining differential treatment effects for depression in racial and ethnic minority women: a qualitative systematic review. *Journal of the National Medical Association*, **99**, 265–274.

Weich, S., Nazroo, J., Sproston, K., *et al* (2004) Common mental disorders and ethnicity in England: the EMPIRIC study. *Psychological Medicine*, **34**, 1543–1551.

Wells, K. B., Staunton, A., Norris, K. C., *et al* (2006) Building an academic-community partnered network for clinical services research: the Community Health Improvement Collaborative (CHIC). *Ethnicity and Disease*, **16** (Suppl 1), S3–S17.

Wilson, M. & MacCarthy, B. (1994) GP consultation as a factor in the low rate of mental health service use by Asians. *Psychological Medicine*, **24**, 113–119.

# CHAPTER 22

# Asylum seekers and refugees

Angela Burnett

### Summary

This chapter describes common psychological difficulties experienced by asylum seekers and refugees and discusses how healthcare and social care workers can offer effective support. It is illustrated throughout by practical examples to help contextualise the theory and to give the evidence base substance and meaning.

The term 'asylum seeker' describes a person who has submitted an application for protection under the 1951 Geneva Convention and is awaiting a decision. Those whose claim is accepted are given 'refugee' status. Globally in 2008 an estimated 16 million people sought asylum outside their country of origin, and a further 26 million were internally displaced within their own country (UNHCR, 2008).

Some people may have mental health problems that precede their experiences of conflict and exile. Others develop psychological problems related to violence, detention, torture and bereavement experienced in their home country. Exile itself represents multiple loss – of home, family, friends, familiar places and food, culture and work, as well as support structures – and has been described as a form of 'cultural bereavement' (Eisenbruch, 1990).

The stress of the asylum process, with its uncertainties and hostilities, as well as social isolation, racism, poverty and unemployment, can cause mental health problems (Civis Trust, 2004). Silove *et al* (2000) describe growing evidence that the post-migration stress facing asylum seekers in Australia adds to the effect of previous trauma on their mental health. A study of Iraqi asylum seekers in the UK showed that depression was linked more with poor social support than with a history of torture (Gorst-Unsworth & Goldenberg, 1998).

Some asylum seekers present with psychological problems after having been exiled for some time, after other aspects of life are more settled and secure. Marshall *et al* (2005) describe Cambodian refugees experiencing mental health problems two decades after resettlement in the USA.

## Epidemiology and classification

Studies show a wide range of psychological problems experienced by refugees. Gerritsen *et al* (2004), in a meta-analysis of population-based studies of refugees living in The Netherlands, found prevalence rates of depression ranging from 3% to 88%, of anxiety ranging from 2% to 80% and of post-traumatic stress disorder (PTSD) ranging from 4% to 70%. The huge range in reported prevalence may be accounted for by variance in the studied populations in their country of origin, length of time in exile and legal status, as well as measurement tools (Mann & Fazil, 2006). However, it also brings into question the universal application of Western psychiatric diagnoses. Ballenger *et al* (2001) suggested that differences in classification and a lack of culturally appropriate instruments may explain perceived variations in the prevalence of mental illness cross-culturally.

## Psychological problems commonly experienced by asylum seekers and refugees

Anxiety and depression are common sequelae of torture and other forms of trauma, often exacerbated by the additional pressures of exile and resettlement (Kizito, 2001).

The frequently experienced signs and symptoms of anxiety fall into three categories:

1 *physiological or somatic* – e.g. panic attacks, hypervigilance, psychosomatic symptoms
2 *cognitive* – e.g. poor concentration, poor memory, worries, sleep disturbances (almost universal), flashbacks, dissociation
3 *behavioural* – e.g. avoidance of potentially fear-invoking situations, withdrawal, passivity, aggressive behaviour, self-blame, fear of relationships.

Depression may be linked to a profound sense of loss and hopelessness. A key source of stress and anxiety relates to family members left behind, as this gives rise to guilt and constant worry. (The International Red Cross/Crescent may be able to assist with family tracing; see e.g. http://www.redcross.org.uk or other country website.)

> ### Case 1
> Hassan arrived as an asylum seeker 3 months ago. He was a member of an opposition party and was detained and tortured. While he was in prison government soldiers had gone to his house and had raped his wife

and daughter. He was advised by party members to leave the country. The family left by road together, but subsequently became separated. The agent organising their journey promised they would be reunited but Hassan has not seen them since.

He is very agitated and angry, cannot sleep and keeps crying all the time. He hears the voices of his wife and daughter and cannot concentrate on anything. In the consultation he speaks very animatedly, keeps looking over his shoulder, and struggles to stay in his chair.

Hassan would benefit from several appointments over time, enabling him to develop a trusting relationship with a clinician. A mental state examination and risk assessment will reveal the nature and extent of his symptoms and the appropriate help required. He is likely to be feeling very guilty and responsible for the rape of his wife and daughter; the voices may be a manifestation of this, but he needs assessment to exclude serious mental illness. Psychological and practical support (including Red Cross family tracing and legal advice) may be helpful.

If the room the assessment is taking place in is small, check if he is reminded of prison and, if necessary, your exit route were you to become concerned about your personal safety.

## Assessment, detection and screening

Manifestations of distress and coping strategies differ both between and within cultures, so psychological assessment may be complex. Several sessions may be required in order to explore multiple needs, which can feel overwhelming. Talking or emotional support may be a lesser priority than basic welfare needs or practical necessities.

Understanding a person's explanatory model (how he or she makes sense of the situation) and culturally appropriate responses to distress is crucial, and an interpreter can offer helpful insights. Risk assessments covering suicide and child protection may be indicated, although cultural and religious taboos may inhibit disclosure.

On arrival, asylum seekers are often anxious, frightened, exhausted, overwhelmed, disoriented and confused. Psychological assessment at this time is therefore difficult and often unreliable, and full disclosure of past experiences is unlikely (Patel & Granville-Chapman, 2006). Health workers should still make an assessment, but they should be aware that this may need to be repeated at a later opportunity and as circumstances change.

Attention should be paid to ensuring that the physical environment is unthreatening (e.g. those previously detained in confined spaces may find small rooms uncomfortable) and to the gender of the health worker and the interpreter, particularly if sexual health, rape or torture may be discussed (women should be offered female professionals; a male rape survivor may also prefer females).

An approach should be utilised that not only seeks to identify vulnerability but also recognises potential resilience. It is important to respect autonomy and to allow the person to maintain control over the pace and timing of disclosure (Patel & Granville-Chapman, 2006).

Screening questionnaires may be used, although they may be hard to translate and may not be culturally appropriate or validated when used cross-culturally.

# Diagnosis

Primary care practitioners should be aware of the potential to pathologise natural and culturally appropriate expressions of grief and distress following traumatic experiences, and to diagnose without a reflective period of assessment. Diagnoses such as PTSD should be used cautiously, as they may not reflect communities' experiences of historical, political and social factors (Bracken, 1998). Many 'symptoms' can develop as adaptive reactions; for example, an exaggerated startle reflex could be an appropriate response to living under gunfire. Although inappropriate in a new environment, it does not necessarily represent mental illness (Burnett & Thompson, 2004). In addition, asylum seekers are not 'post-traumatic', but face ongoing concerns regarding their safety, racism, poverty, destitution and their future. Trauma models can undermine traditional coping strategies, leading to increased helplessness and dependence on external agencies (Giller, 1998). This work is inherently political in nature, and focusing on individual psychology while ignoring the political and social context can reduce both understanding of problems and effective relief (Jones, 1998).

# Important principles when working with asylum seekers and refugees

## Cultural competence

Culture influences both health behaviours and expectations of healthcare; it also provides a framework for classifying psychological health and for seeking help. Behaviour defined as mental illness in Western countries may be interpreted differently in other cultures: for example, it may be viewed as spirit possession, divine punishment, genetic weakness or normal behaviour. Educational, socio-economic and individual factors additionally influence personal beliefs and behaviour (Helman, 2000), so practitioners should resist any temptation to make culture-based assumptions. They need to be aware of their own social and cultural background and how it influences their views, interpretations, diagnoses and treatment.

## Building trust

'Refugees are looking for safety – after some time if we feel safe, we will open up.' (Male doctor with refugee status)

Trust is an important component of any relationship. Developing trust may be a challenge and take longer when professionals work with exiled people, as memories of past experiences may be invoked; health workers may have been identified with the ruling state in their home country, or have been directly involved in oppression.

Primary care workers may need to explain how they can help and, importantly, what they are not able to do, to avoid misunderstandings and unrealistic expectations. Confidentiality should be emphasised. Addressing practical issues initially may establish sufficient security to enable psychological issues to be addressed.

## Stigma

Many exiled people come from countries where mental illness is stigmatised and concealed, recovery considered unlikely and services perceived as unsupportive. They may therefore be reluctant to seek help, until a situation is reached which exceeds their ability to cope. Careful explanation is needed of the range of help and treatments available and their chances of success.

## Interpreting

If language is not shared, an interpreter who is not a friend or family member should be used. Without a professional interpreter, issues such as mental health, torture, sexual health or domestic violence may be difficult or impossible to discuss, since disclosure may be inhibited. A professional interpreter not only improves language understanding but can also illuminate political, social, cultural and related issues that may have an important bearing on psychological health.

Some professionals feel uncomfortable about introducing an additional person into the consultation and fear that their relationship with their client will be affected. However, by drawing on an interpreter's knowledge and experience as a resource, their own professional skills can be enhanced (Blackwell, 2005). The presence of an interpreter can reassure (although some people, fearing a breach of confidentiality, feel more relaxed with a telephone interpreter). Continuity may help to engender feelings of trust and safety for the client.

However, communities in exile may be divided along similar political lines as those determining conflict in the country of origin. An interpreter may be viewed with suspicion if seen as belonging to another group or as politically opposed to the client.

Interpreted sessions take longer, so short appointments will need extending. Briefing and debriefing before and after the session are worthwhile investments, as more will be achieved during the consultation. Most interpreters have no specialist training in mental health work and little supervision or support in dealing with re-stimulated feelings about their own similar experiences. Health workers can benefit from training on working with interpreters.

Language classes should be available to enable people to learn the host language.

---

**Box 22.1** Traumatic events experienced by many asylum seekers

- Massacres
- Sexual assault, including rape
- Forced eviction from home
- Forced conscription
- Deprivation of human rights
- Being held under siege
- Torture
- Witnessing torture of others
- Disappearances
- Political repression
- Detention
- Hostage taking

# Common issues when working with refugees and asylum seekers

## Experience of traumatic events

Many people will have experienced traumatic events in the past (Box 22.1).

### Torture

Torture is defined as follows in Article 7.2(e) of the Rome Statute of the International Criminal Court 1998:

> the intentional infliction of severe pain or suffering, whether physical or mental, upon a person in the custody or under the control of the accused.

Estimates of the proportion of those seeking asylum in the UK who are survivors of torture vary from 5% to 30%, depending on the definition of torture used and the country of origin (Burnett & Peel, 2001). Many do not initially disclose torture, often through shame or embarrassment. Common forms of torture are listed in Box 22.2.

The effects of torture are due to physical violence, detention (inadequate hygiene and diet) and the psychological consequences of one's own and witnessing others' experiences of torture and of being powerless to prevent it. Survivors may perceive their body as irreparably damaged, resulting in repeated consultations for chronic pain. They need to be given time and empathy, allowed to maintain control of the pace of work. The family of a survivor of torture may also need support.

#### Rape as a method of torture

Rape has been used throughout the history of conflict to degrade and humiliate. In most cultures, sexual violence and rape are taboo and survivors may feel too ashamed to disclose their experiences. Women may

---

**Box 22.2** Common forms of torture

- Beating, including *falaka* – severe and prolonged beating of the soles of the feet
- Burning with cigarettes, irons, petrol, acid, etc.
- Electric shocks
- Sexual violence and rape
- Water or submarine torture
- Starvation or poor-quality food
- Bodily mutilation
- Being forced into abnormal positions for long periods – suspension, Palestinian hanging
- Psychological torture – brainwashing, humiliation
- Use of psychotropic drugs
- Sham executions
- Witnessing the torture of others

From Kizito (2001).

---

be shunned by their community and family as having been defiled. Men may doubt their sexuality and fear infertility. Both men and women survivors commonly experience sexual difficulties. Persistent unexplained distress, anxiety and physical symptoms may be due to sexual violation.

Although some people may benefit from talking about their experience of sexual violence, others feel uncomfortable. Assisting people to develop their own support networks and addressing current practical difficulties may prove more effective. Sexual violation should be contextualised within the many traumas and losses experienced (Giller, 1998).

### Case 2

Fatima's family were killed by rebel forces, who abducted her and kept her for several months in captivity. In the consultation she looks very sad and withdrawn and sits hunched up. She complains of vague abdominal pains but despite previous extensive investigations, no cause for these has been found.

The male doctor asks what happened during her captivity but she does not answer. A few weeks later she books an appointment with a female partner. The partner gently questions her indirectly: 'I know that some people in your situation have experienced sexual violence and I'm wondering if this happened to you?' Hesitantly she reveals that during her captivity she was repeatedly raped. She has felt so ashamed that she could not bear to talk about it with anyone. Subsequently, counselling helps her to come to terms with what has happened.

## Physical expressions of distress ('somatisation')

'The sorrow that has no vent in tears makes other organs weep.' (Henry Maudsley, 1870)

**325**

People may present with weakness or pain, with no detectable physical cause. They may be experiencing psychological symptoms but be unable to describe them, owing to lack of appropriate language, the stigma of mental health problems, or the belief that health workers are more interested in physical problems. Although people may request investigations and treatment, they are often aware of the interrelations between physical and psychological symptoms.

Primary care practitioners should take such complaints seriously and, after excluding physical pathology, try to elicit the meaning and context of symptoms for the individual. It may be useful to chart the variability of symptoms alongside mood states. If symptoms persist (which may be for some time), a multifactorial approach is useful, trying to address any underlying causes and alleviating social isolation. Counselling or complementary therapies such as massage could be considered, if available.

## Substance misuse

Research is limited on substance misuse among refugees, although it is perceived that drugs and alcohol are increasingly being used as coping mechanisms. Khat/chat is commonly used by people of East African, Middle Eastern and Arab heritage. The effects of khat on mental health, documented predominantly in the Somali community, include khat-induced psychosis (Cox & Rampes, 2003). However, the social effects, which include financial hardship and family breakdowns, are more visible.

## Experience of detention

Some asylum seekers in the UK are placed in detention or removal centres and prisons. Such detention is distressing. For those who have been detained in their own country, the experience of subsequent detention can be devastating. Silove *et al* (2000) in Australia reported allegations of abuse, untreated medical and psychiatric conditions, suicidal behaviour, hunger strikes and outbreaks of violence among detained asylum seekers. The experience of being locked up will generally evoke powerful memories and these may persist for a long time after release from detention.

## Suicide

There are numerous anecdotal reports of suicides and attempted suicides among asylum seekers, particularly those detained. The risk is heightened by refusal of a claim and threatened deportation. However, since information on immigration status is not collected by coroners, accurate data are difficult to collate (Cohen, 2008).

## Issues for specific groups

Women may have assumed an unfamiliar position as family head and breadwinner, while lacking the support of family and community networks.

Men may find it harder to adjust to the lower status and powerlessness experienced in exile and may rely on alcohol and drugs.

Children may be living in a fragmented family, or may be unaccompanied. They may be survivors of violence or torture, or may have witnessed such acts. Some may have been forced as child soldiers to commit acts of violence. Consequently, they may believe that adults are untrustworthy and that their parents are unable to protect them (Dawes, 1992). They need multifaceted support, aimed at establishing for them as normal a life as possible, promoting education and self-esteem and supporting parents (Melzak & Kasabova, 1999). The most therapeutic event for refugee children, whether living with familiar carers or strangers, is to become part of the local school community, to learn and to make friends. However, they may experience bullying and racial abuse at school.

**Case 3**
Azad is a 16-year-old Turkish Kurd who left his country 2 years ago, having been separated from his family during an attack on his village by police. He is living in a hostel and attends frequently with abdominal pain, which he attributes to the food in the hostel. There are often difficulties at reception as he usually demands to be seen urgently and becomes angry if this is not possible. He is in trouble with the police as has been accused of stealing. He has also been involved in a fight at the hostel and they are threatening to evict him.

During the consultation he becomes very quiet, although the Turkish-speaking interpreter tries to encourage him to talk. The practitioner asks him if he would prefer a Kurdish-speaking interpreter, and he says that he would. At his next appointment, with a Kurdish-speaking interpreter, more at ease, he says that he misses his family terribly and feels that he is wasting his life, as he has nothing to do all day. The practitioner gives him information on the Red Cross/Crescent family tracing service, and on local English and computing classes.

Older people, a minority among newly arrived asylum seekers, face particular difficulties. They may be in poor health and challenged by new surroundings, which may provoke confusion and disorientation.

# Addressing psychological distress: principles of management

## Psychosocial factors

The most valuable inputs for many people are supportive listening and practical assistance to rebuild their lives – restoration of normal activities as far as possible can be the most effective promoter of mental health and can do much to relieve sadness and anxiety. Some, however, may experience guilt or shame regarding their experiences and may not wish to talk.

Many gain support from their community and religious faith. As survivors, their resilience can be a strength to utilise (Burnett & Gebremikael, 2005).

**327**

The following factors promote mental health for exiled people, and interventions should aim to enhance these (C. Watters, personal communication, 1997):

- contact with family/family reunion
- social support – links to integrated community groups
- strong religious or political ideology
- having a proactive, problem-solving approach.

A meta-analysis of the literature on the mental health of refugees has shown that refugee status confers an overall increase in psychological ill health (Porter & Haslam, 2005), which is not an inevitable consequence of conflict and trauma but, rather, reflects the socio-political conditions in host countries. It concludes that improving such conditions could improve mental health outcomes.

### Case 4

Aimee, an African woman in her 40s, was the sole survivor of her family following a massacre in her village by rebel soldiers. She was subsequently held in detention for a year, during which she was repeatedly kicked, punched and hit on the head with wooden batons and iron bars, which often rendered her unconscious for several hours. She was also multiply raped.

She has been living on the streets for the past 2 years after losing her asylum claim. She has to register with the authorities every week, for which she walks a round journey of 10 miles, as she has no money for transport.

She is profoundly depressed and is tearful most of the time. She experiences daily headaches, associated with dizziness.

Her lawyer asks the general practitioner to write a medical report in support of a community care assessment, as a result of which she is deemed to be vulnerable and is offered temporary housing. Subsequently her headaches and dizziness subside, although her situation remains far from secure. She declines counselling, saying that she does not wish to revisit her experiences, but responds positively to information about a local group for refugee women.

## Psychological therapies and counselling

Many people wish to talk about their experiences and find the process of testimony itself to be therapeutic. However, for some exiled people, discussing problems and past traumatic events with a relative stranger may feel inappropriate, embarrassing and humiliating (Helman, 2000). Western therapies prioritising control, personal autonomy and problem-solving may not sit comfortably within cultures valuing acceptance, harmony and contemplation (Fernando, 1995). Some refugees trained in counselling skills adapt them in culturally appropriate ways. Storytelling and narrative may also be helpful. Rather than restricting services to those deemed suitable for counselling and psychotherapy, it is more appropriate to think about how counselling and psychotherapy services can be made more suitable for clients (Blackwell, 2005).

Group work can offer support and reduce isolation, whether therapeutic or more social and practical in nature. For many people, hearing that they are not alone in their struggle and stress can normalise their feelings and provide reassurance. Adult and child psychotherapy, family therapy and cognitive–behavioural therapy may also be considered.

This sort of work is best done when the social situation is relatively stable and clients are feeling 'safe'. If this is not the case, it may be better to focus on improving their social situation and strengthening their coping skills to help with distressing memories. If such memories are addressed, it is important that the client feels in control of the process, and that the counsellor keeps checking whether the pace and content feel comfortable.

The client may be searching for the meaning of an apparently meaningless event. It may be helpful for the counsellor to locate this within the client's political or religious belief system, if present. Survivors of torture who have a political understanding of what happened to them may be less troubled than those who have no such understanding.

Sometimes a person who has previously disclosed a painful past event becomes unwilling to talk about it. It may be more helpful in such cases to talk about current concerns rather than pressing the client on that point. It is also important that the health worker feels safe and confident about being able to manage the disclosures that might be made.

With children, additional considerations need to be taken into account, including age, level of understanding and the context in which they are living.

## Prescribing

'Because of my worries my doctor gives me tablets but my worries are due to my immigration problems and my loneliness.' (Female asylum seeker, dispersed to the north-west of England)

Although drugs may be helpful in some circumstances, many of the problems which refugees and asylum seekers experience are not amenable to medication. Practical psychosocial interventions, counselling and alternatives such as massage should be considered, if available. Antidepressants may help, if used in conjunction with practical and social support; selective serotonin reuptake inhibitors are the first-line agents, but mirtazapine and trazodone can be beneficial if insomnia is marked. When prescribing, the doctor should ensure that information about the drug and its possible side-effects are clearly understood, and should carefully monitor symptoms, side-effects and suicide risk.

## Other forms of therapy and healing

Massage and aromatherapy, used in conjunction with relaxation techniques and self-massage, have been shown to reduce pain among asylum seekers and refugees and to increase their ability to manage their health problems (Negron, 2004). Physiotherapy has been identified as providing a vital link in restoring the personality of survivors of torture, through fostering trust in the context of physical contact (Hough, 1992). Herbal medicine has achieved success with torture survivors – for example, chamomile tea for anxiety and thyme for lower back pain (Linden & Grut, 2002).

Art (Kalmanowitz & Lloyd, 1999), movement psychotherapy (Callaghan, 1993) and music (Dixon, 2002) offer a variety of channels of communication in which to engage with psychological issues. Therapists, who have a professional training, may combine one or more psychological frameworks (e.g. psychodynamic, systemic) with the creative dimension of their art form. An evaluation of a school drama therapy programme for refugee and migrant adolescents in Canada showed that those taking part reported lower mean levels of impairment by emotional symptoms than those in a control group (Rousseau *et al*, 2007). Creative therapies may benefit people who have lived through political conflict, in conjunction with practical support and healthcare (Dokter, 1998). Theatre (Community Arts North West, 2006), music (Akhtar, 1994), writing (Write to Life, 2007), storytelling (Hopkins, 1996) and horticulture (Linden & Grut, 2002) may also help to combat isolation, communicate meaning, enhance self-esteem and strengthen identity and belonging.

# Support services

## Mental health services

Services have a statutory responsibility to provide care to refugees and those seeking asylum, and services should be accessible, flexible and culturally appropriate. Because of stigma, services within the community may be more acceptable and close links should be established with community mental health teams and the voluntary sector, including refugee community organisations.

## Refugee community organisations and other voluntary organisations

Refugee community organisations are often the first port of call for refugees facing crisis, because of their accessibility and empathy (Gebremikael, 2004). Both these and other voluntary organisations may assist with practical issues, befriending schemes, early identification of mental health problems and referral for formal assessment (Burnett & Gebremikael, 2005). Isolation increases the risk of mental health problems and voluntary organisations have an important preventive role through helping people to re-establish social support networks and a sense of context and purpose (Watters & Ingleby, 2002). However, political divisions may exist within refugee communities, deterring some people from contact with such organisations.

# Service gaps

Many asylum seekers and refugees experience difficulties in accessing health services, both in the community and in detention. Many health workers lack experience and training in working with asylum seekers and refugees, cultural competence and access to interpreters. In order to address some of the training issues, guidelines have been developed; these are listed at the end of the chapter, along with suggestions for further reading.

Involving refugees in planning, developing and implementing services is likely to improve their appropriateness and acceptability. Service evaluations should include the views of users (Burnett & Fassil, 2002).

# Reflective practice

Working with refugees and asylum seekers is both rewarding and challenging. Hearing people's experiences and dealing with their current situation can arouse strong emotions. When working with people who have few resources, it is important not to set up unreal expectations. Practitioners should encourage independence, although people may require help to access services. They should be aware of their own health needs, and take care not to become isolated or take on too much; they should also ensure that they themselves get adequate support, supervision, rest and recuperation.

---

Key points

- The stress of the asylum process, social isolation, racism, poverty and unemployment can cause significant mental health problems.
- The appropriateness of a universal application of Western psychiatric diagnoses is questionable.
- Understanding a person's explanatory model and culturally appropriate responses to distress is crucial.
- Practitioners should avoid pathologising natural and culturally appropriate expressions of distress following trauma and diagnosing without reflective assessment.
- Anxiety and depression are common sequelae of torture, other trauma and separation from family, exacerbated by additional pressures of exile and resettlement.
- Drugs may help, but many problems are not amenable to medication.

---

# Further reading and e-resources

Ballenger, J. C., Davidson, J. R. T., Lecrubier, T., *et al* (2001) Consensus statement on transcultural issues in depression and anxiety from the International Consensus Group on Depression and Anxiety. *Journal of Clinical Psychiatry*, **62** (suppl. 13), 47–55.

CVS Consultants & Migrant and Refugee Communities Forum (1999) *A Shattered World – The Mental Health Needs of Refugees and Newly Arrived Communities*. Lavenham Press. (Available from CVS Consultants, 27–29 Vauxhall Grove, London SW8 1SY.)

Eisenbruch, M. (1990) From post traumatic stress disorder to cultural bereavement: diagnosis of Southeast Asian refugees. *Social Science and Medicine*, **33**, 673–680.

Gebremikael, L. (2004) *The Role of Refugee Community Organisations – The Experience of the Ethiopian Health Support Association*. Dissertation for an MA in Migration, Mental Health and Social Care, University of Kent (unpublished).

Gerritsen, A., Bramsen, I., Deville, W., *et al* (2004) Health and health care utilisation among asylum seekers and refugees in The Netherlands: design of a study. *BioMedCentral Public Health*, **4**, 7.

Kleber, R. J., Figley, C. R. & Gersons, B. P. R. (eds) (1995) *Beyond Trauma. Cultural and Societal Dimensions*. Plenum.

Sainsbury Centre for Mental Health (2002) *Breaking the Circles of Fear: A Review of the Relationship between Mental Health Services and African and Caribbean Communities*. SCMH. Downloadable from http://www.scmh.org.uk.

Sashidharan, S. (2003) *Inside Outside: Improving Mental Health Services for Black and Minority Ethnic Communities in England*. National Institute for Mental Health in England.

Watters, C. (1998) The Mental Health Needs of Refugees and Asylum Seekers: Key Issues in Research and Service Development. In *Current Issues of Asylum Law and Policy* (ed. F. Nicholson), pp. 270–285. Avebury.

Webster, A. & Rojas Jaimes, C. (2000) *The Mental Health Needs of Refugees in Lambeth, London*. Available from Refugee Health Team, Masters House, Dugard Way, off Renfrew Rd, London SE11 4TH.

## Guidelines

### UK focused

Burnett, A. & Fassil, Y. (2002) *Meeting the Health Needs of Refugees and Asylum Seekers in the UK: An Information and Resource Pack for Health Workers*. London Directorate for Health and Social Care/Department of Health, downloadable from http://www.dh.gov.uk/en/Publicationsandstatistics/Publications/PublicationsPolicyAndGuidance/DH_4010199

Evelyn Oldfield Unit (1998) *Guidelines for Providers of Counselling Training to Refugees and Guidelines for Refugee Community Organisations Providing Counselling Services*. London Evelyn Oldfield Unit. Available from the Evelyn Oldfield Unit, 356 Holloway Road, London N7 6PA.

Fine, B. & Cheal, C. (2004) *Resource Pack to Help GPs and Other Primary Health Care Professionals in Their Work with Refugees and Asylum Seekers*. Refugee Health Team, Lambeth, Southwark and Lewisham.

Patel, N. & Granville-Chapman, C. (2006) *Assessing Vulnerable Survivors of Torture: Guidelines for Good Practice*. Medical Foundation for the Care of Victims of Torture.

### Australia focused

Bramwell, F. (1998*) Refugee Health and General Practice*. Victoria Foundation for Survivors of Torture.

### New Zealand focused

Kizito, H. (2001) *Refugee Healthcare: A Handbook gor Health Professionals*. New Zealand Ministry of Health and Folio Communications.

### Ireland focused

Irish Refugee Council (2002) Fact sheet on health care for asylum seekers. Social policy information note no. 2. Downloadable from http://www.irishrefugeecouncil.ie/factsheets/healthinfo2.doc

# References

Akhtar, P. (1994) Project report: therapeutic effects of music on torture survivors and refugees. *Torture*, **4**(4), 121–123.

Ballenger, J. C., Davidson, J. R. T., Lecrubier, T., *et al* (2001) Consensus statement on transcultural issues in depression and anxiety from the International Consensus Group on Depression and Anxiety. *Journal of Clinical Psychiatry*, **62** (suppl. 13), 47–55.

Blackwell, D. (2005) *Counselling and Psychotherapy with Refugees*. Jessica Kingsley.

Bracken, P. (1998) Hidden agendas: deconstructing post traumatic stress disorder. In *Rethinking the Trauma of War* (eds P. Bracken & C. Petty), pp. 38–59. Free Association Books.

Burnett, A. & Fassil, Y. (2002) *Meeting the Health Needs of Refugees and Asylum Seekers in the UK: An Information and Resource Pack for Health Workers*. London Directorate for Health and Social Care, Department of Health. Downloadable from http://www.dh.gov.uk/en/Publicationsandstatistics/Publications/PublicationsPolicyAndGuidance/DH_4010199

Burnett, A. & Gebremikael, L. (2005) Expanding the primary mental health team for asylum seekers and refugees. *Journal of Primary Care Mental Health*, **3**, 77–81.

Burnett, A. & Peel, M. (2001) The health of survivors of torture and organised violence. *BMJ*, **322**, 606–609.

Burnett, A. & Thompson, K. (2004) Enhancing the psychological well-being of asylum seekers and refugees. In *Race, Culture, Psychology and Law* (eds K. Barrett & B. George), pp. 205–224. Sage.

Callaghan, K. (1993) Movement psychotherapy with adult survivors of political torture and organised violence. *Arts in Psychotherapy*, **20**, 411–421.

Civis Trust (2004) *Refugees and Mental Health: A Good Practice Guide for Primary Care Workers*. Civis Trust.

Cohen, J. (2008) Safe in our hands? A study of suicide and self-harm in asylum seekers. *Journal of Forensic and Legal Medicine*, **15**, 235–244.

Community Arts North West (2006) Untitled document downloadable from http://www.baringfoundation.org.uk/Profilecanw.pdf (accessed 1 February 2008).

Cox, G. & Rampes, H. (2003) Adverse effects of khat: a review. *Advances in Psychiatric Treatment*, **9**, 456–463.

Dawes, A. (1992) Psychological discourse about political violence and its effects on children. Paper prepared for meeting on the Mental Health of Refugee Children Exposed to Violent Environments, Refugee Studies Programme, University of Oxford.

Dixon, M. (2002) Music and human rights. In *Music, Music Therapy and Trauma* (ed. J. Sutton), pp. 119–132. Jessica Kingsley.

Dokter, D. (1998) *Arts Therapists, Refugees and Migrants. Reaching Across Borders*. Jessica Kingsley.

Eisenbruch, M. (1990) From post traumatic stress disorder to cultural bereavement: diagnosis of Southeast Asian refugees. *Social Science and Medicine*, **33**, 673–680.

Fernando, S. (1995) *Mental Health in a Multi-ethnic Society*. Routledge.

Gebremikael, L. (2004) *The Role of Refugee Community Organisations – The Experience of the Ethiopian Health Support Association*. Dissertation for an MA in Migration, Mental Health and Social Care, University of Kent (unpublished).

Gerritsen, A., Bramsen, I., Deville, W., *et al* (2004) Health and health care utilisation among asylum seekers and refugees in The Netherlands: design of a study. *BioMedCentral Public Health*, **4**, 7.

Giller, J. (1998) Caring for victims of torture in Uganda: some personal reflections. In *Rethinking the Trauma of War* (eds P. Bracken & C. Petty), pp. 128–145. Free Association Books.

Gorst-Unsworth, C. & Goldenberg, E. (1998) Psychological sequelae of torture and organised violence suffered by refugees from Iraq: trauma related factors compared with social factors in exile. *British Journal of Psychiatry*, **172**, 90–94.

Helman, C. (2000) *Culture, Health and Illness*. Hodder Arnold.

Hopkins, B. (1996) Transforming tales: exploring conflict through stories and storytelling. In *Arts Approaches to Conflict* (ed. M. Liebmann), pp. 275–295. Jessica Kinsgsley.

Hough, A. (1992) Physiotherapy for survivors of torture. *Physiotherapy*, **78**, 323–328.

Jones, L. (1998) The question of political neutrality when doing psychosocial work with survivors of political violence. *International Review of Psychiatry*, **10**, 239–247.

Kalmanowitz, D. & Lloyd, B. (1999) Fragments of art at work: art therapy in the former Yugoslavia. *Arts in Psychotherapy*, **26**, 15–25.

Kizito, H. (2001) *Refugee Healthcare: A Handbook for Health Professionals*. New Zealand Ministry of Health and Folio Communications.

Linden, S. & Grut, J. (2002) *The Healing Fields: Working with Psychotherapy and Nature to Rebuild Shattered Lives*. Frances Lincoln.

Mann, C. & Fazil, Q. (2006) Mental illness in asylum seekers and refugees. *Primary Care Mental Health*, **4**, 57–66.

Marshall, G., Schell, T., Elliott, M., *et al* (2005) Mental health of Cambodian refugees two decades after resettlement in the United States. *JAMA*, **294**, 571–579.

Maudsley, H. (1870) *Body and Mind: An Inquiry into Their Connection and Mutual Influence*. MacMillan.

Melzak, S. & Kasabova, S. (1999) *Working with Children and Adolescents from Kosavo*. Medical Foundation for the Care of Victims of Torture.

Negron, A. (2004) *Refugee Health Team Lambeth, Southwark and Lewisham Complementary Therapy Project Final Report and Evaluation*. Downloadable from http://www.threeboroughs.nhs.uk (accessed 1 February 2008).

Patel, N. & Granville-Chapman, C. (2006) *Assessing Vulnerable Survivors of Torture: Guidelines for Good Practice*. Medical Foundation for the Care of Victims of Torture.

Porter, M. & Haslam, N. (2005) Pre-displacement and post-displacement factors associated with the mental health of refugees and internally displaced persons: a meta-analysis. *JAMA*, **294**, 602–612.

Rousseau, C., Benoit, M., Gauthier, M., *et al* (2007) Classroom drama therapy program for immigrant and refugee adolescents: a pilot study. *Clinical Child Psychology and Psychiatry*, **12**, 451–465.

Silove, D., Steel, Z. & Watters, C. (2000) Policies of deterrence and the mental health of asylum seekers. *JAMA*, **284**, 604–611.

UNHCR (2008) UNHCR annual report shows 42 million people uprooted worldwide. Downloadable from http://www.unhcr.org/print/4a2fd52412d.html (accessed 10 August 2009).

Watters, C. & Ingleby, D. (2002) *Good Practice in Mental Health and Social Care for Refugees and Asylum Seekers*. University of Kent and Utrecht University.

Write to Life (2007) The power of the written word. Downloadable from http://www.torturecare.org.uk/print/21 (accessed 1 February 2008).

# CHAPTER 23

# Sexual problems

## Michael King

Summary

This chapter outlines the difficulties in defining sexual dysfunction, in particular in women. It describes the epidemiology of sexual problems, drawing on original research by the author's group which has shown that many problems remain undetected in primary care. Specific helpful advice on taking a history, defining the problem and undertaking investigations is followed by a summary of the evidence for various interventions for problems of desire, arousal, orgasm and painful intercourse.

People consulting their family doctors are more prepared than ever before to ask for help with sexual problems. Furthermore, the English *National Strategy for Sexual Health and HIV* acknowledged sexual fulfilment and equitable relationships as 'essential elements of good sexual health' and called for consistent standards of care to ensure appropriate management of patients with sexual dysfunction (Department of Health, 2002). Liberalisation of sexual attitudes, behaviour and lifestyles since the 1960s and the introduction of new treatments for sexual dysfunction since the 1980s, particularly for men, have made it more acceptable to seek help for sexual difficulties. Nonetheless, although most people with sexual problems regard their general practitioners (GPs) as appropriate sources of help, many remain uncertain whether or not they have a problem or even whether to bring up the subject (Nazareth *et al*, 2003), and GPs do not always have the skill or time to treat sexual disorders (Humphery & Nazareth, 2001).

## Classification

There is considerable debate about how to measure or define sexual difficulties. Part of the problem lies in the definitions of 'normality', which have evolved with changes in attitudes and behaviour in society. Whereas behaviours such as masturbation or sexual contact between people of the same gender were once seen as sexual perversions (Davenport-Hines, 1990), they are now regarded as part of the range of normal sexual response. Nevertheless, defining disorder remains subjective and depends on the values, wishes and sexual knowledge of each person and his or her partner. For example, when is ejaculation considered premature? How quick is too quick? Although distress about the problem is often a guide to, or a prerequisite for, the diagnosis of a sexual problem, distress may occur exclusively in the partner. For example, in women with low sexual desire or in men who ejaculate quickly, it may be only the partner who complains and is responsible for the help-seeking that transpires. Furthermore, concepts of usual sexual behaviour in women are changing and there have been claims that the pharmaceutical industry is building a pseudo-science out of female sexual dysfunction (Moynihan, 2003). A woman-centred definition of sexual problems has recently been recommended as an alternative to concepts of sickness and health (Tiefer, 2000; Moynihan, 2005) and international classifications of sexual dysfunction are being reviewed (Basson *et al*, 2004). In contrast to men, women's sexual function appears to be more responsive than spontaneous and more dependent on emotional closeness with their partner (Basson, 2001). In fact we need further evidence that the common complaints of lack or loss of sexual desire in *either* men or women are impediments to satisfying sexual relations or that a medical approach is indicated. Reduced sexual interest or response may be an adaptation to stress or an unhappy relationship (King *et al*, 2007).

With these caveats in mind, Table 23.1 summarises the commonest classification of sexual problems, that of DSM–IV (American Psychiatric Association, 1994). The two international classification systems, DSM–IV and ICD–10 (World Health Organization, 1992), have similar systems of classification. Both emphasise that aetiological factors may be psychological, or due to a combination of psychological and medical reasons but where the psychological predominate. This means that careful attention is needed to exclude purely medical factors or substances (prescribed, recreational or illicit) that may be causing the sexual dysfunction. DSM–IV and the research edition of ICD–10 (World Health Organization, 1993) also stipulate that the sexual disorder has to cause marked distress or interpersonal difficulty and that the dysfunction is not accounted for by another major mental disorder, such as anxiety or depression.

# Epidemiology

Sexual dysfunction is common but prevalence estimates vary because of doubts about the validity of diagnoses, particularly in women. In a study of general practice attendees in London, up to 40% of women had a diagnosable sexual dysfunction (Table 23.2). However, when those with lack or loss of sexual desire were excluded, prevalence fell to 27% for

**Table 23.1** Difficulties of sexual function not explained by medical disorders

| Problem area | Condition | Characteristics |
|---|---|---|
| Desire | Hypoactive sexual desire disorder | Persistently or recurrently deficient (or absent) sexual fantasies and desire for sexual activity |
| | Sexual aversion disorder | Persistent or recurrent extreme aversion to, and avoidance of, all (or almost all) genital sexual contact with a partner |
| Arousal | Female sexual arousal disorder | Persistent or recurrent inability to attain, or maintain until completion of sexual activity, an adequate lubrication/swelling response of sexual excitement |
| | Male erectile disorder | Persistent or recurrent inability to attain, or maintain until completion of sexual activity, an adequate erection |
| Orgasm | Female orgasmic disorder | Persistent or recurrent delay in, or absence of, orgasm following a normal sexual excitement phase |
| | Male orgasmic disorder | Persistent or recurrent delay in, or absence of, orgasm following a normal sexual excitement phase |
| | Premature ejaculation (PE) | Persistent or recurrent ejaculation before, on, or shortly after penetration and before the person wishes it |
| Pain | Dyspareunia (not due to a medical condition) | Recurrent or persistent genital pain associated with sexual intercourse in men or women |
| | Vaginismus (not due to a medical condition) | Recurrent or persistent spasm of the musculature of the outer third of the vagina that interferes with sexual intercourse. There may be associated spasm of the internal adductor muscles of the thighs |

(Based on DSM–IV (American Psychiatric Association, 1994).

**Table 23.2** Prevalence (%) of sexual dysfunction

| Sexual dysfunction (ICD–10 classification) | Men | Women |
|---|---|---|
| Lack or loss of sexual desire | 6.7 | 16.8 |
| Sexual aversion | 2.5 | 4.1 |
| Failure of genital response | | |
| Male erectile dysfunction (failure at insertion during intercourse) | 8.5 | |
| Female sexual arousal dysfunction | | 3.6 |
| Orgasmic dysfunction | | |
| Male orgasmic dysfunction (inhibited orgasm during intercourse) | 2.5 | |
| Premature ejaculation (at insertion during penetration) | 3.6 | |
| Inhibited female orgasm (during intercourse) | | 18.6 |
| Non-organic vaginismus | 11.3 | 4.5 |
| Non-organic dyspareunia | 1.1 | 2.9 |
| At least one diagnosis | 21.7 | 39.6 |

Data from Nazareth *et al* (2003).

women and 16% for men (Nazareth *et al*, 2003). A subsequent study in the same setting in women only confirmed the perception that, for many, loss of sexual desire was mainly a response to personal or relationship difficulties (King *et al*, 2007). Thus, careful assessment of women with loss of sexual desire is necessary in order to be clear about who it is who complains and the origins of the distress.

Although most medical or psychological disorders tend to be commoner in general practice attendees than people in the general population, this does not seem to be the case with sexual dysfunction. An oft quoted study of a national probability sample of people in the USA reported overall rates of 43% for women and 31% for men (Laumann *et al*, 1999). However, population studies are often unable to use detailed diagnostic criteria, which may explain the higher figures (Mercer *et al*, 2003). In Laumann *et al*'s study and the one in UK general practice (Nazareth *et al*, 2003), sexual problems were associated with older age and poorer physical health. Reporting a sexual problem was also associated with greater psychological distress in the latter study.

# Detection and screening

A very large number of questionnaires designed to detect sexual problems are available (David *et al*, 1998) but few are practical to use in general practice because they are either too long or specific. Once a sexual problem has been detected, however, there are one or two instruments that may be helpful in defining the problem more specifically. For men, there is the International Index of Erectile Function (Rosen *et al*, 1997), which is a short measure of mainly erectile function, or the Brief Sexual Function Questionnaire for Men (Reynolds *et al*, 1988), which takes a more comprehensive approach to the range of possible sexual difficulties. For women, two instruments that might be considered are the McCoy Female Sexuality Questionnaire, which assesses sexual interest and responsiveness (McCoy & Matyas, 1996), and the Self-Report Assessment of Female Sexual Function (Taylor *et al*, 1994), which is adapted from the Brief Sexual Function Questionnaire for Men and is the only questionnaire to be validated in post-menopausal women.

## Taking a sexual history

As for all clinical complaints, it is important to know how long the difficulty has been present, in which circumstances it improves or worsens and to what extent the preferred sexual life is impaired. Other factors that might be considered in a brief sexual history are:

- Is the problem lifelong or has there been a period of satisfactory sexual function?
- Is the difficulty situational? For example, is there normal function in masturbation but difficulties with partners?

- What are the circumstances in which sex is attempted? For example, is there adequate privacy?
- Are there any particular factors in the sexual relationship that make it difficult? For example, is the patient guilty, resentful or fearful when with a partner?
- When concern about sexual drive is not the presenting problem, it is still useful to ask whether interest in sex has changed and, if so, whether it is global or specific to a particular partner(s) or setting(s).

Given more time, a GP might wish to explore the patient's:

- sexual development and experiences in adolescence and young adulthood
- sexual function in previous relationships
- experiences of sexual trauma in childhood or later life
- sexual orientation.

If GPs feel confident they might tactfully explore the patient's sexual fantasies. However, this can be tricky for them and the patient alike and embarrassment (particularly the GP's) is to be avoided at all costs, as nothing is more likely to hinder a frank consultation. Sexual fantasies may provide an indication of whether there is a major divide between the patient's actual and desired sexual behaviour or even whether a paraphilia (sexual deviation) is behind the problem. Current prescribed and recreational drugs need to be considered (see below).

## Investigations

The simplest screening investigations in men are serum testosterone and sex hormone binding globulin. They are mainly useful when there is low sexual drive and/or testicular abnormality (e.g. low volume) on examination. The so-called androgen index, which is the ratio of serum testosterone to sex hormone binding globulin, should exceed 30%. If it does not, it suggests there is insufficient free, or unbound, testosterone in the plasma for full physiological activity. Serum testosterone is unlikely to be low in erectile dysfunction or any other disorder when sexual drive is unaffected.

The most productive initial test in women is serum prolactin level, which if raised may be related to low sexual drive and requires further investigation. The normal range for serum testosterone in women is not yet well delineated.

## Prescribed drugs

The commonest medications to impair sexual function are those that affect the dopamine, noradrenaline and serotonin pathways in the brain (pathways related to the sexual response) and those that affect endocrine function (particularly exogenous steroids) or vascular function. Contrary to popular belief, antihypertensive drugs (including the older generation of drugs, developed from 1970 onwards) have little specific impact on sexual function (Beto & Bansal, 1992). If a side-effect is suspected, judicious reduction in dosage of the offending drug may be worth a try, but this is not always possible without losing adequate control of blood pressure. Sildenafil (see 'Erectile dysfunction', below) may be useful in such circumstances.

Although antidepressants affect sexual arousal and orgasm, it is difficult to decide whether the drugs, as distinct from the depressed mood, are impairing sexual responsiveness. Whatever the reason, it is risky to reduce or withdraw antidepressants in order to reduce sexual dysfunction because of the possibility of self-harm or other adverse effects of the depressive illness. Although a syndrome of low arousal and erectile dysfunction is popularly believed to persist *long after* courses of selective serotonin reuptake inhibitors, the evidence for this is hard to accumulate, as the problem will not usually appear in post-marketing surveillance studies of people currently taking the drug. Again, sildenafil may be useful.

## Management of common sexual problems

Unsurprisingly, the approach to management of sexual dysfunction involves medical or psychological treatments or a combination of both. The pioneers of sexual therapy, William Masters and Virginia Johnson, who eventually became famous enough to appear on the cover of *Time* magazine in 1970, were the first to develop a short, intensive sex therapy for couples that combined sexual education with a mainly behavioural intervention aimed at reducing anxiety about sexual performance and increasing the focus on mutually pleasurable sexual arousal (Masters & Johnson, 1970). However, there is little evidence for the effectiveness of their approaches. In fact, despite their long history, psychological treatments have considerably less evidence of effectiveness than physical treatments for sexual dysfunction. Furthermore, research into the effectiveness of psychological treatments has been declining. The principal reasons for this gap in the evidence are an apparent low priority for funders of research, particularly given the advent of physical therapies, and the relative complexity of the undertaking. Estimating efficacy of a complex psychological intervention for a condition that may be the result of physical, psychological and cultural factors is difficult. However, there is also a lack of adequate, testable theories about psychological mechanisms; in particular, there is a lack of evidence for the efficacy of the various components of sex therapy (Weiderman, 1998). However, there are grounds for assuming that cognitive–behavioural therapy or interpersonal psychotherapy, both of which have evidence for their efficacy in other related domains, are effective in this one.

### Erectile dysfunction

Erectile dysfunction is the inability to initiate or sustain a penile erection hard enough for penetrative sex until orgasm. The dysfunction may depend on the type of penetration attempted, be it oral, vaginal or anal. The phospohodiesterase-5 inhibitor sildenafil has become the first line of treatment (*Drugs and Therapeutics Bulletin*, 2004). By inhibiting breakdown of cyclic guanosine monophosphate in penile tissues, it prolongs smooth muscle relaxation and facilitates erection. Side-effects are headache, flushing of the skin, stomach upsets and nasal stuffiness. However, only 1% of men stop taking the drug because of such effects (Goldstein *et al*, 1998). The blue visual tinge that sometimes occurs is due to its weak action on phosphodiesterase-6 activity in the retina. Although response rates against placebo in clinical trials were above 80%, in clinical practice its efficacy is about 50% (Morgentaler, 1999). Nitrate drugs are the main contraindication as, in combination with sildenafil, they may cause profound hypotension.

Tadalafil is another phosphodiesterase-5 inhibitor, with a half-life at least twice that of sildenafil and equal efficacy (Carson *et al*, 2004). Its potential advantage is that it is effective for up to 36 hours after dosing, a longer effect than for sildenafil. Vardenafil has equivalent efficacy and duration of action to sildenafil (Markou *et al*, 2004).

The ready availability of these drugs means that major psychological factors are often overlooked or bypassed when they are prescribed. Although sildenafil may be helpful as an adjunct to psychological treatment for younger men with erectile dysfunction, my clinical impression is that men easily become anxious about initiating sex without it. The drug also has street value and is misused by men with normal erectile function (Smith & Romanelli, 2005).

Psychological management focuses on the almost universal performance anxiety (a form of stage fright), challenges myths about sexual performance, educates about sex, emphasises the negative consequences of avoidance, encourages exposure to sexual situations and helps the man to distance himself from his distressing thoughts about inadequacy or failure. When performance anxiety is very high, however, sildenafil can reduce tension enough to encourage relaxation and help the man to distance himself from his anxious thoughts. Sometimes it may be helpful to bring in the partner, who may have unrealistic expectations of the man's sexual performance or blame herself or himself for the difficulties.

## Hypoactive sexual desire in women

Lack of sexual desire is the commonest reason women seek help for sexual dysfunction (Warner *et al*, 1987). It is associated with anxiety, depression, discord with the spouse or partner (Dunn *et al*, 2000) and use of psychotropic medication (Segraves, 2002). There is a persistent lack of sexual thoughts or fantasies and desire for a partner, which leads to personal distress. The diagnosis may not apply to women who lack desire in certain situations such as marital conflict or at times such as menstruation but not at others. Nor is it a disorder when due simply to an imbalance between the woman's desire and that of her partner (Basson *et al*, 2000). Loss of sexual desire may occur in the year after childbirth, although few affected couples regard it as a serious problem (Dixon *et al*, 2000).

Sildenafil has no role in women with arousal disorder (Berman *et al*, 2003). However, androgens are responsible for sexual drive in women as well as men (Shifren, 2004) and testosterone patches appear to have beneficial effects on hypoactive sexual desire in postmenopausal women (Buster *et al*, 2005) and possibly even in older premenopausal women (Goldstat *et al*, 2003). However, use of testosterone in women runs the risk of masculinising side-effects (Modelska & Cummings, 2003). Furthermore, the normal physiological range of serum testosterone in women is still unclear. Hormone replacement therapy enhances sexual function in postmenopausal women through its action on the vaginal epithelium and the vulval and clitoral erectile tissues. Tibolone, a synthetic steroid that has oestrogenic, progestogenic and androgenic activity, is used to treat menopausal symptoms and may enhance sexual function in postmenopausal women (Modelska & Cummings, 2003).

Psychological therapy for women with low sexual desire, and their partners, focuses on improving communication, dealing with anger and resentment and the identification of insecurity (Bancroft, 2002). Couple therapy may also take the form of a systemic approach to improve sexual desire in long-term relationships (Clement, 2002). Although these therapies are widely used as pragmatic approaches, little is known about their efficacy. Cognitive–behavioural therapy may enable the woman to identify and manage negative thoughts about her sexual feelings, let go of psychological control, address beliefs about her attractiveness and responsiveness as a partner and manage her anxiety about love-making. These approaches need not be highly complex and considerable relief can be experienced by women who are helped to recognise that their thoughts do not define them or the nature of their sexual lives, and can be challenged (Hayes & Smith, 2005).

## Orgasmic disorders in men

### Premature ejaculation

A common sexual problem in men is ejaculation before, on or shortly after penetration, before he wishes it and over which he has little or no voluntary control (McMahon *et al*, 2004). The aetiology of most cases of premature ejaculation is unclear; potential physical causes are chronic prostatitis, neurological disease, pelvic injury, vascular disease, prostatic hypertrophy and hypogonadal hypertrophy (Richardson *et al*, 2006). Premature ejaculation may occur when the man is highly sexually aroused and/or anxious. It may be primary or can begin after years of normal sexual function. Rapid ejaculation is a process that is likely to be selected for in evolution and it seems that primary premature ejaculation in men may simply be one extreme on a physiological spectrum which impairs sexual pleasure and sometimes prevents insemination.

Medical approaches to premature ejaculation are daily, or as needed, treatment with serotonergic antidepressants. Evidence from randomised trials shows little difference in efficacy between sertraline, fluoxetine, paroxetine and clomipramine (Mendels *et al*, 1995; Waldinger *et al*, 1998; Montague *et al*, 2004). Nefazodone, citalopram, fluvoxamine and mirtazapine are ineffective and may be helpful for treatment of depression in men *not* wanting ejaculatory impairment (Montejo *et al*, 2001; Montague *et al*, 2004). Intermittent administration (on the day of intercourse) is as effective as daily administration for most men (Kolomaznik, 2004). I find low-dose clomipramine (10–20 mg daily) is effective, with minimal side-effects. Sildenafil is not helpful but topical anaesthetics may be, such as lidocaine or prilocaine cream (2.5 g applied 20–30 min before sex) (Montague *et al*, 2004).

A behavioural technique developed by Masters and Johnson is the squeeze technique, when the penis is pressed lightly just below the glans, inducing a reflex that retards ejaculation. In the stop–start technique (Semans, 1956; Kaplan, 1974) the man stops moving or withdraws his penis when close to orgasm. However, there is little evidence for efficacy of either the squeeze or stop–start technique. Cognitive–behavioural therapy with a particular focus on anxiety management is useful but good evidence for efficacy is lacking. Developing increased tone in the pubococcygeous muscles (Kegel exercises, in which the man clenches his perineal area as if to stop the flow of urine) may improve ejaculatory control (La & Nicastro, 1996) but no definitive trial has been published (Richardson *et al*, 2006).

## Retarded ejaculation and anorgasmia

Delayed is a much less common dysfunction than early orgasm. Sufferers include men who can never achieve orgasm, those who reach orgasm (or emission without orgasm) only when asleep, those who reach orgasm only in masturbation and those who are orgasmic with a partner but only during non-penetrative sex. Causes include testosterone deficiency, spinal cord injury, pelvic floor injury or disease, diabetes mellitus, a number of prescribed drugs, severe anxiety, lack of desire for the partner, and other psychological factors, such as recurrent obsessive and compulsive thoughts and behaviours in men who need to feel emotionally in control. It is also more prevalent with increasing age (McMahon *et al*, 2004).

Drugs that facilitate ejaculation act via central dopaminergic or anti-serotonergic mechanisms. Although alpha-adrenergic agonists such as phenylpropolamide, pseudo-ephedrine and ephedrine have been suggested, their efficacy is uncertain (Jannini *et al*, 2002; McMahon *et al*, 2004). Complete anorgasmia is a rare and usually primary condition that is also unlikely to respond to drug treatment, unless occurring in men with spinal cord injuries (Kamischke & Nieschlag, 2002).

Delayed ejaculation or anorgasmia that is not secondary to testosterone deficiency or other identified physical causes may respond to increased stimulation from a vibrator applied to the frenulum area of the penis.

Achieving an orgasm first in masturbation can facilitate orgasm later, when with a partner. If he has a partner, the man is encouraged to reach orgasm in his or her presence and then begin insertive sexual intercourse just before or at the point of ejaculation. There are many published case reports on psychodynamic, behavioural and cognitive approaches to retarded ejaculation (e.g. Catalan, 1993) but little empirical evidence to support any particular treatment (McMahon *et al*, 2004).

## Sexual arousal disorder in women

This is a disorder in which there is lack of mental excitement or interest and deficient genital engorgement and vaginal lubrication. There may be two subtypes of women with arousal dysfunction. In the first and apparently more common subtype are women who seem unaware that physical arousal is occurring. In the second are women who find arousal unpleasant (Carson *et al*, 2004). The main physical aetiologies are vascular impairment in disorders such as diabetes mellitus and changes associated with reduction of oestrogen at the menopause (Berman *et al*, 1999).

Pharmaceutical industry trials of sildenafil involving about 3000 women have produced mixed results and Pfizer has not pursued a licence for the drug in women (Mayor, 2004). Two small trials have suggested that sublingual administration of apomorphine may be helpful (Bechara *et al*, 2004; Carson *et al*, 2004).

Psychological approaches have concentrated on the woman's relationship with her partner or on issues of loss in terms of menopausal or surgical changes in later life. Individual approaches which focus on relaxation and self-focusing to reduce anxiety are also used. For example, use of a vibrator, alone or with a partner, may be helpful in bringing about orgasm in some women. However, qualitative research has shown that women may be less concerned with achieving orgasm through heterosexual intercourse than with pleasing their partner (Nicolson & Burr, 2003).

## Vaginismus

An inability to allow vaginal penetration because of involuntary spasm of vaginal and adductor muscles of the thighs may occur as a primary problem in women who have never achieved a satisfactory penetrative sexual relationship or may occur after sexual assault or other trauma. There are no known physical causes and the exact psychological aetiology is unknown. Sexual arousal and interest are often normal but the woman may dislike or feel sensitive about her body, particularly the perineal area and its functions. It can be difficult to distinguish from dyspareunia (Meana *et al*, 1997).

There are no drug treatments for vaginismus, although vaginal lubricants may help penetration. Behavioural treatments are offered on the basis that the muscle spasm appears to be a phobic response to a normal stimulus. The woman can be helped by encouraging her to view her genital area in a mirror and teaching her to examine herself. We have had good results with this desensitisation approach and quite rapid improvements may occur. There is little good trial evidence for the approach, although one trial comparing desensitisation using dilators or in imagination showed both were helpful (Schnyder *et al*, 1998). We avoid the use of dilators, as the term itself implies there is something narrow or constricted about the vagina that requires widening, when this is not the case. Unfortunately, a Cochrane review of only two randomised trials of treatments for vaginismus published up to 2002 (McGuire & Hawton, 2003) showed no effectiveness for any particular type of intervention.

## Guidelines for the management of sexual dysfunction

There are many national and international guidelines, recommendations and standards available for the treatment of sexual dysfunction and associated problems, the vast majority of which apply only to men. These range from management of erectile dysfunction in the UK (Ralph & McNicholas, 2000) to premature ejaculation in the USA (Montague *et al*, 2004) and the UK (Richardson *et al*, 2006). General guidance on the management of sexual dysfunction in women was developed in New Zealand and published in the *American Family Physician* (Phillips, 2000).

---

Key points

- Sexual dysfunction is common but prevalence estimates vary because of doubts about the validity of diagnoses, particularly in women.
- Reporting of sexual problems is associated with psychological distress; most problems go undetected in primary care.
- Structured questionnaires are not recommended for screening but may help in defining a problem once detected.
- In men with low sex drive, serum testosterone and sex hormone binding globulin may be useful tests.
- In women with low sex drive, prolactin levels should be measured.
- Psychological treatments have considerably less evidence of their effectiveness than physical treatments for sexual dysfunction.
- The phospohodiesterase-5 inhibitor sildenafil has become the first line of treatment for erectile dysfunction.
- Premature ejaculation may respond to a selective serotonin reuptake inhibitor.
- Cognitive–behavioural therapy may help women identify and manage negative thoughts about sexual feelings, and reduce anxiety about love making.

---

# Further reading and e-resources

Geneva Foundation for Medical Education and Research, Sexual dysfunction: Guidelines, reviews, statements, recommendations, standards, http://www.gfmer.ch/Guidelines/Sexual_dysfunction/Sexual_dysfunction_mt.htm

# References

American Psychiatric Association (1994) *Diagnostic and Statistical Manual of Mental Disorders* (4th edn) (DSM–IV). APA.

Bancroft, J. (2002) The medicalization of female sexual dysfunction: the need for caution. *Archives of Sexual Behavior*, **31**, 451–455.

Basson, R. (2001) Female sexual response: the role of drugs in the management of sexual dysfunction. *Obstetrics and Gynecology*, **98**, 350–353.

Basson, R., Berman, J., Burnett, A., *et al* (2000) Report of the international consensus development conference on female sexual dysfunction: definitions and classifications. *Journal of Urology*, **163**, 888–893.

Basson, R., Leiblum, S., Brotto, L., *et al* (2004) Revised definitions of women's sexual dysfunction. *Journal of Sexual Medicine*, **1**, 40–48.

Bechara, A., Bertolino, M. V., Casabe, A., *et al* (2004) A double blind randomized placebo control study comparing the objective and subjective changes in female sexual response using sublingual apomorphine. *Journal of Sexual Medicine*, **1**, 209–214.

Berman, J. R., Berman, L. A., Werbin, T. J., *et al* (1999) Clinical evaluation of female sexual function: effects of age and estrogen status on subjective and physiologic sexual responses. *International Journal of Impotence Research*, **11** (Suppl. 1), S31–S38.

Berman, J. R., Berman, L. A., Toler, S. M., *et al* (2003) Safety and efficacy of sildenafil citrate for the treatment of female sexual arousal disorder: a double-blind, placebo controlled study. *Journal of Urology*, **170**, 2333–2338.

Beto, J. A. & Bansal, V. K. (1992) Quality of life in treatment of hypertension. A metaanalysis of clinical trials. *American Journal of Hypertension*, **5**, 125–133.

Buster, J. E., Kingsberg, S. A., Aguirre, O., *et al* (2005) Testosterone patch for low sexual desire in surgically menopausal women: a randomized trial. *Obstetrics and Gynecology*, **105**, 944–952.

Carson, C. C., Rajfer, J., Eardley, I., *et al* (2004) The efficacy and safety of tadalafil: an update. *BJU International*, **93**, 1276–1281.

Catalan, J. (1993) Primary male anorgasmia and its treatment: three case reports. *Sexual and Marital Therapy*, **8**, 275–282.

Clement, U. (2002) Sex in long-term relationships: a systemic approach to sexual desire problems. *Archives of Sexual Behavior*, **31**, 241–246.

Davenport-Hines, R. P. T. (1990) *Sex, Death, and Punishment: Attitudes to Sex and Sexuality in Britain Since the Renaissance*. Collins.

David, C. M., Yarber, W. L., Bauserman, R., *et al* (1998) *Handbook of Sexuality-Related Measures*. Sage.

Department of Health (2002) *The National Strategy for Sexual Health and HIV*. Department of Health.

Dixon, M., Booth, N. & Powell, R. (2000) Sex and relationships following childbirth: a first report from general practice of 131 couples. *British Journal of General Practice*, **50**, 223–224.

Drugs and Therapeutics Bulletin (2004) New oral drugs for erectile dysfunction. *Drugs and Therapeutics Bulletin*, 42.

Dunn, K. M., Croft, P. R. & Hackett, G. I. (2000) Satisfaction in the sex life of a general population sample. *Journal of Sexual and Marital Therapy*, **26**, 141–151.

Goldstat, R., Briganti, E., Tran, J., *et al* (2003) Transdermal testosterone therapy improves well-being, mood, and sexual function in premenopausal women. *Menopause*, **10**, 390–398.

Goldstein, I., Lue, T. F., Padma-Nathan, H., *et al* (1998) Oral sildenafil in the treatment of erectile dysfunction. Sildenafil Study Group. *New England Journal of Medicine*, **338**, 1397–1404.

Hayes, S. C. & Smith, S. (2005) *Get Out of Your Mind and Into Your Life: The New Acceptance and Commitment Therapy*. New Harbinger Publications.

Humphery, S. & Nazareth, I. (2001) GPs' views on their management of sexual dysfunction. *Family Practice*, **18**, 516–518.

Jannini, E. A., Simonelli, C. & Lenzi, A. (2002) Sexological approach to ejaculatory dysfunction. *International Journal of Andrology*, **25**, 317–323.

Kamischke, A. & Nieschlag, E. (2002) Update on medical treatment of ejaculatory disorders. *International Journal of Andrology*, **25**, 333–344.

Kaplan, H. S. (1974) *The New Sex Therapy: Active Treatment of Sexual Dysfunctions*. Brunner Mazel.

King, M., Holt, V. & Nazareth, I. (2007) Women's views of their sexual difficulties: agreement and disagreement with clinical diagnoses. *Archives of Sexual Behavior*, **36**, 281–288.

Kolomaznik, M. (2004) Intermittent administration of sertraline in premature ejaculation. *Psychiatrie*, **8**, 100–103.

La, P. G. & Nicastro, A. (1996) A new treatment for premature ejaculation: the rehabilitation of the pelvic floor. *Journal of Sexual and Marital Therapy*, **22**, 22–26.

Laumann, E. O., Paik, A. & Rosen, R. C. (1999) Sexual dysfunction in the United States: prevalence and predictors. *JAMA*, **281**, 537–544.

Markou, S., Perimenis, P., Gyftopoulos, K., *et al* (2004) Vardenafil (Levitra) for erectile dysfunction: a systematic review and meta-analysis of clinical trial reports. *International Journal of Impotence Research*, **16**, 470–478.

Masters, W. H. & Johnson, V. (1970) *Human Sexual Inadequacy*. Little Brown.

Mayor, S. (2004) Pfizer will not apply for a licence for sildenafil for women. *BMJ*, **328**, 542.

McCoy, N. L. & Matyas, J. R. (1996) Oral contraceptives and sexuality in university women. *Archives of Sexual Behavior*, **25**, 73–90.

McGuire, H. & Hawton, K. (2003) Interventions for vaginismus. *Cochrane Database of Systematic Reviews*, (1), CD001760.

McMahon, C. G., Abdo, C., Incrocci, L., *et al* (2004) Disorders of orgasm and ejaculation in men. *Journal of Sexual Medicine*, **1**, 58–65.

Meana, M., Binik, Y. M., Khalife, S., *et al* (1997) Dyspareunia: sexual dysfunction or pain syndrome? *Journal of Nervous and Mental Diseases*, **185**, 561–569.

Mendels, J., Camera, A. & Sikes, C. (1995) Sertraline treatment for premature ejaculation. *Journal of Clinical Psychopharmacology*, **15**, 341–346.

Mercer, C. H., Fenton, K. A., Johnson, A. M., *et al* (2003) Sexual function problems and help seeking behaviour in Britain: national probability sample survey. *BMJ*, **327**, 426–427.

Modelska, K. & Cummings, S. (2003) Female sexual dysfunction in postmenopausal women: systematic review of placebo-controlled trials. *American Journal of Obstetrics and Gynecology*, **188**, 286–293.

Montague, D. K., Jarow, J., Broderick, G. A., *et al* (2004) AUA guideline on the pharmacologic management of premature ejaculation. *Journal of Urology*, **172**, 290–294.

Montejo, A. L., Llorca, G., Izquierdo, J. A., *et al* (2001) Incidence of sexual dysfunction associated with antidepressant agents: a prospective multicenter study of 1022 outpatients. Spanish Working Group for the Study of Psychotropic-Related Sexual Dysfunction. *Journal of Clinical Psychiatry*, **62** (Suppl 3), 10–21.

Morgentaler, A. (1999) Male impotence. *Lancet*, **354**, 1713–1718.

Moynihan, R. (2003) The making of a disease: female sexual dysfunction. *BMJ*, **326**, 45–47.

Moynihan, R. (2005) The marketing of a disease: female sexual dysfunction. *BMJ*, **330**, 192–194.

Nazareth, I., Boynton, P. & King, M. (2003) Problems with sexual function in people attending London general practitioners: cross sectional study. *BMJ*, **327**, 423.

Nicolson, P. & Burr, J. (2003) What is 'normal' about women's (hetero)sexual desire and orgasm? A report of an in-depth interview study. *Social Science and Medicine*, **57**, 1735–1745.

Phillips, N. A. (2000) Female sexual dysfunction: evaluation and treatment. *American Family Physician*, **62**, 127–132.

Ralph, D. & McNicholas, T. (2000) UK management guidelines for erectile dysfunction. *BMJ*, **321**, 499–503.

Reynolds, C. F., Frank, E., Thase, M. E., *et al* (1988) Assessment of sexual function in depressed, impotent, and healthy men: factor analysis of a Brief Sexual Function Questionnaire for Men. *Psychiatry Research*, **24**, 231–250.

Richardson, D., Goldmeier, D., Green, J., *et al* (2006) Recommendations for the management of premature ejaculation: BASHH Special Interest Group for Sexual Dysfunction. *International Journal of STD and AIDS*, **17**, 1–6.

Rosen, R. C., Riley, A., Wagner, G., *et al* (1997) The International Index of Erectile Function (IIEF): a multidimensional scale for assessment of erectile dysfunction. *Urology*, **49**, 822–830.

Schnyder, U., Schnyder-Luthi, C., Ballinari, P., *et al* (1998) Therapy for vaginismus: in vivo versus in vitro desensitization. *Canadian Journal of Psychiatry*, **43**, 941–944.

Segraves, R. T. (2002) Female sexual disorders: psychiatric aspects. *Canadian Journal of Psychiatry*, **47**, 419–425.

Semans, J. H. (1956) Premature ejaculation: a new approach. *Southern Medical Journal*, **49**, 353–358.

Shifren, J. L. (2004) The role of androgens in female sexual dysfunction. *Mayo Clinic Proceedings*, **79**, S19–S24.

Smith, K. M. & Romanelli, F. (2005) Recreational use and misuse of phosphodiesterase 5 inhibitors. *Journal of American Pharmaceutical Association*, **45**, 63–72.

Taylor, J. F., Rosen, R. C. & Leiblum, S. R. (1994) Self-report assessment of female sexual function: psychometric evaluation of the Brief Index of Sexual Functioning for Women. *Archives of Sexual Behavior*, **23**, 627–643.

Tiefer, L. (2000) Sexology and the pharmaceutical industry: the threat of co-optation. *Journal of Sex Research*, **37**, 273–283.

Waldinger, M. D., Hengeveld, M. W., Zwinderman, A. H., *et al* (1998) Effect of SSRI antidepressants on ejaculation: a double-blind, randomized, placebo-controlled study with fluoxetine, fluvoxamine, paroxetine, and sertraline. *Journal of Clinical Psychopharmacology*, **18**, 274–281.

Warner, P., Bancroft, J. & Members of the Edinburgh Sexuality Group (1987) A regional clinical service for sexual problems: a three year survey. *Sexual and Marital Therapy*, **2**, 115–126.

Weiderman, M. W. (1998) The state of the theory in sex therapy. *Journal of Sex Research*, **35**, 99.

World Health Organization (1992) *The ICD–10 Classification of Mental and Behavioural Disorders. Clinical Descriptions and Diagnostic Guidelines*. WHO.

World Health Organization (1993) *The ICD–10 Classification of Mental and Behavioural Disorders: Diagnostic Criteria for Research*. WHO.

# Part III: Policy and practice

Clinicians do not work in a vacuum or a time capsule. Even if they practise alone, there is a professional imperative to consider methods of improving the quality of care that they are providing for people with mental health problems, an issue that is increasingly in the gaze of international policy-makers. Many primary care professionals work in extended teams, and all clinicians have to collaborate with other providers of care, particularly across the primary–specialist interface. How this interface should be organised for optimal efficiency remains a topic of hot debate.

The five chapters in Part III address themes that cut across clinical problems and conditions. They are concerned with mental health promotion, improving the quality of mental healthcare, the roles of different professionals, particularly practice nurses, and the expanding variety of psychological therapies that may be or should be accessible from primary care. Particular attention is also given to novel approaches to organising and configuring the interface: stepped and collaborative care.

Part III: Policy and practice

# CHAPTER 24

# Mental health promotion

Andre Tylee and Annie Wallace

Summary

The chapter looks at mental health promotion in its broadest context, including links to the wider public health agenda. It provides an overview of mental health promotion within the primary care setting and gives examples of health promotion practice within the context of patients with common mental health problems.

## Attempting a definition of mental health promotion

Defining mental health promotion (MHP) is at least as difficult a task as defining health promotion. In order to define it you need to be clear about where you sit in terms of how you define mental health. Confusingly, as with health generally, we define our mental health services as a place where we treat mental ill health. Unsurprisingly, the public still tend to think of mental health in terms of schizophrenia and depression. The World Health Organization (WHO), in defining 'health' in 1947, included mental health as part of an attempt at a holistic vision of health. In 2001, the WHO published the following definition of positive mental health:

> a state of well-being in which the individual realises his or her own abilities, can cope with normal stresses of life, can work productively and fruitfully and is able to make a contribution to his or her own community. (WHO, 2001)

This definition, while capturing what many may view as good mental health, reflects the same arguments as physical well-being versus disability and leaves the survivors of mental health issues, to some extent, outside of the definition. Health and illness, however, can coexist. They are mutually exclusive only if health is defined in a restrictive way as the absence of disease (Sartorius, 1990). Lay beliefs about health vary across culture, gender, age and social circumstance; for example, young people in high-income countries tend to think in terms of fitness or healthy diet, older people in terms of inner strength and coping with life's challenges. However, the definitions of mental health we routinely use are culturally skewed, individualised and expert-led versions of what it means to be mentally healthy. For example, what these Westernised definitions fail to take account of might be the reliance on fate or a deity, or on some other belief system present in other cultural representations.

The prevention model which is defined as interventions designed to avert mental ill health pays no heed to the structural and political features of mental health. Narrowly defining MHP as prevention misses the opportunity to see mental health as a positive attribute and its measurement becomes reduction in ill-health rather than increases in positive well-being. Latterly, the WHO has looked at MHP as a human rights issue. In *Promoting Mental Health: Concepts, Emerging Evidence and Practice* (WHO, 2004) it is suggested that a 'climate that respects and protects basic civil political, economic, social and cultural rights is fundamental to the promotion of mental health'.

A broad definition of MHP from the UK Health Education Authority (HEA) included in the document *Making It Happen: A Guide to Delivering Mental Health Promotion* developed by Mentality (Department of Health, 2001a) is 'any action to enhance the mental well-being of individuals, families or communities'. However, it makes no attempt to explore either what actions are more effective than others or to illustrate the very real dilemma that action to enhance one community's well-being could be to the detriment of another.

Mental health promotion tends to be conceptualised into its component parts. One such conceptualisation might be:

1    strengthening individuals – increasing emotional resilience, and promoting self-esteem, life and coping skills, parenting, stress management, communication skills
2    strengthening communities – increasing social inclusion and participation, improving environments, increasing access to and improving services, and improving organisational settings like schools and workplaces
3    reducing structural barriers – reducing discrimination, and increasing access to education, meaningful employment and housing.

## Mental health promotion as disease prevention

The disease prevention model tends to focus on health promotion at a level of the individual and is bound up with ideas of risk and resilience; the health promotion focuses on risk reduction and building strategies to enhance resilience in much the same way as a heart disease prevention programme may work. There is a structural element to this view of MHP; however, it tends to focus on better services and better access to services. The risks are viewed in terms of how they might be reduced at an individual level; for example, homeless people may be regarded as an 'at risk' population as opposed to regarding homelessness as a risk situation. Defining MHP in this way means we tend to give resources to supporting people living in inadequate situations rather than resourcing efforts to remove the inadequate situations. The measurement of MHP in this sense is similar, in that, for instance, reductions in levels of depression would be a long-term outcome. This model of MHP is certainly reflected in UK policy. For example, while purporting to be aimed at tackling inequality, one of the main foci of *Our Health, Our Care, Our Say*, the Department of Health White Paper published in 2006 (Department of Health, 2006), in terms of mental health is 'Mental health promotion as enhancing well-being'. This has some features in common with disease prevention, in the sense that it can concentrate on individual coping strategies. However, the recipients of this MHP are universal, from stress reduction in the workplace to school programmes like SEAL ('social and emotional aspects of learning'), which takes a whole-school approach to promoting social and emotional well-being (SEAL, 2007). MHP as enhancing well-being also tends to acknowledge the role of structures in MHP; for example, within an organisation or institution there is a recognition of the role of environment and policy to enhance the mental health and well-being of individuals. An added complication, however, has been to use the term 'well-being' rather than 'mental health' in an attempt to move away from notions of mental illness.

## Social capital and mental health promotion

> On the one hand, millions of dollars are committed to alleviating ill-health through individual intervention, meanwhile we ignore what our everyday experience tells us (i.e. the way we organise our society, the extent to which we encourage interaction among the citizenry and the degree to which we trust and associate with each other in caring communities is probably the most important determinant or our health). (Lomas, 1998)

Social capital refers to a set of resources within communities, usually a variant on the following categories (Cooper *et al*, 1999):

- social resources (e.g. informal arrangements between neighbours)
- collective resources (e.g. self-help groups, credit unions, community safety schemes)
- economic resources (e.g. levels of unemployment, access to green open spaces)
- cultural resources (e.g. libraries, art centres, schools).

It embodies notions of respect, feeling safe and the visual environment, together with structural issues like access to all kinds of services and economic development. Social capital includes notions of how people feel about their neighbourhood and is a useful concept within a broad health promotion framework, since addressing social capital addresses a number of health issues in a holistic way and goes some way to moving MHP from an individualised concept to something that occurs within communities and organisations.

## Mental health promotion and public health

Mental health promotion in the context of a broader public health agenda is concerned with the wider determinants of health. Mental health becomes part of tackling inequalities and the focus is on regeneration, participation and social inclusion. This way of looking at MHP fits well with notions of a mentally healthy community.

Looking beyond the individual and unpicking the features of a mentally healthy community, the whole notion of what MHP covers becomes clearer. The list of factors influencing the mental well-being of communities in Box 24.1 is taken from *Making It Happen: A Guide to Delivering Mental Health Promotion* (Department of Health, 2001a).

Public mental health looks beyond prevention and calls for a greater understanding of the values and strategic priorities underpinning a broader public health agenda – partnerships, community involvement, regeneration, social inclusion and reducing inequalities

The VicHealth framework (WHO, 2004) illustrates in practice how MHP sits within a public health context (Fig. 24.1). The framework was developed by the Victorian Health Promotion Foundation in 1999 to illustrate the need to view MHP as public MHP. The three main themes identified by the VicHealth framework are:

1    a clear focus on the social and economic determinants of health
2    the involvement of the full range of health promotion methods, working at population and sub-population levels
3    the engagement of a range of sectors working across settings.

---

**Box 24.1** Factors influencing the mental well-being of communities

- Housing
- Local democracy
- Employment
- Self-help
- Neighbourhood and voluntary agencies
- Friendship and social networks
- Advocacy and user groups
- Statutory services
- Confiding relationships
- Discrimination
- Information
- Income distribution

From Department of Health (2001a).

---

**Social inclusion**
Supportive relationships
Involvement in group activities
Civic engagement

**Freedom from discrimination and violence**
Valuing diversity
Physical security
Self-determination and control of one's life

**Economic participation**
Work
Education
Housing
Money

**Population groups and action areas**

**Population groups**
Children
Young people
Women and men
Older people
Indigenous communities
Culturally diverse communities
Rural communities

**Health promotion action**
Research, monitoring and evaluation
Individual self-development
Organisational development
Community engagement
Communication and marketing
Advocacy of legislative and policy reform

**Sectors and settings for action**
Housing
Transport
Community
Corporate
Education
Public
Workplace
Academic
Sports, arts and recreation
Local government
Health
Justice

**Intermediate outcomes**

**Individual**
Increased sense of
belonging, self-esteem,
self-determination
and control

**Organisational and community**
Accessible and responsive organisations
Safe, supportive and inclusive environments

**Societal**
Integrated and supportive
public policy and
programmes
Strong legislative platform
Resource allocation

**Improved mental health**

**Long-term benefits**
Less anxiety and depression
Less substance misuse
Improved physical health
Improved productivity at work, home or school
Less violence and crime
Reduced health inequalities
Improved quality of life and life expectancy

**Fig. 24.1** Key determinants of mental health and themes for action. Reproduced with permission from the Victorian Health Promotion Foundation.

# Does mental health promotion add value?

It should be clear that defining MHP is difficult: it is easy to narrow it right down to a prevention agenda or to make it so broad as to make it meaningless as a separate concept. It is beyond the scope of this chapter to detail the evidence base for MHP; however, the WHO (2004) report *Promoting Mental Health* gives an overview of the emerging evidence base for MHP, with further references.

# Policy context

To suggest that there can be a single policy for MHP misses the point somewhat; on the other hand, to have no dedicated focus can mean MHP is overlooked as an outcome. The WHO (2004) suggests that:

> Mental health promotion requires multi-sectoral action, involving a number of government sectors such as health, employment/industry, education, environment, transport and social and community services as well as non-governmental or community-based organisations such as health support groups, churches, clubs and other bodies.

We have no argument in principle with this as an aspirational goal; however, it should be clear from the above discussion that what MHP is and what it means will vary considerably across organisations, across communities and across individuals in those communities. Introducing the concept of enhancing mental health through policy is therefore open to a variety of interpretations. The concept of health impact is a useful one in thinking about how this huge policy agenda could possibly be met. Addressing the components of MHP (and indeed health promotion) – like social inclusion, poverty, access to services – is common to many policy areas. Health impact as a basic premise asks what impact a particular policy will have on mental health. The health impact assessment process then seeks to address policy from a positive health perspective, including maximising health benefit, minimising negative effects and prioritising areas for investment to enhance mental health.

Mental health promotion in health policy has a mixed degree of success in terms of getting to grips with the wider public health agenda. In UK policy, the *National Service Framework for Mental Health* (Department of Health, 1999) had its 'standard 1' as promoting mental health across the whole population. The success of standard 1 was by and large to be judged across a mental health services community. This highlights the difficulty in implementing MHP. The mechanism for achieving standard 1 was unclear, calling for the kind of cooperation the WHO statement aspires to but without the cross-government links required to achieve it. More recent UK health policy, set out in *Our Health, Our Care, Our Say* (Department of Health, 2006), focuses on some elements of MHP, such as more choice and a stronger voice, but misses the point in the wider context, since the policy concentrates on health and social services and ignores the level of collaboration required to embed MHP in other sector cultures. For example, within sexual health, targets like reducing teenage conception rates are shared by the National Health Service and local authorities. If MHP had the same level of commitment, shared targets across sectors would start to emerge.

In the introduction to this section, we quoted the WHO aspiration for inter-sectoral collaboration as the ideal. If MHP is about social capital and the wider public health agenda, then policy that addresses inequalities will have the greatest impact on public mental health. The WHO suggests three main components for successful inter-sectoral collaboration:

1   the adoption of a unifying language with which to work across sectors
2   a partnership approach to allocation and sharing of resources
3   a strengthening of capacity across the individual, organisational and community dimensions.

# Mental health promotion as civil and human rights

Many of the features of the United Nations Declaration on Human Rights, first published in 1948, are common to MHP, particularly in the context of building social capital and the wider determinants of health. For example, the principles of equality and freedom from discrimination reflect human rights and are factors in the promotion of good mental health. The right of people to participate and have their views regarded in the decision-making process is a further example of the links. Using a human rights framework as illustrated by the United Nations Declaration also has a clear advantage in terms of accountability and therefore the monitoring of success.

# MHP and primary care

> Mental well-being is influenced by many factors, including genetic inheritance, childhood experiences, life events, individual ability to cope and social support, as well as factors such as adequate housing, employment, financial security and access to health facilities. (Department of Health, 2001a)

The promotion of mental health in primary care plays out in micro the issues highlighted above. Much of the focus at a primary care level has been about identifying, managing and treating mental health conditions. There has been an emphasis on early intervention, particularly in relation to high-risk populations, like young men in suicide prevention. However, a more radical approach can be taken, adopting the features of MHP and the wider determinants of health. There are several frameworks that could be adopted; for example, the Ottawa Charter (WHO, 1986) provides a health promotion framework that includes action at individual, community and policy levels. Table 24.1 gives one example of how a practice within the primary care setting might address MHP. It is not intended to be exhaustive, but rather to give a flavour of the factors affecting mental health across a practice population.

# Links between mental health problems and physical problems

In general practice populations, many people with mental health problems will also have comorbid physical problems. It is increasingly known that poor mental health is associated with the development of poor physical health. For instance, depression may be an independent risk factor for ischaemic heart disease in men, but not in women. In a study in one general practice, 188 men with ischaemic heart disease were matched by age to 485 men without ischaemic heart disease The risk of ischaemic heart disease was three times higher among men with a recorded diagnosis of depression than among controls of the same age (odds ratio 3.09; 95% confidence interval 1.33 to 7.21; $P = 0.009$). This association persisted when smoking status, diabetes, hypertension and underprivileged area (UPA 8) score were included in a multivariate model (adjusted odds ratio 2.75; 95% confidence interval 1.13 to 6.69; $P = 0.03$). Men with depression within the preceding 10 years were three times more likely to develop ischaemic heart disease

**Table 24.1** Framework for mental health promotion in the primary care setting

| Increasing participation | Social inclusion | Strengthening individuals | Information needs | Supportive environment |
|---|---|---|---|---|
| Forums for patient and public involvement | Equity audit utilised to ensure practice population is being served | Social prescriptions like exercise, learning and arts | Accessible health information | An environment that respects cultural diversity and the requirements of those with enhanced needs |
| Forums for staff involvement | Practice has an ethos of welcome | Concordant relationships in treatment | Help for individuals with poor health literacy | Services brought into practices, for example benefits advice |
| Participatory methods used | Equality and diversity policy | Workplace measures in place like stress audits, general workplace health | | Personal safety of staff and public considered |

than were the controls (odds ratio 3.13; 95% confidence interval 1.27 to 7.70; $P = 0.01$) (Hippisley-Cox *et al*, 1998).

The association between mental health problems such as depression and chronic physical health problems led to the introduction in the General Medical Services (GMS) contract of payment to practices across the UK for screening patients with coronary heart disease and diabetes for depression. Most general practitioners (GPs) know that sustained mental health problems are associated with a wide range of physical health problems in their patients and MHP cannot be separated from physical health promotion. Primary care teams may often be in positions where they can practise primary prevention rather than just secondary prevention (i.e. early recognition) or tertiary prevention (treatment).

## Practice role in 'signposting' services and support groups

An important aspect of MHP involves 'signposting' relevant voluntary organisations for patients. In a study of facilitated referral to local voluntary organisations, referral to the Amalthea Project and subsequent contact with the voluntary sector resulted in clinically important benefits compared with usual GP care in managing psychosocial problems, but at a higher cost (Grant *et al*, 2000). The Amalthea Project was a liaison organisation that facilitated contact between voluntary organisations and patients in primary care, and this was compared with patients receiving routine GP care in 26 general practices in Avon.

Practices themselves can be a true community resource and a site for community groups, voluntary agencies and so on to meet and provide education and support to the local population (e.g. benefits advice, housing advice, exercise, talks on nutrition, alcohol).

Suggestions for practices to consider when addressing MHP are shown in Box 24.2. Some are easily within the control of the GP (e.g. having a high index of awareness for domestic violence and opportunistically asking about it when appropriate). Other aspects, such as local housing and employment, are more difficult for the GP to influence, but nevertheless important. Access to psychological interventions may improve in the near future if pilot schemes in Doncaster in the north of England and Newham in London are successful under the new Improved Access to Psychological Therapies (IAPT) programme within the Department of Health (Department of Health, 2007) (see www.dh.gov.uk).

At the level of the primary care trust, MHP activity in recent years has taken into account Department of Health guidance on how to implement standard 1 of the *National Service Framework for Mental Health* (Department of Health, 1999). This included considering in any plans how best to combat discrimination and the social exclusion of people with mental health problems and how best to promote mental health in schools, workplaces

Box 24.2 A checklist of ten key areas for practices to consider in terms of mental health promotion

1 Enhancing confidence and self-esteem
2 Talking things over
3 Encouraging physical activity
4 Encouraging access to learning opportunities
5 Support with child care
6 Opportunities for creativity
7 Opportunities to gain employment and income
8 Support with domestic violence
9 Addressing mental health of people with chronic physical health problems
10 Access to psychological interventions

Developed by Dr Maryanne Freer, Dr Dave Tomson and colleagues, MHP in Primary Care, contact Maryanne.freer@pcpartners.org.

and neighbourhoods for individuals at risk and vulnerable groups. These might include people sleeping rough, people in prison, victims of abuse or domestic violence, refugees, people with alcohol and drug problems, looked-after children, Black and ethnic minority populations, and low-income and excluded groups (Department of Health, 2006).

# Key skills for primary care providers

The Care Services Improvement Partnership (CSIP) and National Institute for Mental Health (NIMH) in England have produced a competency guide for primary care and community services (CSIP & NIMHE, 2006). This resource describes a key skill, which is to promote positive mental health and emotional well-being by respecting diversity and challenging inequality. This is important to improve the health and well-being of the practice population, to reduce the stigma associated with mental health problems and to increase the social inclusion of disadvantaged groups. To achieve this, it is essential to recognise and appreciate people's diverse backgrounds, including age, race, culture, gender, disability, spirituality and sexuality. It is important to know how to access interpreter services when appropriate. It is necessary to be able to offer support to people seeking advice about issues of discrimination or injustice; an example may be helping asylum seekers find accommodation. It is important to identify and challenge discriminatory attitudes and practices towards people with mental health problems and to be self-aware in this regard and ensure an appropriate level of support for local needs. Another key skill is to have an awareness of the factors that protect against mental health problems and those that make people more vulnerable. This is important to help strengthen the individual's emotional resilience to adverse life events. The Commonwealth Department of Health and Aged Care in Canberra, Australia, has described in detail the possible protective factors and risk factors for mental health problems (Commonwealth Department of Health and Aged Care, 2000).

Skills that are important in promoting emotional well-being and social inclusion are those of being able to apply a person-centred approach, unique to each individual patient, to plan care that is physical, psychological and social and identifies individual needs, strengths and coping strategies. This means believing in and acknowledging each individual's uniqueness, positive attributes and potential to contribute to society. It means delivering support that promotes the service users' citizenship and community participation and enhances their independence from services wherever possible. It is important to remember that people's lives are much bigger than the services they receive, and to provide just enough support when needed yet to encourage self-reliance and autonomy.

# Health promotion practice – patients with common mental health problems

It is important for practices to consider the health promotion potential of working with patients presenting with common mental health problems, typically depression and anxiety. The aims of developing a health promotion strategy with these patients would be to enhance mental well-being, improve social networks (and therefore reduce social exclusion) and improve general physical health.

Meeting the general information needs of patients experiencing a common mental health problem is crucial to increase their well-being. The practice may choose to organise psycho-education individually or in groups. Groups would have the added benefit of encouraging social networking, which can in itself enhance social support and social capital. 'Social prescribing' may include arranging for advice to be provided, again, individually or in groups, on areas such as housing, finances, nutrition and exercise.

## Exercise and mental health

Using the example of exercise and mental health, the Department of Health published a quality assurance framework for exercise in 2001 (Department of Health, 2001b). The authors suggest that:

> Physical activity reduces the risk of depression and has positive benefits for mental health, including reducing anxiety and enhancing mood and self-esteem.

In addition, there are clear physical benefits, in relation to type II diabetes, obesity, falls prevention, bone density and blood pressure. There are equally obvious social advantages to some types of exercise: gardening and walking

**361**

groups, for example, have the added bonus of enabling people to become less socially isolated and to engage with wider supportive networks.

The framework concludes that the primary care setting is ideally placed to promote physical activity:

> 95% of the population will see a medical practitioner within any 3 year period yet only 1:4 is likely to be physically active on a regular basis.

The framework suggests four areas the practitioner can engage in:

1  a knowledge of what activity is available in the local community, including information leaflets
2  advice on particular activities and their benefits
3  help and in some cases referral to others for support and motivation
4  specific referral to an exercise scheme.

The first two areas require the practice to have up-to-date and accessible information for patients.

One of the issues with recommending exercise, like any other healthy lifestyle activity, might be the motivation to engage and to keep on engaging with a lifestyle change. This involves a more detailed input than simply giving information; for example, barriers to exercise, exercise benefits and motivations may be discussed. There may be local initiatives such as health trainers, children's centres or community support schemes where people can support patients in making behavioural changes. The local public health department should be able to advise.

## Social prescribing opportunities and mental health

The literature cites other examples of social prescribing for people with common mental health problems, typically social groups, arts and learning. The common aims are to increase social interaction, to improve emotional literacy and communication skills, and to engage in problem-solving activity. White (2003), for example, in talking about arts and mental health says that art is 'a medium for participants to explore and understand feelings and develop alternative coping strategies'.

## Food and mood

Good advice about a healthy diet is not only helpful for preventing obesity, diabetes and heart disease. Fresh fruit and vegetables and oily fish can provide omega fats and folic acid, both of which may be beneficial to mood (see under Mental Health Foundation in the list of Further reading and e-resources).

## Better access to psychological treatment

The Improved Access to Psychological Therapies programme (Department of Health, 2007) includes work-focused counselling to assist people who have been out of work because of mental health problems to regain employment (where appropriate), as being in work is likely to improve ongoing mental state. This pilot work is being evaluated.

## Conclusion

Mental health promotion is about facilitating the well-being of individuals, families and communities. Well-being is qualitatively more than the absence of disease. Strengthening individuals involves increasing their emotional resilience, and promoting their self-esteem, life and coping skills, parenting skills, stress management and communication skills. Strengthening communities involves: promoting social inclusion and participation; improving environments; increasing access to and improving services; and improving organisational settings like schools and workplaces. Reducing structural barriers involves: reducing discrimination; improving access to education; improving meaningful employment; and providing housing where necessary. While this needs collaboration between many relevant government departments, the Department of Health plays a key role. At a more micro level, practices and primary care trusts have a key role in supporting and providing a range of activities that promote mental health. This involves professionals in primary care, prisons, schools (via school nurses) and so on. Parenting skills and support for new mothers and babies through schemes such as SureStart (http://www.surestart.gov. uk) may help promote well-being in mothers and their children. This may be particularly important for teenage single parents.

Stress management skills and cognitive–behavioural strategies are increasingly provided by primary care mental health workers, who were initially known as 'graduate mental health workers' in practices and primary care trusts. In addition, these new workers in primary care can provide self-help materials or recommend or loan appropriate books to patients with mild common mental health problems ('bibliotherapy'). They can also provide brief therapy, either individually or to groups (CSIP & NIMHE, 2006). The National Health Service tends to be more reactive than proactive where mental health is concerned and if it is going to respond to the challenge set by the WHO ('there is no health without mental health'), there needs to be huge systemic change. All generalists and non-mental health professionals in primary or secondary care will need to have MHP at the front of their own minds (including their own mental health) if this is to become a reality.

## Further reading and e-resources

The Department of Health's *Making It Happen* is probably the best and most comprehensive document about mental health promotion and can be found at http://www.publications. doh.gov.uk/pdfs/makingithappen.pdf

Key points

- Mental health promotion is about facilitating the well-being of individuals, families and communities.
- Well-being is qualitatively more than the absence of disease.
- Strengthening individuals involves increasing emotional resilience, and promoting self-esteem, life and coping skills, parenting skills, stress management and communication skills.
- Strengthening communities involves promoting social inclusion and participation, improving environments, increasing access to and improving services, and improving organisational settings like schools and workplaces.
- Mental health promotion requires structural barriers to be overcome, by reducing discrimination and increasing access to education, meaningful employment and housing.
- Practices and primary care trusts have a key role in supporting and providing these activities.
- The National Health Service should embrace and properly resource these activities.

Mental Health Foundation, Exercise and depression: Information for GPs and healthcare practioners, http://www.mentalhealth.org.uk/campaigns/exercise-and-depression/information-for-gps/?locale=en

Mental Health Foundation, Healthy eating and depression: how diet may help protect your mental health, http://www.mentalhealth.org.uk/campaigns/food-and-mental-health/healthy-eating/

Victorian Health Promotion Foundation (1999) Mental Health Promotion Framework 2005–2007. Downloadable from http://www.vichealth.vic.gov.au/~/media/ProgramsandProjects/MentalHealthandWellBeing/Attachments/vhp%20framework-print.ashx

# References

Commonwealth Department of Health and Aged Care (2000) *Promotion, Prevention and Early Intervention for Mental Health. A Monograph.* Mental Health and Special Programs Branch, Commonwealth Department of Health and Aged Care.

Cooper, H., Arber, S., Fee, L., *et al* (1999) *The Influence of Social Support and Social Capital on Health.* London Health Education Authority.

CSIP & NIMHE (2006) *Improving Primary Care Mental Health Services. A Practical Guide.* Department of Health.

Department of Health (1999) *National Service Framework for Mental Health.* Department of Health.

Department of Health (2001a) *Making It Happen: A Guide to Delivering Mental Health Promotion.* Mentality, Sainsbury Centre for Mental Health. Downloadable from http://www.publications.doh.gov.uk/pdfs/makingithappen.pdf

Department of Health (2001b) *Exercise Referral Systems: A National Quality Assurance Framework.* Department of Health.

Department of Health (2006) *Our Health, Our Care, Our Say.* Department of Health.

Department of Health (2007) *Commissioning a Brighter Future. Improving Access to Psychological Therapies (IAPT).* Department of Health.

Grant, C., Goodenough, T., Harvey, I., *et al* (2000) A randomised controlled trial and economic evaluation of a referrals facilitator between primary care and the voluntary sector. *BMJ*, **320**, 419–423 .

Hippisley-Cox, J., Fielding, K. & Pringle, M. (1998) Depression as a risk factor for ischaemic heart disease in men: population based case–control study. *BMJ*, **316**, 1714–1719.

Lomas, J. (1998) Social capital and health – implications for public health and epidemiology. *Social Science and Medicine*, **47**, 1181–1188.

Sartorius, N. (1990) Preface. In *The Public Health Impact of Mental Disorders* (eds D. Goldberg & D. Tantam). Hogrefe and Huber.

SEAL (2007) Social and emotional aspects of learning. At http://www.standards.dfes.gov.uk

White, M. (2003) *Addressing the Evidence Base for Participation in Arts and Cultural Activity – A Report to the Social Inclusion Unit, Durham*. University of Durham.

WHO (1986) *Ottawa Charter*. World Health Organization.

WHO (2001) Mental health: strengthening mental health promotion. World Health Organization. At http://www.who.int/mediacentre/factsheets/fs220/en/index.html

WHO (2004) *Promoting Mental Health – Concepts, Emerging Evidence and Practice*. World Health Organization. At http://www.who.int/mental_health/evidence/MH_Promotion_Book.pdf

# Improving the quality of primary care mental health: what does and does not work?

Linda Gask, Simon Gilbody and Tony Kendrick

## Summary

Most of the literature on quality improvement for primary care mental health has focused on the common mental disorders, primarily on depression. However, recent literature has also emphasised the role of primary care in improving the quality of both physical and mental healthcare for those with more severe and enduring mental health problems (such as schizophrenia). This chapter reviews the evidence for quality improvement through professional, financial, and organis-ational interventions.

## What do we mean by quality of care?

Campbell *et al* (2000) have usefully defined two principal dimensions of quality of care for individual patients: *access* and *effectiveness*. In essence, do users of services get the care they need, and is the care effective when they get it? Within effectiveness, they define two key components – effectiveness of *clinical care* and effectiveness of *interpersonal care*.

The effectiveness of *clinical care* depends on the effective application of knowledge-based care. Knowledge-based care refers to both evidence-based medicine (Sackett *et al*, 1996) and care that is regarded as legitimate (Donabedian, 1990). The latter relates to aspects of care that may be widely accepted without necessarily having scientific evidence of effectiveness. Knowledge-based care incorporates the extent to which a treatment or service is consistent with patients' reasonable expectations and contemporary professional standards of care, reflecting both societal and professional norms. Care is described as 'evidence based' only when there is good scientific evidence of a link between process and outcome.

However, effective care also requires appreciation of the quality of *interpersonal care*, the patient's personal experience of illness (Stewart *et al*, 1995) and the perceived quality of the communication with the health professional. Care should be planned for and agreed with individual patients through negotiation with the doctor; such 'shared decision making' (Elwyn *et al*, 1999) means that truly 'patient-centred care' (Stewart *et al*, 1995; Mead & Bower, 2000) may sometimes seem to be at odds with the implementation of 'evidence-based' care (Bensing, 2000).

*Coordination* or *integration* of care for individual patients is also an important attribute of effectiveness of care, and is particularly relevant to primary care (Starfield, 1998). Coordination refers to the effectiveness with which health professionals deal with other organisations, or other professionals within the same organisation, which directly or indirectly affect patient care. *Relational continuity of care,* that is, the existence of an ongoing therapeutic relationship with a health professional, is also of key importance to people with mental health problems (Haggerty *et al*, 2003).

# Improving the quality of mental healthcare in primary care

Bower & Gilbody (2005) have suggested that services delivering primary care mental health should be aiming to achieve:

- effectiveness – services should improve health and well-being
- efficiency – limited resources should be distributed to maximise health gains to society.

They acknowledge, however, that other aims are also important and are less often dealt with explicitly in systematic reviews:

- access – service provision should meet the need for services in the community
- equity – resources should be distributed according to need.

They describe four 'models', which represent qualitatively different ways of improving the quality of primary care mental health services (Box 25.1 and see Chapter 27). This, they suggest, helps to reduce the complexity faced by policy makers, who need to try to implement 'what works' in routine healthcare settings. The four models map (imperfectly) onto Boxes 25.2 and 25.3. For example, *collaborative care* (see below) has features of both professional-level and organisation-level interventions. A wider range of professional interventions is described in the quality improvement literature than simply training primary care staff, although these are often used in combination with training. We will broadly utilise this typology, with some additions, in reviewing what does and does not seem to work.

## Interventions to improve quality of care

The Cochrane Collaboration Effective Practice and Organisation of Care Review Group (EPOC) include in their typology of quality improvement

---

**Box 25.1** Four models for improving quality of primary care mental health

**Training primary care staff**
- General practitioners and other members of the primary care team
- Recognition
- Pharmacological and psychological management

**Consultation–liaison**
- Focus on improving skills of general practitioners
- Regular specialist contact for support and feedback
- Referral only after discussion
- Management by primary care

**Collaborative care**
- Training
- Consultation
- Case management
- Direct patient contact
- Education, monitoring, psychological treatment, medication management

**Replacement**
- General practitioner has overall clinical responsibility
- Referral passes responsibility for mental healthcare to specialist in primary care
- Specialist treatment as psychological therapy

---

**Box 25.2** Professional interventions to improve quality of care

- Distribution of educational materials (published or printed recommendations for clinical care, including clinical practice guidelines, audio-visual materials and electronic publications)
- Educational meetings (conferences, lectures, workshops, traineeships)
- Local consensus processes (inclusion of providers in discussions to ensure that they have agreed that a chosen clinical problem is important and that the approach to managing it is appropriate)
- Educational outreach visits (use of a trained person to meet with providers in their practice settings to give information with the intent of changing practice; the information given may include feedback on performance)
- Local opinion leaders (use of providers nominated by colleagues as 'educationally influential')
- Patient-mediated interventions (new clinical information collected directly from patients and given to the provider, such as scores from a rating scale for depression)
- Audit and feedback (any summary of clinical performance of healthcare over a specified period, which may include recommendations for clinical action, with information obtained, for example, from medical records, computerised databases, or observations from patients)

---

**Box 25.3** Organisational interventions to improve quality of care

- Revision of professional roles (also known as 'professional substitution'; it includes the shifting of roles among health professionals)
- Clinical multidisciplinary teams (creation of a new team of health professionals of different disciplines or additions of new members to the team who work together to care for patients)
- Formal integration of services (bringing together of services across sectors or teams or the organisation of services to bring all services together at one time; also sometimes called 'seamless care')
- Changes to the skill mix (changes in numbers, types or qualifications of staff)
- Continuity of care, with arrangements for follow-up and case management (including coordination of assessment, treatment and arrangement for referrals)
- Communication and case discussion between distant health professionals (e.g. telephone links; telemedicine)

---

interventions (see http://www.epoc.cochrane.org) the following categories:

1  *professional interventions* (Box 25.2), including educational sessions, audit
2  *financial interventions*, including fee-for-service payments, financial incentives or penalties – the Quality and Outcomes Framework (QOF), which has recently been instituted in the UK for general practitioners (GPs), can be included here (British Medical Association & NHS Confederation, 2003)
3  *organisational interventions* (Box 25.3), which can be further divided into provider-oriented, patient-oriented and structural interventions.

The following sections focus in greater detail on the educational, financial, and organisational (other professionally focused, but patient-mediated) interventions, such as use of screening. Other models of quality improvement are discussed in greater detail in specific chapters within this book.

# Educational interventions: does training improve quality of care?

## Depression management

The key systematic review on educational interventions for the management of depression, carried out by Gilbody *et al* (2003), found that most types of training (such as passive dissemination of guidelines and short-term courses) were ineffective alone in improving outcome for patients. A broader review on mental health education, by Hodges *et al* (2001), arrived at similar conclusions: that attitudinal and organisational barriers were 'equally or more important for educators to consider than the selection of educational methods'. This is not to say that education is not essential to improve mental healthcare, but it seems alone to be insufficient to do this in settings that have thus far been researched.

Probably the most influential research on educational interventions was the Gotland study (Rutz *et al*, 1989, 1992), which used local opinion leaders, and was conducted on the Swedish island of Gotland in the 1980s. An interrupted time-series analysis showed an apparent reduction in suicide rates and an increase in antidepressant prescription. However, this study had a weak methodological design and, although there are other examples of studies which show that educational interventions can influence prescribing behaviour (van Eijk *et al*, 2001; Freemantle *et al*, 2002), the other outcomes of the Gotland study have never been replicated using more robust designs (e.g. the Hampshire Depression Project, discussed below) and the STORM study in the UK, which did not demonstrate an effect of training on the suicide rate in a single English region (Morriss *et al*, 2005).

One of the best-known negative studies of training was the Hampshire Depression Study, carried out in the UK. This involved a well-developed clinician education and guideline implementation strategy. Education involved videotapes, written materials, small-group teaching sessions and role-play provided by a multidisciplinary team. However, the intervention had no effect on either recognition rates for depression or clinical improvement (Thompson *et al*, 2000; Kendrick *et al*, 2001).

A second UK study, which had previously successfully demonstrated that training *did* achieve change in doctor behaviour (Gask *et al*, 1998), was similarly unable to demonstrate an impact on patient outcomes (Gask *et al*, 2004). A nested qualitative study (Gask *et al*, 2005) suggested three major barriers to the effectiveness of the intervention: the lack of the GP's belief that he or she could have an effect on the outcome of depression, the appropriateness of the training, and the organisational context in which doctors had to implement what they had learned.

Even when educational sessions are accompanied by other *professional* interventions, such as audit and feedback or academic detailing (see Box 25.2), they do not seem to have an impact on depression, quality of life or adherence to medication (Brown *et al*, 2000). Educational meetings, the commonest educational intervention universally provided to doctors, have an effect on knowledge of and attitudes to mental illness (Andersen & Harthorn, 1990) but not on practice or outcomes (Worrall *et al*, 1999).

There are a large number of studies of guideline implementation in the literature. For example, Croudace *et al* (2003) attempted an unsuccessful local implementation of guidelines based on the *International Classification of Diseases* mental health guidelines for primary care (ICD–10–PC). Such studies often include active dissemination and clinician education, academic detailing, peer review and the use of opinion leaders. They appear to be successful only when the educational interventions are accompanied by organisational interventions (see below) (Gilbody *et al*, 2003).

## Psychosocial interventions

Huibers *et al* (2004) specifically examined the effectiveness of psychosocial interventions delivered by GPs. They found that the available evidence addressed five distinct disorders or health complaints (depression, somatisation, smoking addiction, excessive alcohol consumption and fatigue). They concluded that there was some evidence that problem-solving treatment (PST) by a GP is effective in the treatment of major depression. However, they noted that these findings should be interpreted with considerable caution: the two studies on PST (Mynors-Wallis *et al*, 1995, 2000) were conducted by the same research team and groups consisting of only 30 to 40 patients were treated by a small number of experienced and highly trained research GPs, which limits the translation to routine general practice. In most of the studies that they reviewed there was limited information provided about the training actually provided to the (highly selected) group of doctors. They concluded that the evidence concerning the remaining interventions for other health complaints (reattribution or cognitive–behavioural group therapy for somatisation, cognitive–behavioural therapy for unexplained fatigue, counselling for smoking cessation, behavioural interventions to reduce alcohol intake) was either limited or conflicting.

## Care of people with severe and enduring mental illness

Research in the 1990s showed that many patients with serious mental illness (SMI), such as schizophrenia, had no contact with specialist services but saw only their GP (King, 1992; Kendrick *et al*, 1994). However, GP care of the patients' mental health was clearly suboptimal. Evidence of review of elements of the formal mental state examination within the preceding 12 months was found in only 32% of patients and GP-initiated changes in psychotropic drug regimens were recorded in only 20% of cases (Kendrick *et al*, 1994).

A randomised controlled trial of setting up registers of SMI patients and teaching GPs to carry out structured assessments of these patients led to significant improvements in the process of care (Kendrick *et al*, 1995). Changes in psychotropic medication, particularly the major tranquillisers, and referrals for psychosocial problems, particularly to community psychiatric nurses, were increased in the intervention group. However, most of the study GPs, despite being self-selected for their interest in mental health, reported there was not enough time in routine consultations to carry out the structured assessments, and the number of assessments carried out soon dwindled after the first year of the intervention (Kendrick *et al*, 1995).

A second approach was a trial of teaching practice nurses, who frequently give depot neuroleptic injections to SMI patients, to carry out brief structured assessments during injection appointments and to bring any problems to their GP's attention (Burns *et al*, 1998). The nurses were keen to learn more about the problems of people with SMI, but the training failed to lead to demonstrable improvements in care, apparently because problems uncovered by the nurses were not always dealt with by the GP. It was concluded that joint GP and nurse assessments would be best, in special clinic sessions. Nazareth *et al* (1996) had previously carried out a controlled trial of such an approach in four practices and found it to be feasible, and to lead to small but measurable improvements in patient outcomes in terms of symptoms and functioning. Setting up patient registers and instituting regular recall and special clinic sessions competes with numerous other obligations in general practice, and needs resourcing. It seemed, therefore, that these initiatives needed to be promoted through targeted remuneration. Burns & Cohen (1998) went on to show that more practices would set up joint GP/practice nurse assessments in response to the introduction of trial item-of-service payments for the initiative.

# Financial interventions

## The UK GP contract Quality and Outcomes Framework

The new General Medical Services contract for GPs in the UK, agreed in 2003, allowed practices to earn more money if they adopted two quality indicators related to the care of SMI patients (British Medical Association & NHS Confederation, 2003). Practices could earn points for producing a register of people with SMI who required regular follow-up, and points related to the percentage of patients on the register with a review recorded in the preceding 15 months, which included a check on the accuracy of prescribed medication, a review of physical health, and a review of coordination arrangements with secondary care. In 2004–05, the first year of the new contract, 99% of practices in the UK set up SMI patient registers, and more than three-quarters reviewed more than 90% of their SMI patients (NHS Information Centre, 2005; see also Chapters 14 and 15).

So, financial incentives can dramatically increase the number of patient reviews carried out, but further research is needed to determine whether such changes in the process of care lead to better patient outcomes.

# Organisational interventions

## Screening for mental illness in primary care

Screening is an example of a 'patient-mediated' professional intervention (see Box 25.2). The professional is provided with information about 'caseness' collected when the patient completes a questionnaire while waiting to see the doctor. In the USA, screening for common mental health problems is thought to be effective and is a cornerstone of the agenda to improve mental health (New Freedom Commission on Mental Health, 2003), and population-level screening programmes are supported by the drug industry. Similar national programmes have been advocated in Australia (Hickie *et al*, 2001) through the Beyond Blue initiative (see under Further reading and e-resources at the end of the chapter). In England and Wales, screening for depression has been supported more cautiously by the National Institute for Health and Clinical Excellence (NICE), which recommends that it is offered to people at high risk of depression (e.g. the elderly, those who are physically ill and after childbirth), although 'case finding' by asking two screening questions for depression has been rewarded in people with diabetes and coronary heart disease under the Quality and Outcomes Framework of the new GP contract (see below).

Despite early suggestions of effectiveness, the most recent systematic review of screening for depression has concluded that it should be considered only as part of a package with other organisational interventions to improve care (Gilbody *et al*, 2006).

## Consultation–liaison

Consultation–liaison with primary care, sometimes also known as 'shared care', particularly in the Canadian and Australian literature (Craven & Bland, 2002), developed out of consultation–liaison practice in the general hospital setting. Health professionals, usually psychiatrists but sometimes psychologists and nurses, discuss patients with GPs before referral (see Box 25.1) and see a limited number of patients following this discussion. Although theoretically it seems very attractive (Gask *et al*, 1997), there is unfortunately no evidence that it leads to any change in outcome for patients in the primary care setting, despite some evidence that it can change professional behaviour (Bower & Sibbald, 2000, 2004).

## Collaborative care

The origins of collaborative care and approaches to the management of depression, in particular using 'case management', are dealt with in detail in Chapter 27. Several systematic reviews have now demonstrated the effectiveness of this complex intervention in depression. Collaborative care has also been utilised successfully in panic disorder (Roy-Byrne *et al*, 2001).

## Replacement and referral

In this model, the primary responsibility for the management of the presenting problem is passed on to the mental health specialist for the duration of treatment. This model is most often associated with psychological therapy, such as counselling or cognitive–behavioural therapy.

**373**

Specific evidence for different types of replacement and referral interventions, such as counselling and cognitive–behavioural therapy, can be found in Chapters 26 and 27.

# Conclusions

Educational and training interventions alone do not improve the quality of care. Most educational interventions that have been systematically evaluated and reported in the literature have been carried out in Western European or North American settings, with doctors who have already received a basic training in mental health, and who are largely self-selected. We do not know what the impact would be of providing training to doctors in other settings who have little knowledge of mental healthcare, even though the delivery of such interventions is widely supported by bodies such as the World Health Organization, as research has not yet been carried out. The practical aspects of teaching and learning about mental health in primary care are discussed in Chapter 29.

Financial incentives can change the process of care, but so far there is little evidence that such changes translate into improvements in patient outcomes. Complex interventions incorporating organisational change, such as 'collaborative care', seem to hold the most promise in improving the quality of primary care mental health.

---

Key points

- Educational and training interventions do not, alone, or in combination with audit, feedback or academic detailing, improve quality of care.
- Financial incentives such as the Quality and Outcomes Framework in the UK can change the process of care, such as regularly reviewing patients with severe mental illness, but evidence that such changes translate into improvements in patient outcomes is lacking.
- There is no evidence, despite extensive research, that simply providing doctors with feedback about patient's scores on a mental health screening questionnaire actually alters doctor behaviour or changes outcomes for patients.
- Complex interventions incorporating organisational change, such as 'collaborative care' for depression, seem to hold the most promise in improving the quality of care for mental health problems in the primary care setting.

---

# Further reading and e-resources

Beyond Blue, the Australian national initiative for depression, http://www.beyondblue.org.au

National Institute for Health and Clinical Excellence guidelines, http://www.nice.org.uk

# References

Andersen, S. M. & Harthorn, B. H. (1990) Changing the psychiatric knowledge of primary care physicians. The effects of a brief intervention on clinical diagnosis and treatment. *General Hospital Psychiatry*, **12**, 177–190.

Bensing, J. (2000) Bridging the gap. The separate worlds of evidence-based medicine and patient-centered medicine. *Patient Education and Counselling*, **39**, 17–25.

Bower, P. & Gilbody, S. (2005) Managing common mental health disorders in primary care: conceptual models and evidence base. *BMJ*, **330**, 839–842.

Bower, P. & Sibbald, B. (2000) Do consultation–liaison services change the behaviour of primary care providers? A review. *General Hospital Psychiatry*, **222**, 84–96.

Bower, P. & Sibbald, B. (2004) On-site mental health workers in primary care: effects on professional practice. *Cochrane Database of Systematic Reviews*, (2), CD000532.

British Medical Association & NHS Confederation (2003) *Investing in General Practice: The New General Medical Services Contract*. BMA & NHS Confederation.

Brown, J. B., Shye, D., McFarland, B. H., *et al* (2000) Controlled trials of CQI and academic detailing to implement a clinical practice guideline for depression. *Joint Commission Journal on Quality Improvement*, **26**, 39–54

Burns, T. & Cohen, A. (1998) Item-of-service payments for general practitioner care of severely mentally ill persons: does the money matter? *British Journal of General Practice*, **48**, 1415–1416.

Burns, T., Millar, E., Garland, C., *et al* (1998) Randomised controlled trial of teaching practice nurses to carry out structured assessments of patients receiving depot antipsychotic injections. *British Journal of General Practice*, **48**, 1845–1848.

Campbell, S., Roland, M. O. & Buetow, S. A. (2000) Defining quality of care. *Social Science and Medicine*, **51**, 1611–1625.

Craven, M. A. & Bland, R. (2002) Shared mental health care: a bibliography and overview. *Canadian Journal of Psychiatry*, 47 (Suppl. 1), iS–viiiS, 1S–103S.

Croudace, T., Evans, J., Harrison, G., *et al* (2003) Impact of the ICD–10 Primary Health Care (PHC) diagnostic and management guidelines for mental disorders on detection and outcome in primary care. Cluster randomised controlled trial. *British Journal of Psychiatry*, **182**, 20–30.

Donabedian, A. (1990) The seven pillars of quality. *Archives of Pathology and Laboratory Medicine*, **114**, 1115–1118.

Elwyn, G., Edwards, A. & Kinnersley, P. (1999) Shared decision-making in primary care: the neglected second half of the consultation. *British Journal of General Practice*, **49**, 477–482.

Freemantle, N., Nazareth, I., Eccles, M., *et al* (2002) A randomised controlled trial of the effect of educational outreach by community pharmacists on prescribing in UK general practice. *British Journal of General Practice*, **52**, 290–295.

Gask, L., Sibbald, B. & Creed, F. (1997) Evaluating models of working at the interface between mental health services and primary care. *British Journal of Psychiatry*, **170**, 6–11.

Gask, L., Usherwood, T., Thompson, H., *et al* (1998) Evaluation of a teaching package for the assessment and management of depression in general practice. *Medical Education*, **32**, 190–198.

Gask, L., Dowrick, C., Dixon, C., *et al* (2004) A pragmatic cluster randomised controlled trial of an educational intervention for GPs in the assessment and management of depression. *Psychological Medicine*, **34**, 63–72.

Gask, L., Dixon, C. & May, C. (2005) Qualitative study of an educational intervention for general practitioners in the assessment and management of depression. *British Journal of General Practice*, **55**, 854–859.

Gilbody, S., Whitty, P., Grimshaw, J., *et al* (2003) Educational and organisational interventions to improve the management of depression in primary care: a systematic review. *JAMA*, **289**, 3145–3151.

Gilbody, S., Sheldon, T. & Wessely, S. (2006) Should we screen for depression? *BMJ*, **332**, 1027–1030.

Haggerty, J., Reid, R., Freeman, G., *et al* (2003) Continuity of care: a multidisciplinary review. *BMJ*, **327**, 1219–1221.

Hickie, I. B., Davenport, T. A., Naismith, S. L., *et al* (2001) Conclusions about the assessment and management of common mental disorders in Australian general practice. SPHERE National Secretariat. *Medical Journal of Australia*, **175**, 52–55.

Hodges, B., Inch, C. & Silver, I. (2001) Improving the psychiatric knowledge, skills, and attitudes of primary care physicians, 1950–2000: a review. *American Journal of Psychiatry*, **158**, 1579–86.

Huibers, M., Beurskens, A., Bleijenberg, G., *et al* (2004) The effectiveness of psychosocial interventions delivered by general practitioners. *Cochrane Database of Systematic Reviews*, (**3**), CD003494.

Kendrick, T., Burns, T., Sibbald, B., *et al* (1994) Provision of care to general practice patients with disabling long-term mental illness: a survey in 16 practices. *British Journal of General Practice*, **44**, 301–305.

Kendrick, T., Burns, T. & Freeling, P. (1995) Randomised controlled trial of teaching general practitioners to carry out structured assessments of their long-term mentally ill patients. *BMJ*, **311**, 93–98.

Kendrick, T., Stevens, L., Bryant, A., *et al* (2001) Hampshire Depression Project: changes in the process of care and cost consequences. *British Journal of General Practice*, **51**, 911–913.

King, M. B. (1992) Management of patients with schizophrenia in general practice (editorial). *British Journal of General Practice*, **42**, 310–311.

Mead, N. & Bower, P. (2000) Patient-centredness: a conceptual framework and review of the empirical literature. *Social Science and Medicine*, **51**, 1087–1110.

Morriss, R., Gask, L., Webb, R., *et al* (2005) The effects on suicide rates of an educational intervention for front-line health professionals with suicidal patients (the STORM Project). *Psychological Medicine*, **35**, 957–960.

Mynors-Wallis, L. M., Gath, D. H., Lloyd-Thomas, A. R., *et al* (1995) Randomised controlled trial comparing problem solving treatment with amitriptyline and placebo for major depression in primary care. *BMJ*, **310**, 441–445.

Mynors-Wallis, L. M., Gath, D. H., Day, A., *et al* (2000) Randomised controlled trial of problem solving treatment, antidepressant medication and combined treatment for major depression in primary care. *BMJ*, **320**, 26–30.

Nazareth, I., King, M. & See Tai, S. (1996) Monitoring psychosis in general practice: a controlled trial. *British Journal of Psychiatry*, **169**, 482–487.

New Freedom Commission on Mental Health (2003) *Achieving the Promise: Transforming Mental Health Care in America – Final Report*. DHHS Pub. No. SMA-03-3832. Department of Health and Human Services.

NHS Information Centre (2005) *National Quality and Outcomes Framework Statistics for England 2004/05*. Downloadable from http://www.ic.nhs.uk

Roy-Byrne, P. P., Katon, W., Cowley, D. S., *et al* (2001) A randomized effectiveness trial of collaborative care for patients with panic disorder in primary care. *Archives of General Psychiatry*, **58**, 869–876.

Rutz, W., von Knorring, L. & Walinder, J. (1989) Frequency of suicide on Gotland after systematic postgraduate education for general practitioners. *Acta Psychiatrica Scandinavica*, **80**, 151–54.

Rutz, W., von Knorring, L. & Walinder, J. (1992) Long-term effects of an educational programme for general practitioners given by the Swedish Committee for the Prevention and Treatment of Depression. *Acta Psychiatrica Scandinavica*, **85**, 83–88.

Sackett, D. L., Rosenberg, W. M. C., Gray, J. A. M., *et al* (1996) Evidence based medicine: what it is and what it isn't. *BMJ*, **312**, 71–72.

Starfield, B. (1998) *Primary Care: Balancing Health Needs, Services and Technology*. Oxford University Press.

Stewart, M., Brown, J. B., Weston, W. W., *et al* (1995) *Patient Centred Medicine: Transforming the Clinical Method*. Sage.

Thompson, C., Kinmonth, A. L., Steven, L., *et al* (2000) Effects of a clinical practice guideline and practice-based education on detection and outcome of depression in primary care: Hampshire Depression Project randomized controlled trial. *Lancet*, **355**, 50–57.

van Eijk, M. E., Avorn, J. & Porsius, A. J. (2001) Reducing prescribing of highly anticholinergic antidepressants for elderly people: a randomised trial of group versus individual academic detailing. *BMJ*, **322**, 654–657.

Worrall, G., Angel, J. & Chaulk, P. (1999) Effectiveness of an educational strategy to improve family physicians' detection and management of depression: a randomized controlled trial. *Canadian Medical Association Journal*, **161**, 37–40.

# CHAPTER 26

# Psychological treatments

Frances Cole and Karina Lovell

Summary

Psychological treatments are a valuable option when managing common mental health problems in primary care. The evidence base for their role in everyday primary care practice continues to emerge from both research and clinical practice; it suggests these approaches can improve patient care and empowerment and reduce distress.

Psychological treatment covers a wide range of different approaches which have an increasing evidence base for their effectiveness. The aim of treatment based on talking therapy is a reduction in emotional distress, and changes in behaviours and patterns of thinking which lead to partial or complete resolution of the impact of mild to severe psychological difficulties. The improvement of emotional, physical and social role function, including a return to work, is a valued outcome.

The wide range of treatments can make choosing one to suit a particular patient and condition a challenge for the primary care practitioner. This challenge can be complicated by access to treatment, in terms of both location and length of waiting list.

The choice runs from self-help interventions, in a range of media and written form, to individual therapy or group-based therapy, for more complex cases with multiple psychological problems. This chapter focuses on the more commonly accessible treatment options within local services, and self-help interventions.

## Access to psychological treatment

Psychological treatments are recommended for a range of mental health difficulties (Department of Health, 2001). However, the demand for psychological therapies currently outstrips supply, at least in the UK, resulting in long waiting times for therapy and often precluding access to treatment (Lovell & Richards, 2000). The issue of increasing access to psychological therapies, particularly in primary care, has led to recent UK mental health policy demanding more accessible and effective treatments. In response to this, alternative models of interventions are emerging including Improving Access to Psychological Therapies (IAPT) services.

The National Institute for Health and Clinical Excellence (2004*a,b*) has proposed the use of a 'stepped-care approach' for depression and anxiety. Guidelines for a stepped-care approach (Scogin *et al*, 2003) are intended to provide evidence-based and best-practice pathways to services. Stepped care is designed to increase the efficiency of service provision, with an overall benefit to patient populations. The basic principle is that patients presenting with a common mental health disorder will 'step through' progressive levels of treatment as necessary, with the expectation that many of these patients will recover during the less intensive phases. Such a system seeks to enhance the efficiency and effectiveness of service delivery by providing low-intensity 'minimal interventions' to a proportion of patients in the first instance. The stepped-care model for depression is shown in Fig. 26.1 (see also Chapter 8).

## What are the types of psychological treatments?

There are many types of treatment and linking individual patients to the most appropriate treatment for their difficulties (Table 26.1) means

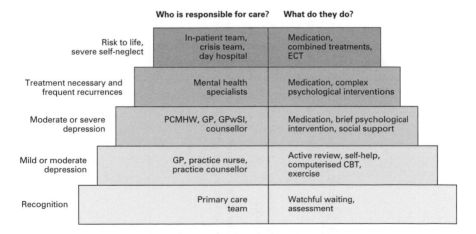

**Fig. 26.1** Stepped care model for depression. ECT, electroconvulsive therapy; PCMHW, primary care mental health worker; GP, general practitioner; GPwSI, GP with Special Interest; CBT, cognitive–behavioural therapy.

**Table 26.1** Summary of psychological treatments and mode of delivery based on severity and complexity

|  | Mild impact on health functioning | Mild–moderate impact on health functioning | Severe impact on health functioning |
|---|---|---|---|
| Who is responsible for leading therapy? | Patient led or client self-help | Primary care: general practitioner, practice nurse, counsellor | Specialist individual and/or therapist groups |
| What psychological treatments options are provided | Self-help resources; books, workbooks, audiovisual materials; programmes based on cognitive–behavioural therapy | Brief intervention therapy options<br>Counselling<br>Problem-solving<br>Solution-focused therapy<br>Behavioural activation<br>Motivational interviewing | Longer duration, 10–20+ sessions<br>Cognitive–behavioural therapy<br>Psychodynamic therapy<br>Cognitive analytical therapy<br>Acceptance and commitment therapy |

adopting a person-centred approach, with collaboration with the individual. Each treatment has a particular approach and theoretical framework and the people choosing to pursue treatment will need commitment. Initially, this will be to gain an understanding of their psychological issues and to make choices about their needs. They may seek to make changes and in some therapies be prepared to implement significant changes within their thinking, behaviours and life context. Individuals have a range of emotional literacy, from those with very little understanding of their psychological issues and needs to those who may have extensive experience, for various reasons.

Health functioning is based on the social model of health, with a focus on emotional roles, social functioning and mental health.

The range of problems or conditions in which psychological treatments can be of value are summarised in Box 26.1.

# A psychological or five-areas framework and guide to treatment

The model shown in Fig. 26.2 explains the person-centred interrelationship of the five areas of the individual presenting in primary care. Crucially, it guides *both* the practitioner and patient to identify the main area(s) that need to be addressed by those psychological treatments that offer more than empathic listening (Cape, 1996). This model also has a role in helping the patient to understand the impact of both physical and mental health disorders. This means interventions need to focus on the management of both physical and mental health symptoms, rather than either alone.

Three key steps to using the five-areas model and guide to treatment (Williams & Garland, 2002) are:

1    sharing the model with the individual
2    supporting the individual in identifying the areas where there are

---

**Box 26.1** Conditions in which psychological treatments can help

- Mental health problems such as depression, anxiety disorders, stress at work or home, alcohol or drug misuse, body image disorders
- Medically unexplained symptoms, acute and chronic, and somatisation
- Significant life-threatening physical health problems such as cancer, organ failure (e.g. heart or respiratory failure)
- Persistent disabling physical health symptoms – chronic pain, persistent fatigue
- Reduced health functioning due to accidents, stroke, heart disease or significant illnesses, autoimmune diseases, rheumatoid arthritis
- Change in stages of life such as pregnancy and childbirth, unemployment or returning to work, bereavement

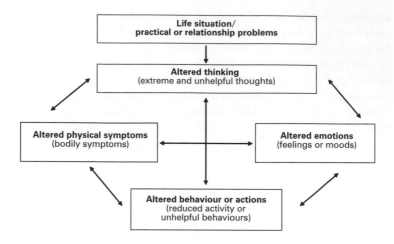

**Fig. 26.2** Person-centred five-areas model.

difficulties and in making priorities (for which there is the option of using the motivational interviewing approach)

3     using the map to guide the choice of interventions (see Case 1 below and accompanying map, Fig. 26.3).

### Case 1. Example of the five-areas model in practice

Annie is 49 and was a school meals cook until a fall at work 2 years ago. She was retired because of persistent back pain and depression and now lives alone. She was recently diagnosed with mild Parkinson's disease and has a tremor in her right hand and feels constantly tired. An appointment card from the hospital precipitated altered thoughts about herself, other people and her future, and her mood more generally. This linked with her altered behaviours because of her pre-existing body symptoms.

## Psychological treatments

The following section covers the commoner types of treatments which a practitioner can access either within primary care or in mental health services. These are generally 'minimal interventions', focused on mild and moderate levels of severity, and include guided self-help, CCBT (computerised cognitive–behavioural therapy), brief psychological interventions and exercise. They are designed to provide effective care and reduce the need for high input from specialist therapists. In addition, these interventions can sometimes be provided in ways that promote access for those unable to attend scheduled face-to-face clinical appointments, including over the telephone, and via the internet and email. These interventions range from those based

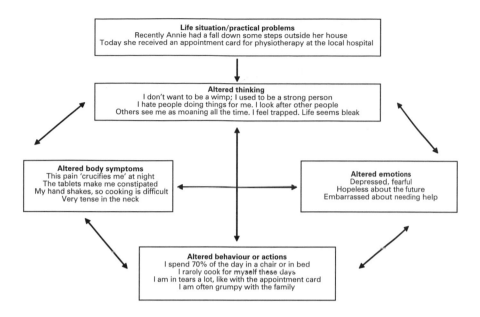

**Fig. 26.3** Use of the person-centred five-areas model in practice: Annie from Case 1.

on cognitive–behavioural principles, such as behavioural activation, cognitive techniques, exposure therapy and relaxation techniques, motivational interviewing, and other psychological interventions, such as counselling, exercise and solution-focused therapy. Examples of these interventions are detailed below.

## Self-help

These interventions may be guided or not and differ from traditionally delivered cognitive–behavioural therapy (CBT) by the use of a health technology (e.g. book, computer, audiotape); the focus is on patient self-management (Box 26.2). The key role of the mental health worker or trained primary care practitioner is to guide, support, review and monitor the patient through the material. Guidance sessions are usually brief, 15–30 minutes, and are preferably delivered according to patient preference (e.g. face-to-face, telephone or email).

### Case 2. Example of guided self-help

Tom is a 19-year-old man whose depression improved with guided self-help. A patient-centred semi-structured interview with a mental health worker (MHW) revealed that he had been moderately depressed for 6 months following the break-up of a long-term relationship. He described a poor sleeping pattern, with difficulty falling to sleep, irritability and a loss of interest in previously enjoyed activities (e.g. playing rugby and socialising). His attendance at college had fallen to below 30% and exclusion from college

---

**Box 26.2** Key principles of guided self-help

- A self-administered intervention
- Involves a health technology (book, workbook, computer, audiotape)
- Interventions based on cognitive–behavioural principles
- Facilitated (1–3 hours of contact)
- Role of the mental health worker is to guide, support, review and monitor

---

was consequently imminent. He had been offered medication by his general practitioner but had refused. The MHW explained the rationale of guided self-help, that he would be given a book which outlined the nature of depression and ways in which he could help improve his mood and that he would be supported in using the book by the MHW either face to face or by telephone over approximately 8 weeks.

After reading the book, which included a range of CBT interventions, Tom felt that behavioural activation was something he could work with. With the support of material in the book (which gave step-by-step instructions on how to use behavioural activation) and from the MHW, Tom gradually planned and increased his level of activities, so that over a few weeks his attendance at college had returned to full and he had started to socialise and play rugby again. The main role of the MHW was to help Tom set realistic and practical activities and to help problem-solve difficulties as they arose; a further key role was liaising with student support services at the college to help Tom to avoid exclusion. Tom had four 30-minute sessions with the MHW over the 8 weeks and on completion of the intervention his mood had returned to normal.

The health technology options available for mental health problems range in format from leaflets by organisations such as MIND, interactive workbooks, and books on CBT to specifically designed CBT courses on overcoming depression or anxiety (see Further reading and e-resources at the end of the chapter). It is important to assess patients' language and literacy skills to maximise their potential benefit from self-help.

Despite the current widespread use of minimal interventions and guided self-help, the overall evidence base remains inconclusive. There is preliminary evidence that self-help interventions can be effective (McKendree-Smith *et al*, 2003; Anderson *et al*, 2005). However, evidence for the effectiveness of self-help interventions is not uniformly positive. Some studies have shown significant benefits (Proudfoot *et al*, 2004), whereas others have not (Richards *et al*, 2003; Mead *et al*, 2005). A systematic review of self-help interventions with depression (Gellatly *et al*, 2007) showed a significantly greater effect with studies that had used guided self-help (rather then pure self-help). No differences in clinical outcome were found between different health technologies, suggesting that patient preference combined with service resources should determine the ones used.

## Bibliotherapy

This is available in some areas, often with books on prescription service, and can facilitate improved health literacy. Trained librarians in local libraries can provide a listening ear and guide individuals to relevant self-help materials and internet resources; creative writing, reading groups and poetry may also help individuals understand their condition and engage in social activities.

## Exercise

Evidence (NICE, 2004a) shows that exercise can be valuable for depression and can have a place in anxiety, as well as physical health problems. Practitioners can usually make referrals to local exercise schemes.

## Motivational interviewing

This effective brief intervention offers relatively few (usually less than six) 15- to 30-minute sessions with a skilled therapist. Motivational interviewing helps people recognise and do something about their present or potential problems. It is valuable with people who are reluctant to change or who are ambivalent about changing. Research by Prochaska & Diclemente (1986) has shown that individuals pass through six changes, including relapse, in changing unhelpful or problem behaviours (Fig. 26.4).

Accepting that relapse is part of the cycle of change is helpful, as it leads back into the cycle, often at the contemplation stage, and the discovery of how not to change is equally valuable in the process of change. This client-centred therapy is directive and follows five guiding principles (Box 26.3) (Miller, 1983).

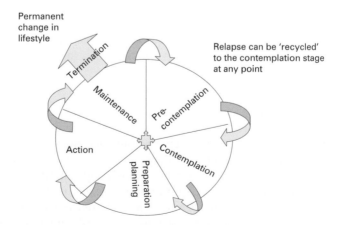

**Fig. 26.4** Stages of change (Prochaska & Diclemente, 1986).

---

**Box 26.3** Principles of motivational interviewing

1  The practitioner should express empathy, as acceptance facilitates change; skilful reflective listening is crucial and ambivalence is normal.
2  The practitioner should 'develop discrepancy'. That is, in exploring where the individual is at present and where he or she wishes to be, an awareness of consequences of current behaviours should present arguments for change.
3  The practitioner should avoid argumentation, as this is counterproductive and breeds defensiveness. Resistance is a signal to change strategies; labelling is unnecessary.
4  The practitioner should 'roll with resistance'. Momentum within interviewing can be used to advantage, to shift perspectives and develop new perspectives; the individual is a resource for finding solutions.
5  The practitioner should support individuals' self-efficacy to motivate them; individuals are responsible for choosing and implementing change.

---

## Counselling

Counselling is a widely available talking therapy in primary care. It can take many forms; commonest is Rogerian or person-centred counselling, in which a trained counsellor uses a reflective, empathic style of communication to enable individuals to explore their emotional or life issues, for example bereavement or relationship issues, with the counsellor passively following their offerings. Patients value those who listen and enable them to disclose mental health problems and so help them to understand and gain realistic perspectives (Kadam *et al*, 2001).

Counselling can:

- give more time than brief consultations in primary care
- offer a limited number of 30- to 60-minute sessions
- be useful in specific problems or life events difficulties (e.g. bereavement, postnatal depression)
- be valuable when a patient has a life-threatening illness ( e.g. cancer)
- be useful when a patient is coping with a long-term health condition (e.g. diabetes, stroke)
- have a role in relationship difficulties (e.g. within the family or workplace).

The individual's reflection upon and processing of the issues may lead to new insights and understandings, and acceptance of the unchangeable aspects of themselves or their lives.

Person-centred counselling has limited applicability to common mental health conditions, such as depression and anxiety, particularly with severe or recurrent episodes, as it does not offer a shared and clearly understandable framework or formulation to allow the individual to understand the persistence or recurrence of the condition; or the development of skills to develop patient confidence to self-manage their mental health condition and facilitate valued changes in their unhelpful belief systems about their self, the world and the future, and so reduce relapse. Counselling can prove unhelpful in two ways: when there are long delays to treatment and when a person with depression repeatedly focuses on negative past life events, which can worsen depressed mood.

Counselling can reduce distress in the short term but it remains unclear which patients benefit from this intervention. It is more effective than usual care and has favourable patient satisfaction, possibly linked to its focus on an empathic, caring approach (Bower et al, 2000; Ward et al, 2000).

## Solution-focused therapy

Therapists trained in this brief intervention enable patients to use themselves as their own resources; they help them identify their current strengths and possible solutions to life issues or mental health difficulties. Solution-focused therapy uses or refines patients' inherent skills for current difficulties to build confidence and well-being. It is a skills-based therapy in which individuals learn to question themselves to identify what enables them to cope with problems and build on these solutions and resources.

## Problem-solving

This is another brief intervention therapy, based on three principles (Mynors-Wallis et al, 2002):

1    Patients' symptoms are caused by practical problems facing them in their daily life situations.
2    If these problems are resolved or improved, then patients' psychological symptoms will improve.
3    Problem-solving techniques can help resolution.

Problem-solving is an effective treatment for depression. Here, it is based on a collaborative five- or seven-stage approach, in which individuals gain a sense of achievement and purpose to manage their difficulties (Mynors-Wallis et al, 1995, 2002). Box 26.4 outlines the five-stage approach.

## Exposure therapy

Exposure therapy involves planned, regular and graded therapeutic confrontation of the feared stimuli (object, situation) until anxiety decreases.

## Behavioural activation

Behavioural activation is a therapeutic process that focuses on a gradual, structured and regular plan to increase routine, pleasurable and necessary activities that will bring individuals into contact with reinforcing environmental contingencies and thus produce improvements in mood.

---

**Box 26.4** Five-stage approach to problem-solving therapy

**Step 1: Define the problem**
- What is the specific problem or goal?
- Talk it through, make notes for yourself until it is clearer.
- Break it down into smaller parts if necessary.

**Step 2: List all possible solutions, so as many ideas as you can**
- What helpful ideas would other people suggest?
- What have you tried that worked in the past?
- What would you suggest to a friend in similar position?
- What ridiculous or silly solutions can you include?

**Step 3: Advantages and disadvantages of solutions**
- Highlight the pros and cons of each idea.

**Step 4: Choose the 'best solution'**
- Choose which idea you are going to try first.
- Remember to take into account your resources – time, money, skills, circumstances.
- How will you carry it out?
- When will you check your progress on this problem/goal?
- How will you know if it worked? What will be different?
- What problems might there be with it?
- How will you overcome them?
- Are there any things you need to practise first?

**Step 5: Review the solution**
- Remember to give yourself a pat on the back for having a go!
- What went well? Did it help the problem? What could you try to use again?
- Write down how well the plan worked, and which parts need to be changed.

---

## Cognitive–behavioural therapy

Cognitive–behavioural therapy (CBT) has a robust evidence base (Churchill *et al*, 2001; Department of Health, 2001) and is defined as an active, directed, time-limited, structural approach that treats a variety of mental health disorders by trained therapists. It is based on the rationale that an individual's emotions and behaviour are determined by the way in which that person structures the world through thoughts or cognitions (Beck *et al*, 1979). Beck's model proposes that maladaptive cognitions, that is verbal thoughts and pictorial thoughts or images in a stream of consciousness, are based on schemas or core beliefs developed in childhood and based on previous experience. These maladaptive beliefs affect people's own perceptions of themselves, other people, the world and their future. These beliefs can lead to a range of automatic thinking patterns that are mistaken or distorted with negative content. These negative, automatic, involuntary thoughts lead to depressed mood and altered, self-defeating patterns of behaviour (Box 26.5).

Again, the five-areas model can be used (Fig. 26.5), so both practitioner and individual can see connections between the areas. This leads to awareness of how events and experiences are interpreted and link to altered or distorted automatic thinking and its behavioural consequences. CBT is both a knowledge-based and a skills-based therapy that enables individuals to test out their thinking, identify maladaptive thinking styles or cognitive distortions and challenge their validity using an automatic thought record process. This process can result in reducing depression or other moods and changing unhelpful behavioural patterns. CBT uses behavioural approaches to introduce flexibility and change in thinking patterns using behavioural experiments or techniques such as daily logs to observe and change behavioural patterns. These self-discovery approaches can test the perceived or predicted versus actual experience of events and their emotional consequences. Often the focus of CBT is on negative thinking or beliefs and the need to challenge these effectively.

This therapy is an active collaboration between the therapist and individual and usually will offer limited sessions, typically 10–20 hour-long sessions. The evidence base for this therapy for a range of conditions is extensive and guidelines from the National Institute for Health and Clinical Excellence (2004a, 2004b) indicate it has a key role in the common disorders in primary care – depression, anxiety disorders, post-traumatic stress, and so on. Its availability is limited partly by a lack of therapists.

## Other cognitive–behavioural techniques or approaches

These can be used by practitioners within primary care, using the five-areas model and an empathic collaborative questioning style that increases

---

**Box 26.5** The cognitive model

By way of illustration, the cognitive model is here applied to a person experiencing depression and faced with the situation at work of getting a report done (see also Fig. 26.5).

- Core belief (e.g. I am a failure)
- Intermediate belief or underlying assumption (If I do not get this all done and right, then I am useless)
- Automatic thoughts (I never get this right on time)
- Reactions
  - altered emotion (depressed)
  - altered behaviour (put off until later)
  - physical symptoms (feel very tired)

Based on Beck *et al* (1979).

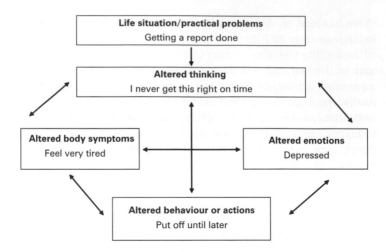

**Fig. 26.5** The cognitive model applied to an example involving depression (see also Box 26.5).

individuals' awareness of unhelpful thinking patterns when depressed or altered behaviours aggravate their problems. These techniques can help support or prepare patients to commit themselves to full therapy. It can be confusing and unhelpful for patients to mix cognitive approaches or techniques with the full therapy as described above. Being explicit or providing patients with information (from sources such as the British Association for Behavioural and Cognitive Psychotherapies) about this therapy can be helpful (see also www.patient.co.uk).

Cognitive analytic therapy (CAT) is a brief integrative therapy that combines elements of cognitive–behavioural and psychodynamic psycho-therapy. This is a long-term therapy (16–24 sessions) that requires considerable commitment by the individual. CAT focuses on discovering how problems have evolved and how the procedures devised to cope with them may be ineffective. It is designed to enable clients to gain an understanding of how the difficulties they experience may be made worse by their habitual coping mechanisms. Problems are understood in the light of clients' personal histories and life experiences. The client is encouraged to recognise how these coping procedures originated and how they can be adapted and improved. Then, mobilising the client's own strengths and resources, plans are developed to bring about change.

Acceptance and commitment therapy (ACT) is another branch of CBT, an empirically based psychological intervention that uses acceptance and mindfulness strategies, together with commitment and behaviour change strategies, to increase psychological flexibility. Originally this approach was referred to as 'comprehensive distancing'. ACT differs from traditional CBT in that, rather than trying to teach people to be balanced in their thoughts, feelings, sensations, memories and other private events, ACT focuses on what they can control more directly: their arms, legs and mouth. ACT teaches them to 'just notice', accept and embrace their private events, especially previously unwanted ones. ACT helps the individual get in contact with a 'transcendent' sense of self, known as 'self-as-context' – the 'you' that is always there, observing and experiencing and yet distinct from thoughts, feelings, sensations and memories. ACT aims to help individuals clarify their personal values and to take action on them, bringing more vitality and meaning to their life in the process.

# Roles and skills of practitioners

The key principle of psychological treatment in primary care is to work with the best evidence, offer information on choice and support patient preference. The practical role of practitioners is therefore:

- to help patients identify their needs using communication skills such as problem-based interviewing and the five-areas model
- to improve health literacy by enabling access to relevant self-help materials and resources (e.g. books on prescription that help individuals makes sense of their mental health problem)
- to identify the severity of the mental health problem using scales or questionnaires (see Chapters 8 and 10 for examples)
- to conduct a risk assessment
- jointly to make the choice from treatments available locally using a stepped-care approach and based on severity and the context of the patient
- to offer brief interventions if the practitioner is skilled and trained in problem-solving, solution-focused therapy or motivational interviewing
- in depression or anxiety disorders, to offer referral to a local exercise programme or bibliotherapy or to suggest national or local self-help groups
- in complex cases, to refer patients to the local psychological therapies service for assessment for the best fit for the individual and the problems and context
- to monitor improvement using measures of health outcomes
- to support individuals' maintenance of improvement
- in relapse, to identify jointly with the patient contributing factors and to support the relapse plan or interventions
- to ensure that where counselling is offered as an intervention from primary care practice, the counsellors are fully qualified according to recognised national guidelines. (In addition, it is important to clarify whether counsellors have regular supervision of their case-load rather than practising unsupported.)

# Conclusion

Psychological problems are frequently seen in primary care and we have discussed a number of evidence-based psychological approaches, at different levels, ranging from high-intensity approaches (e.g. CBT) to low-intensity approaches (e.g. guided self-help). Comprehensive patient-centred assessment, working in partnership, regular monitoring using outcome measures, and offering and promoting patient choice and preference with evidence-based interventions are the key principles to delivering accessible, effective and acceptable psychological approaches.

---

### Key points

- The presenting psychological problems can be identified and their severity rated using patient interviews.
- Psychological problems are likely to accompanied by physical health problems, especially where patients have long-term health conditions.
- The person-centred model means that both practitioner and patient can gain a common understanding of issues presented and see potential solutions.
- Mental health problems of mild to moderate severity are amenable to psychological interventions like problem-solving, motivational interviewing and behavioural activation.
- Counselling can have value for individuals with life events or relationship issues.
- Referral for assessment to specialist services is essential if the impact is both severe and complex.
- Self-help resources (written, audiovisual, computer based or web based) are helpful. Patients can choose to use these unaided or supported.
- Guided self-help is a brief intervention with the active support of a mental health worker over several sessions, lasting in total 1–3 hours.

---

# Further reading and e-resources

## *Practitioner resources*

Beck, A., Rush, A. J., Shaw, B. J., *et al* (1979) *Cognitive Therapy of Depression*. Guilford Press.

Miller, W. & Rollnick, S. (1991) *Motivational Interviewing*. Guilford Press.

World Health Organization (2004) *WHO Guide to Mental and Neurological Problems in Primary Care* (2nd edn). RSM Press.

## *Patient resources*

Butler, G. & Hope, T. (2007) *Manage Your Mind*. Oxford University Press.

Gilbert, P. (2000) *Overcoming Depression*. Constable Robinson.

Padesky, C. A. & Greenberger, D. (1995) *Clinicians' Guide to Mind Over Mood*. Guilford Press.

Stallard, P. (2007) *Think Good Feel Good CBT Workbook for Children and Young People*. Wiley.
Williams, C. (2001) *Overcoming Depression. A Five Areas Approach*. Arnold.
Williams, C. (2003) *Overcoming Anxiety. A Five Areas Approach*. Arnold.

## Websites

http://www.overcoming.co.uk. This offers wide range of CBT self-help guides and workbooks for many mental and physical health problems, including depression, anxiety, post-traumatic stress, sleep, pain and chronic fatigue. Materials can be partially perused by listening or reading on the site. It offers information on useful self-help organisations and books on prescription.

http://www.livinglifetothefull.com. This is an accessible site for patients for CBT self-help.

http://www.healthtalkonline.org.uk. This unique patient-experience site covers physical and mental health problems like depression. It provides experience in written, audio and visual formats.

http://www.patient.co.uk. This site offers very useful information resources and is extensively used in primary care.

http://www.babcp.com. This professional organisation is for CBT-based therapies in the UK and offers patient and professional information resources.

http://www.fiveareas.com. This offers CBT information and resources for work with patients.

http://www.mentalhealth.org.uk. This site offers information about mental health and new developments and written information for a wide range of mental health disorders, including self-help resources.

# References

Anderson, L., Lewis, G., Araya, R., *et al* (2005) Self-help books for depression: how can practitioners and patients make the right choice? *British Journal of General Practice*, **55**, 387–392.

Beck, A. T., Rush, A. J., Shaw, B. F., *et al* (1979) *Cognitive Therapy of Depression*. Guilford Press.

Bower, P., Byford, S., Sibbald, B., *et al* (2000) Randomised controlled trial of non-directive counselling, cognitive–behaviour therapy, and usual general practitioner care for patients with depression. II: Cost effectiveness. *BMJ*, **321**, 1389–1392.

Cape, J. (1996) Psychological treatment of emotional problems by general practitioners. *British Journal of Medical Psychology*, **69**, 85–99.

Churchill, R., Hunot, V., Corney, R., *et al* (2001) A systematic review of controlled trials of the effectiveness and cost-effectiveness of brief psychological treatments for depression. *Health Technology Assessment*, **5** (35).

Department of Health (2001) *Treatment Choice in Psychological Therapies and Counselling: Evidence Based Clinical Practice Guideline*. Department of Health.

Gellatly, J., Bower, P., Hennessy, S., *et al* (2007) What makes self-help interventions effective in the management of depressive symptoms? Meta-analysis and meta-regression. *Psychological Medicine*, **37**, 1217–1228.

Kadam, U. T., Croft, P., McLeod, J., *et al* (2001) A qualitative study of depression and anxiety. *British Journal of General Practice*, **51**, 375–380.

Lovell, K. & Richards, D. (2000) Multiple access points and levels of entry (MAPLE): ensuring choice, accessibility and equity for CBT services. *Behavioural and Cognitive Psychotherapy*, **28**, 379–391.

McKendree-Smith, N., Floyd, M. & Scogin, F. (2003) Self administered treatments for depression: a review. *Journal of Clinical Psychology*, **59**, 275–288.

Mead, N., MacDonald, W., Bower, P., *et al* (2005) The clinical effectiveness of guided self-help versus waiting list control in the management of anxiety and depression: a randomised controlled trial. *Psychological Medicine*, **35**, 1633–1643.

Miller, W. (1983) Motivational interviewing with problem drinkers. *Behavioural Psychotherapy*, **11**, 147–172.

Mynors-Wallis, L., Gath, D., Lloyd-Thomas, A., *et al* (1995) Randomised controlled trial comparing problem solving treatment with amitriptyline and placebo for major depression in primary care. *BMJ*, **310**, 441–445.

Mynors-Wallis, L., Moore, M., Maguire, J., *et al* (2002) *Shared Care in Mental Health*. Oxford University Press.

National Institute for Health and Clinical Excellence (2004a) *Depression: Management of Depression in Primary and Secondary Care*. Clinical guideline 23. NICE.

National Institute for Health and Clinical Excellence (2004b) *Anxiety: Management of Anxiety (Panic Disorder, With or Without Agoraphobia, and Generalized Anxiety Disorder) in Adults in Primary, Secondary and Community Care*. Clinical guideline 22. NICE.

Prochaska, J. O. & Diclemente, C. C. (1986) Towards a comprehensive model of change. In *Treating Addictive Behaviours: Processes of Change* (eds W. R. Miller & N. Heather), pp. 3–27. Plenum Press.

Proudfoot, J., Ryden, C., Everitt, B., *et al* (2004) Clinical efficacy of computerised cognitive–behavioural therapy for anxiety and depression in primary care: randomised controlled trial. *British Journal of Psychiatry*, **185**, 46–54.

Richards, A., Barkham, M., Cahill, J., *et al* (2003) PHASE: a randomised, controlled trial of supervised self-help cognitive behavioural therapy in primary care. *British Journal of General Practice*, **53**, 764–770.

Scogin, F., Hanson, A. & Welsh, D. (2003) Self-administered treatment in stepped-care models of depression treatment. *Journal of Clinical Psychology*, **59**, 341–349.

Ward, E., King, M., Lloyd, M., *et al* (2000) Randomised controlled trial of non-directive counselling, cognitive–behaviour therapy, and usual general practitioner care for patients with depression. II: Clinical effectiveness. *BMJ*, **321**, 1383–1388.

Williams, C. & Garland, A. (2002) A cognitive–behavioural therapy assessment model for use in everyday clinical practice. *Advances in Psychiatric Treatment*, **8**, 172–179.

# CHAPTER 27

# Collaborative care and stepped care: innovations for common mental disorders

David Richards, Peter Bower and Simon Gilbody

Summary

Mental health problems such an anxiety and depression are highly prevalent and are a major burden on patients, families and health systems. Systems for the care of common mental health problems need to meet a number of aims: to provide rapid access to effective services in a way that is efficient, equitable and responsive to the needs and preferences of patients. A number of different models for the delivery of services for common mental problems have been described, but the current models fail to meet all these aims. Collaborative care and stepped care are innovations that should help to meet the demand for care for common mental disorders.

## Competing demands in the management of common mental health problems

The individual and public health burden of mental ill health is dominated by 'common mental health problems' such as depression and anxiety. Prevalence estimates from around the globe suggest that around 16% of the adult population experience depression and anxiety in any one year, with common or 'high prevalence' mental health problems constituting 97% of the total population prevalence (Singleton *et al*, 2001; Andrews & Tolkein II Team, 2006). These problems cause such significant disability (World Health Organization, 2001) that in Australia it is estimated that at least 50% of days lost to disability through all types of mental illness are caused by the experience of depression or anxiety (Andrews *et al*, 2001). Many patients do not present for help; of those who do, as many as 50% will report purely physical symptoms and not be recognised as suffering from anxiety and depression. Even so, somewhere between 1% and 3.5% of the adult population are likely to be diagnosed with a common mental health problem annually (National Institute for Health and Clinical Excellence, 2004a,b, 2005).

In the UK, the prevalence of these problems and the lack of effective services to deal with them have been blamed for a multi-billion pound cross-subsidy from the welfare budget. It has been estimated that the UK spends £7–£10 billion per year on benefit payments to support people with anxiety and depression through the payment of incapacity benefit to the long-term sick (Centre for Economic Performance, 2006). With more people on incapacity benefits owing to mental illness than unemployment benefit, mental health problems were cited as 'the biggest causes of misery' in Britain (Centre for Economic Performance, 2006).

Ameliorating the burden of common mental health problems presents a major challenge for primary care. The challenge is particularly significant because primary care services are expected to meet a number of goals:

- *Access*. Service provision should meet the need for services in the community. The right to obtain treatment should depend on need for services, not ability to pay or geographic location.
- *Effectiveness*. Mental health services should do what they are intended to do: improve health. Health may be defined in terms of health status, or broader definitions may involve wider function and quality of life.
- *Efficiency and equity*. Given that resources for any healthcare system are limited, they should be distributed in such a way as to maximise health gains to society, and should be distributed fairly across the population at large.
- *Patient-centred services*. Although the precise definition of patient-centredness varies, one definition is that patient-centred services are services 'closely congruent with, and responsive to patients' wants, needs and preferences' (Laine & Davidoff, 1996).

Clearly, there are potential tensions between these goals. For example, prioritising access to care may improve equity but compromise efficiency. There may be clashes between patients' preferences and evidence of effectiveness. Dealing with these multiple, competing demands has been a major challenge for those designing and delivering primary care mental health services.

# Models of service delivery for common mental health problems

Clearly, there are many different ways of delivering services for common mental health problems to meet the goals outlined above, and making sense of them is a significant challenge. One method that can help is to describe 'models' of services. Models are abstract representations of complex areas, 'inventions of the human mind to place facts, events and theories in an orderly manner' (Siegler & Osmond, 1974). In the current context, models represent broad descriptions of alternative approaches to service delivery, which vary in important ways and have different advantages and disadvantages.

The structure of mental healthcare in primary care is generally understood in terms of the 'pathways to care' model (Goldberg & Huxley, 1980), where accessing mental healthcare involves passing through a series of levels and filters between the community and specialist care (see Table 1.2, p. 10). The pathways model highlights the importance of the primary care professional, whose ability to detect disorder in presenting patients and refer them to specialist care appropriately represent key stages in the pathway.

To meet the needs of patients with common mental health problems, four broad models have been described (Bower & Gilbody, 2005a; see also Box 25.1, p. 368). Although the models differ in important ways, a key issue is the degree to which the primary care professional takes the lead responsibility for the management of common mental health problems. Primary care professionals are at the forefront of care, and services which improve the quality of care at the primary care level have the greatest potential to increase access and equity, because such a large proportion of the population can access primary care with relative ease. The more that a service delivery model requires input from specialist mental health professionals, the more potential there is for problems with access, efficiency and equity, because specialists are relatively rare and expensive and their input cannot be easily made available for all patients.

Two of these models have received significant research attention. The first model (education and training) involves the provision of knowledge and skills concerning mental healthcare to primary care professionals (Kerwick & Jones, 1996). Generally, this has focused on improving recognition of common mental health problems and appropriate prescribing of medication. Training can involve widespread dissemination of guidelines, or more intensive practice-based education seminars (Gilbody *et al*, 2003) (see Chapters 24 and 29).

The second model (psychological therapy referral) is very different. In this model, primary responsibility for the management of the common mental health problems is passed to a psychological therapy practitioner (such as a counsellor or clinical psychologist). The workforce expansion of counsellors in UK primary care in the 1990s was a result of the enthusiastic adoption of this model (Mellor-Clark *et al*, 2001).

How do these models fare in terms of the goals of primary care? The education and training model scores highly on *access*, *efficiency* and *equity*, because changing the behaviour of primary care professionals has the potential to affect *all* patients with common mental health problems in primary care (Bower & Gilbody, 2005a). However, this model scores low on *effectiveness* and *patient-centredness*. Although there is good evidence that medication itself is effective, trials of interventions to change general practitioners' recognition and prescribing behaviour have generally failed (Thompson *et al*, 2000; Gilbody *et al*, 2003). Furthermore, patient attitudes to medication are often negative (Priest *et al*, 1996; Khan *et al*, 2007), which means that their preferences are not being met.

In contrast, the psychological therapy referral model scores highly on effectiveness and patient-centredness. Psychological therapies such as cognitive–behavioural therapy (CBT) are effective (Churchill *et al*, 2002) and as effective as pharmacological agents in depression (National Institute for Health and Clinical Excellence, 2004*b*) and recommended over medication in most anxiety disorders (National Institute for Health and Clinical Excellence, 2004*a*, 2005). There is also evidence that many patients would like at least the choice of 'talking treatments' and a significant proportion have an outright preference for them (Bird, 2006). However, effectiveness and patient-centredness come at a price. The direct healthcare costs associated with employing a psychological therapist are potentially higher than a prescription for medication. Because of the prevalence of common mental health problems and the finite number of psychological therapists, demand far exceeds supply. Between 24% and 40% of people with common mental health problems worldwide receive any kind of treatment for their difficulties (Singleton *et al*, 2001; Andrews & Tolkein II Team, 2006). In the UK, a mere 9% receive any form of talking treatment, of which only 1% receive evidence-supported treatment such as CBT (Singleton *et al*, 2001). Therefore access is poor, efficiency may be compromised and equity is threatened.

This chapter deals with two major innovations that seek to overcome some of the limitations of these models to better fulfil the multiple and competing goals outlined above. These innovations are *collaborative care* and *stepped care*. Both were originally formulated in the USA and have attracted attention worldwide as both the evidence for their effect has accumulated and their inherent good sense has become apparent.

# Collaborative care

One way of improving access to care while ensuring quality is through more effective use of specialist expertise to support primary care professionals. Originally, the model adopted to achieve this aim was 'consultation–liaison' (Gask *et al*, 1997; Bower & Gask, 2002). The premise behind consultation–liaison was that closer working between specialists and primary care professionals around the care of individual patients would improve the quality of their care, while ensuring that those benefits flowed through changes in the behaviour of primary care professionals and were thus able to benefit all patients accessing those services. Although used by a small number of enthusiasts (Strathdee & Williams, 1984), the consultation–liaison model was never adopted more widely in any primary healthcare setting internationally. However, consultation–liaison served as the basis for a US development known as 'collaborative care' (Bower & Gask, 2002).

Like consultation–liaison, collaborative care seeks to enhance relationships between primary care professionals and specialist staff. However, collaborative care is based on the principles of chronic disease management, and involves the addition of new staff ('case managers') who work with patients and liaise with primary care professionals and specialists in order to improve the quality of care (Katon *et al*, 2001). Case managers provide support, medication management and brief psychotherapies directly to patients, while liaising with the primary care professional and receiving support from a specialist. Collaborative care may also involve screening, patient education, changes to practice routines and developments in information technology (Gilbody *et al*, 2003).

How does collaborative care meet the goals outlined at the start of the chapter? The model attempts to overcome the lack of effectiveness of training and education by increasing the amount of specialist input to primary care professionals, and by employing case managers to work directly with patients and support practitioners in delivering care (e.g. supporting patients to adhere better with medication). It attempts to provide more patient-centred services, because case managers have a supportive role, and many collaborative care models also include brief psychotherapy. In addition, it attempts to preserve the advantages in terms of access, equity and efficiency by ensuring that this increased input of specialists is delivered as efficiently as possible.

## Evidence for the effectiveness of collaborative care

The model has been the subject of a large number of trials. Most were conducted in the USA (many by the Seattle group, led by Wayne Katon) but a number have now been carried out in other countries, such as the UK (Chew-Graham *et al*, 2007; Richards *et al*, 2008) and Chile (Araya *et al*, 2003). These trials have been summarised in a number of systematic reviews, which all agree that the model has shown robust evidence of clinical effectiveness (Badamgarav *et al*, 2003; Gilbody *et al*, 2003; Vergouwen *et al*, 2003; Gilbody *et al*, 2006a; Kates & Mach, 2007; Williams *et al*, 2007). In one of the most recent reviews, 37 randomised studies, with 12 355 patients with depression in primary care, were analysed. Meta-analysis showed that depression outcomes were improved at 6 months and evidence of longer-term benefit was found for up to 5 years (Gilbody *et al*, 2006a). There is evidence that the model is associated with higher costs (Gilbody *et al*, 2006b), however, and it remains to be seen whether the benefits can be delivered effectively *and* efficiently.

Bower *et al* (2006b) explored factors in collaborative care treatments that were directly related to outcomes. Collaborative care models that improved medication compliance were more effective. The background of case managers was also important, with those studies using staff with a mental health background (e.g. psychologists or mental health nurses) more effective than those that used non-specialist staff (e.g. practice nurses). Also, collaborative care was more effective when case managers were regularly supervised by specialists such as psychiatrists. However, the review did not find that the addition of brief psychotherapy substantially improved outcomes, nor did increased numbers of sessions (Bower *et al*, 2006*b*), although some individual trials did show benefits from adding brief psychotherapy (Wells *et al*, 2000). The optimal mix of 'active ingredients' in a collaborative care model remains of key interest among researchers and practitioners.

## Service delivery issues in collaborative care

The key service delivery issues in collaborative care reflect the difficulties of achieving the optimum balance between access, efficiency and equity while delivering effectiveness and patient-centredness. For example, despite the thin evidence that psychological therapy improves outcomes in a collaborative care model, patient preferences for talking treatments (Bird, 2006) render it preferable to include a psychological therapy component within collaborative care. Unfortunately, this may reduce the optimal efficiency of collaborative care, since psychological treatments require both more time and a greater skill in delivery. If case managers are to function only at a basic level – coordinating rather than delivering care – then psychological therapists must be provided within the model, at greater direct cost. Alternatively, training case managers to deliver psychological therapy themselves increases the training costs of these workers.

The finding that scheduled supervision improves patient outcomes requires that case managers and specialists can access the same individual patient record in order to enhance their supervision and consequent decision-making. This is likely to require a shared patient record, something which services may struggle to achieve, particularly where primary care and specialist practitioners are operating different systems. Furthermore, sophisticated decision algorithms may be required to differentiate between patients who are progressing well, those who require additional input and those who can be expected to recover spontaneously. Routinely collected outcome measures, albeit not the only piece of information, are central to such decision-making (Bower *et al*, 2006*a*). Once again, this is a feature of clinical practice that may be hard to enforce comprehensively to ensure accurate and consistent decision-making.

# Stepped care

Whereas the collaborative care model is an attempt to increase the effectiveness and acceptability of the training and education model, stepped care is an attempt to modify the psychological therapy referral model in such a way that the benefits (i.e. effectiveness and patient-centredness) are maintained, while its problems (i.e. access and efficiency) are minimised. Worldwide, guidelines for depression and anxiety recommend that stepped care should be the mechanism whereby treatments for depression and most anxiety disorders are organised (National Institute for Health and Clinical Excellence, 2004*a,b*; Andrews & Tolkein II Team, 2006).

Stepped care is based around two fundamental concepts. The first principle is that of 'least burden'. That is, interventions received by a patient should always be those which deliver good outcomes, while burdening the patient and the healthcare system as little as possible (Sobell & Sobell, 2000). Such a principle underpins most other healthcare interventions; for example, a non-invasive diagnostic or therapeutic procedure may be preferred by patients and healthcare providers alike over more invasive alternatives. In the case of common mental health problems, such interventions are often described as 'self-help' or 'minimal interventions' to contrast them with conventional psychological therapy interventions (such as 6- to 12-hour sessions of CBT). 'Minimal interventions' are designed to provide effective care while reducing the need for input from specialist therapists. Interventions without therapist contact (so-called 'pure self-help') are potentially the most efficient and could have the biggest impact on access, but these may not be optimally effective with depressed and anxious patients, who could lack motivation and confidence. Interventions with a small amount of therapist contact beyond an initial assessment are often called guided self-help, and might include supplying an initial therapeutic rationale or ongoing assessment of progress (Newman *et al*, 2003).

Can minimal interventions maintain the effectiveness of psychological therapies while doing so in a manner that is more efficient, thus increasing access and equity? There is a developing evidence base concerning effectiveness (McKendree-Smith *et al*, 2003; Den Boer *et al*, 2004; Anderson *et al*, 2005; Hirai & Clum, 2006; Gellatly *et al*, 2007). Studies reviewed by the National Institute for Health and Clinical Excellence (2004*b*) for the depression guidelines and other reviews suggest that guided self-help is effective, although there have been difficulties in replicating some of these results in the UK context of the National Health Service (Richards *et al*, 2003; Mead *et al*, 2005; Salkovskis *et al*, 2006).

The second principle is that of 'self-correction' (Newman, 2000). Here, the idea is that if minimal interventions such as guided self-help are not working, there must be a system in place to detect this, which in turn leads to alternative, more intensive treatments being offered (such as conventional psychological therapy). The decision to step up (or otherwise) requires sound information and systems of clinical review which are far from *ad hoc*. Programmed review at clinically relevant intervals requires the regular and systematic collection of outcome measures and clinical information.

In psychological therapies, these two principles are often interpreted as the provision of minimal interventions, such as guided self-help with 'scheduled reviews' of clinical outcomes in place to detect treatment response. Lack of improvement then leads to a 'step up' to more intensive treatment, such as conventional CBT. A narrative review of stepped care concluded that while such systems offer the potential for greater efficiency, the optimal configuration of system elements is unknown. The authors note that the benefits of stepped care are unlikely to be fully realised if significant resources are expended on complex assessments and if a large proportion of patients are allocated to conventional interventions (Bower & Gilbody, 2005b).

## Service delivery issues in stepped care

Although stepped care is of inherently good sense, there is a lack of specific empirical evidence for this system when used with high-prevalence disorders (Andrews & Tolkein II Team, 2006). This causes difficulty when implementing stepped care, since the two principles of least burden and self-correction may be interpreted and implemented in more than one way. If a stepped approach is prioritised, all patients should be offered a minimal intervention as the initial step in a treatment programme. Interventions of greater intensity are reserved for those patients who do not benefit from the initial minimal intervention. In contrast, a stratified approach assesses patients and allocates some to either minimal or conventional interventions. Such allocation requires some judgement to be made as to the likely response patients will make to the treatments available at different steps – so-called 'aptitude treatment interaction' (Sobell & Sobell, 2000).

There are advantages and disadvantages to both systems of implementation. A stratified model requires an ability to predict the likely benefit for an individual patient of different types of interventions. While factors such as severity of disorder, chronicity and disability have predictive power at a population level, they are unreliable indicators of individual patient response to treatment. Workers familiar with operating conventional services may err on the side of caution and favour more intensive treatment without attempting to deliver a minimal intervention first. Such a risk-averse approach could negate the potential efficiencies of the system as a whole.

In contrast, a stepped model runs the risk of prolonging waits for higher-intensity treatments by requiring all patients to spend some time first trying a minimal intervention. If patients who would benefit from a more intensive therapy are not recognised, they may be inappropriately treated. Paradoxically, this may inappropriately extend the duration of their contact with services, once again compromising system efficiency. It may even deter some patients from seeking further treatment (through their experience of treatment failure), although some studies suggest that experience of minimal interventions actually whet patients' appetite for further treatment (MacDonald et al, 2007).

The degree of emphasis on stepped or stratified care will have a major influence on system performance. However, whatever the balance between these two approaches, the vital importance accorded to the principle of clinical review cannot be overstated. Unless health and social outcomes are recorded accurately, regularly and frequently for each patient, stepped care cannot be self-correcting. Despite valiant attempts to set up routine outcome measures as standard in the UK and elsewhere (Barkham *et al*, 1999; Margison *et al*, 2000), outcomes of therapy are often recorded subjectively, irregularly and infrequently. Algorithms which take severity, chronicity and disability into account in a systematic and objective manner are rarely used in clinical decision-making. Furthermore, the availability of different treatments in the stepped care model will affect system performance. There is little point in a review indicating that another treatment is required if this merely leads to a step up to a long wait for such therapy. Stepped care systems need to ensure a smooth transition between steps, so that patient experience is not disjointed.

# A UK case study: the Newham and Doncaster demonstration sites

This case study, undertaken in the UK, is a reflection of worldwide concern to improve access to mental health services (Horton, 2007; Thornicroft, 2007) and reduce the disability caused by disorders such as depression and anxiety (Andrews & Titov, 2007). Two clinical 'demonstration sites' were set up to test the hypothesis that investing in psychological therapies will increase patients' well-being and decrease their reliance on state benefits (Layard, 2006). Doncaster chose a model of care which could be broadly categorised as a stepped model and Newham (a London borough) a stratified model. Many operational lessons have been learned through these sites.

In Newham it was found that the allocation model was not able to deliver the volume of psychological therapy anticipated. Newham was heavily resourced, with experienced and highly trained therapists (mostly clinical psychologists) providing conventional psychological therapy and working in a traditional fashion (one-to-one appointments each lasting about 1 hour). Although minimal interventions were available, these were found to be underresourced. As a consequence, within a year of operation, the management in Newham recruited a significant number of workers to deliver minimal interventions at a lower step. In the first year, assessments were conducted by the therapists providing conventional treatments. It was found, though, that when patients were allocated to a minimal intervention after this initial assessment they became dissatisfied. Assessment is itself an engaging experience for patients and they felt let down by the experience of being handed on to another worker whom they might have perceived as being less 'expert'. Therefore, different, less-qualified workers, albeit specifically trained in low-intensity psychological interventions, were directed to undertake the triage function, directing patients to low- or high-intensity steps, with low-intensity treatment being the default preferred option.

In contrast, Doncaster's stepped care model was combined with telephone-based case management inspired by the collaborative care approach (Richards & Suckling, 2008a,b). Case managers were recruited from community members and educated specifically to support minimal interventions such as computerised CBT and guided self-help, with rigorous and scheduled supervision from mental health specialists. This model was able to deliver the required volume but Doncaster's inability to recruit sufficient conventional therapists limited the ability to deliver a seamless stepped care service. Although less than 5% of patients were 'stepped up', waiting lists still developed at the higher-intensity steps. Importantly, although the proportion of patients receiving conventional treatment was much smaller in Doncaster than in Newham, the overall treatment effect sizes were identical. This was not explained by differences in the initial severity of disorder, which was similar. Although Doncaster treated more recent-onset cases (patients with disorder duration of less than 6 months), outcomes were equivalent for both recent-onset and chronic cases. The two sites were resourced equivalently, but Doncaster treated four times as many patients as Newham in the 1 year of operation. These volumes and outcomes led to the UK Secretary of State for Health announcing an additional £300 million investment for psychological therapy services for 2008–11. This figure represented sufficient funds to treat almost 1 million additional patients with anxiety and depression.

Both demonstration sites found, therefore, that stepped care was more efficient when a greater proportion of patients received minimal interventions. Patient preference could be significantly influenced by the person conducting an initial assessment, but outcomes appeared to be just as good when the default treatment was mainly a minimal intervention, rather than a predominance of conventional psychological therapy. Some of the latter is definitely required, however, and services must be careful to ensure that sufficient is available to prevent waiting lists building up between steps.

In Doncaster, telephone-based collaborative care case management was an effective way of delivering the majority of minimal interventions for both depression and anxiety. While collaborative care is not an essential component of stepped care, it can be used to enhance efficiency (telephone contacts were typically 40–50% shorter than face-to-face appointments) and maintain contact with reluctant attenders for appointments. Providing case managers are adequately trained, providing they receive full case-load supervision from mental health experts and providing evidence-based minimal interventions exist, case managers can support and effectively treat the majority of patients with common mental health problems in stepped care.

# Conclusion

Organising and delivering primary care mental health services in a way that meets the goals of access, effectiveness, efficiency and patient-centredness remains a key challenge for the future. Dissatisfaction with conventional models of delivery has led to the development of innovative new models which may be better suited to meet the multiple goals of primary care mental health. However, delivering these innovations in practice remains a challenge, and researchers and managers are only beginning to develop an understanding of how collaborative care and stepped care can function in routine practice. Future developments may see these two models being integrated further, to provide a more seamless and integrated approach to delivery. The results of ongoing evaluations of these services are eagerly awaited.

---

Key points

- This chapter describes two innovative models which may significantly improve the quality of services for common mental health problems: collaborative care and stepped care.
- Collaborative care is based on chronic disease management principles, and involves the addition of case managers, who work with patients and primary care and specialist professionals to improve quality of care.
- Stepped care is designed to increase the efficiency of service delivery. In this model, patients initially receive 'self-help' or 'minimal interventions'. Patients are subsequently assessed, and only those patients who fail to benefit are then 'stepped up' to more intensive treatments.
- The evidence base concerning both of these models is accumulating, and case studies of the models in action illustrate important service delivery issues.

---

# Further reading and e-resources

Centre for Economic Performance, http://cep.lse.ac.uk/research/mentalhealth/default. asp. This site features influential reports on the economic issues in mental healthcare and the need for investment in psychological therapy.

The chronic care model, http://www.improvingchroniccare.org/index.php?p=The_ Chronic_Care_Model&s=2. This site describes the model that underlies collaborative care models in mental health

Clinical Research Unit for Anxiety and Depression (CRUFAD), http://www.crufad.org. This is a site describing the work of CRUFAD in Australia, including relevant self-help resources.

Improving access to psychological therapies, http://www.iapt.nhs.uk. This is a site describing the Improving Access to Psychological Therapies programme in the UK.

Improving access to psychological therapies research project, University of Sheffield, http://www.iapt.group.shef.ac.uk. This site describes a project (funded by the UK Service Delivery and Organisation programme) evaluating new models for the delivery of psychological therapy in the UK.

UK Care Services Improvement Partnership, *Primary Care Services for Depression*, http:// kc.csip.org.uk/viewdocument.php?action=viewdox&pid=0&doc=35064&grp=1. This is a guide that outlines possible stepped care models for depression.

# References

Anderson, L., Lewis, G., Araya, R., *et al* (2005) Self-help books for depression: how can practitioners and patients make the right choice? *British Journal of General Practice*, **55**, 387–392.

Andrews, G. & Titov, N. (2007) Depression is very disabling. *Lancet*, **370**, 808–809.

Andrews, G. & Tolkein II Team (2006) *A Needs-Based, Costed Stepped-Care Model for Mental Health Services*. CRUFAD, University of New South Wales.

Andrews, G., Henderson, S. & Hall, W. (2001) Prevalence, comorbidity, disability and service utilisation: overview of the Australian Mental Health Survey. *British Journal of Psychiatry*, **178**, 145–153.

Araya, R., Rojas, G., Fritsch, R., *et al* (2003) Treating depression in primary care in low income women in Santiago, Chile: a randomised controlled trial. *Lancet*, **361**, 995–1000.

Badamgarav, E., Weingarten, S., Henning, J., *et al* (2003) Effectiveness of disease management programs in depression: a systematic review. *American Journal of Psychiatry*, **160**, 2080–2090.

Barkham, M., Evans, C., Margison, F., *et al* (1999) The rationale for developing and implementing core outcome batteries for routine use in service settings and psychotherapy outcome research. *Journal of Mental Health*, **7**, 35–47.

Bird, A. (2006) *We Need to Talk: The Case for Psychological Therapy on the NHS*. Mental Health Foundation.

Bower, P. & Gask, L. (2002) The changing nature of consultation–liaison in primary care: bridging the gap between research and practice. *General Hospital Psychiatry*, **24**, 63–70.

Bower, P. & Gilbody, S. (2005a) Managing common mental health disorders in primary care: conceptual models and evidence base. *BMJ*, **330**, 839–842.

Bower, P. & Gilbody, S. (2005b) Stepped care in psychological therapies: access, effectiveness and efficiency. *British Journal of Psychiatry*, **186**, 11–17.

Bower, P., Gilbody, S. & Barkham, M. (2006a) Making decisions about patient progress: the application of routine outcome measurement in stepped care psychological therapy services. *Primary Care Mental Health*, **4**, 21–28.

Bower, P., Gilbody, S., Richards, D., *et al* (2006b) Collaborative care for depression in primary care. Making sense of a complex intervention: systematic review and meta regression. *British Journal of Psychiatry*, **189**, 484–493.

Centre for Economic Performance (2006) *The Depression Report: A New Deal for Depression and Anxiety Disorders*. Centre for Economic Performance, LSE.

Chew-Graham, C., Lovell, K., Roberts, C., *et al* (2007) A randomised controlled trial to test the feasibility of the collaborative care model for the management of depression in the elderly. *British Journal of General Practice*, **57**, 364–370.

Churchill, R., Hunot, V., Corney, R., *et al* (2002) A systematic review of controlled trials of the effectiveness and cost-effectiveness of brief psychological treatments for depression. *Health Technology Assessment*, **5** (35).

Den Boer, P., Wiersma, D. & Van Den Bosch, R. (2004) Why is self-help neglected in the treatment of emotional disorders? A meta-analysis. *Psychological Medicine*, **34**, 959–971.

Gask, L., Sibbald, B. & Creed, F. (1997) Evaluating models of working at the interface between mental health services and primary care. *British Journal of Psychiatry*, **170**, 6–11.

Gellatly, J., Bower, P., Hennessey, S., *et al* (2007) What makes self-help interventions effective in the management of depressive symptoms? Meta-analysis and meta-regression. *Psychological Medicine*, **37**, 1217–1228.

Gilbody, S., Whitty, P., Grimshaw, J., *et al* (2003) Educational and organisational interventions to improve the management of depression in primary care: a systematic review. *JAMA*, **289**, 3145–3151.

Gilbody, S., Bower, P., Fletcher, J., *et al* (2006*a*) Collaborative care for depression: a systematic review and cumulative meta-analysis. *Archives of Internal Medicine*, **166**, 2314–2321.

Gilbody, S., Bower, P. & Whitty, P. (2006*b*) The costs and consequences of enhanced primary care for depression: a systematic review of randomised economic evaluations. *British Journal of Psychiatry*, **189**, 297–308.

Goldberg, D. & Huxley, P. (1980) *Mental Illness in the Community: The Pathway to Psychiatric Care*. Tavistock.

Hirai, M. & Clum, G. (2006) A meta-analytic study of self-help interventions for anxiety problems. *Behavior Therapy*, **37**, 99–110.

Horton, R. (2007) Launching a new movement for mental health. *Lancet*, **370**, 806.

Kates, N. & Mach, M. (2007) Chronic disease management for depression in primary care: a summary of the current literature and implications for practice. *Canadian Journal of Psychiatry*, **52**, 77–85.

Katon, W., Von Korff, M., Lin, E., *et al* (2001) Rethinking practitioner roles in chronic illness: the specialist, primary care physician and the practice nurse. *General Hospital Psychiatry*, **23**, 138–144.

Kerwick, S. & Jones, R. (1996) Educational interventions in primary care psychiatry. *Primary Care Psychiatry*, **2**, 107–117.

Khan, N., Bower, P. & Rogers, A. (2007) Guided self-help in primary care mental health: a meta synthesis of qualitative studies of patient experience. *British Journal of Psychiatry*, **191**, 206–211.

Laine, C. & Davidoff, F. (1996) Patient-centered medicine: a professional evolution. *JAMA*, **275**, 152–156.

Layard, R. (2006) The case for psychological treatment centres. *BMJ*, **332**, 1030–1032.

MacDonald, W., Mead, N., Bower, P., *et al* (2007) A qualitative study of patients' perceptions of a 'minimal' psychological therapy. *International Journal of Social Psychiatry*, **53**, 23–35.

Margison, F., Barkham, M., Evans, C., *et al* (2000) Measurement and psychotherapy: evidence-based practice and practice-based evidence. *British Journal of Psychiatry*, **177**, 123–130.

McKendree-Smith, N., Floyd, M. & Scogin, F. (2003) Self-administered treatments for depression: a review. *Journal of Clinical Psychology*, **59**, 275–288.

Mead, N., MacDonald, W., Bower, P., *et al* (2005) The clinical effectiveness of guided self-help versus waiting list control in the management of anxiety and depression: a randomised controlled trial. *Psychological Medicine*, **35**, 1633–1643.

Mellor-Clark, J., Simms-Ellis, R. & Burton, M. (2001) *National Survey of Counsellors in Primary Care: Evidence for Growing Professionalisation*. Royal College of General Practitioners.

National Institute for Health and Clinical Excellence (2004*a*) *Clinical Guidelines for the Management of Anxiety (Panic Disorder, With or Without Agoraphobia, and Generalised Anxiety Disorder) in Adults in Primary, Secondary and Community Care*. London: HMSO.

National Institute for Health and Clinical Excellence (2004*b*) *Depression: Management of Depression in Primary and Secondary Care*. HMSO.

National Institute for Health and Clinical Excellence (2005) *Post-traumatic Stress Disorder (PTSD): The Management of PTSD in Adults and Children in Primary and Secondary Care*. HMSO.

Newman, M. (2000) Recommendations for a cost-offset model of psychotherapy allocation using generalized anxiety disorder as an example. *Journal of Consulting and Clinical Psychology*, **68**, 549–555.

Newman, M., Erickson, T., Przeworski, A., *et al* (2003) Self-help and minimal-contact therapies for anxiety disorders: is human contact necessary for therapeutic efficacy? *Journal of Clinical Psychology*, **59**, 251–274.

Priest, R., Vize, C., Roberts, A., *et al* (1996) Lay people's attitudes to treatment of depression: results of opinion poll for Defeat Depression Campaign just before its launch. *BMJ*, **313**, 858–859.

Richards, D. & Suckling, R. (2008a) Improving access to psychological therapy: the Doncaster demonstration site organisational model. *Clinical Psychology Forum*, **181**, 9–16.

Richards, D. & Suckling, R. (2008b) Response to commentaries on 'Improving access to psychological therapy: the Doncaster demonstration site organisational model'. *Clinical Psychology Forum*, **181**, 47–51.

Richards, A., Barkham, M., Cahill, J., *et al* (2003) PHASE: a randomised, controlled trial of supervised self-help cognitive behavioural therapy in primary care. *British Journal of General Practice*, **53**, 764–770.

Richards, D., Lovell, K., Gilbody, S., *et al* (2008) Collaborative care for depression in UK primary care: a randomized controlled trial. *Psychological Medicine*, **38**, 279–287.

Salkovskis, P., Rimes, K., Stephenson, D., *et al* (2006) A randomized controlled trial of the use of self-help materials in addition to standard general practice treatment of depression compared to standard treatment alone. *Psychological Medicine*, **36**, 325–333.

Siegler, M. & Osmond, H. (1974) *Models of Madness, Models of Medicine*. Macmillan.

Singleton, N., Bumpstead, R., O'Brien, M., *et al* (2001) *Psychiatric Morbidity Among Adults Living in Private Households, 2000*. The Stationary Office.

Sobell, M. & Sobell, L. (2000) Stepped care as a heuristic approach to the treatment of alcohol problems. *Journal of Consulting and Clinical Psychology*, **68**, 573–579.

Strathdee, G. & Williams, P. (1984) A survey of psychiatrists in primary care: the silent growth of a new service. *Journal of the Royal College of General Practitioners*, **34**, 615–618.

Thompson, C., Kinmonth, A., Stevens, L., *et al* (2000) Effects of a clinical practice guideline and practice-based education on detection and outcome of depression in primary care: Hampshire Depression Project randomised controlled trial. *Lancet*, **355**, 185–191.

Thornicroft, G. (2007) Most people with mental illness are not treated. *Lancet*, **370**, 807–808.

Vergouwen, A., Bakker, A., Katon, W., *et al* (2003) Improving adherence to antidepressants: a systematic review of interventions. *Journal of Clinical Psychiatry*, **64**, 1415–1420.

Wells, K., Sherbourne, C., Schoenbaum, M., *et al* (2000) Impact of disseminating quality improvement programs for depression in managed primary care: a randomized controlled trial. *JAMA*, **283**, 212–220.

Williams, J., Gerrity, M., Holsinger, T., *et al* (2007) Systematic review of multifaceted interventions to improve depression care. *General Hospital Psychiatry*, **29**, 91–116.

World Health Organization (2001) *The World Health Report 2001. Mental Health: New Understanding, New Hope*. WHO.

# CHAPTER 28

# The role of practice nurses

Sue Plummer and Mark Haddad

### Summary

This chapter examines the role of practice nurses, district nurses and to a lesser extent health visitors and midwives in the provision of primary care mental health. Although practice nurses' roles have traditionally been concerned with physical activities, it is evident from the literature that many nurses are seeing patients with common mental disorders. One of the most common reasons for patients to see practice nurses is for review of chronic physical illnesses such as hypertension, asthma, diabetes and coronary heart disease. These conditions are often comorbid with depression and therefore nurses require mental health skills. The detection of depression has been shown to be poor but could be improved with appropriate training and the use of screening instruments validated for use in primary care. Nurses are also well placed to deliver evidence-based interventions. However, all of these have training implications and a clear strategy for the ongoing education and training of all the members of the primary care team needs to be identified. Clinical supervision will then be needed to sustain skills and knowledge.

As has been seen in previous chapters, most mental illness is treated in primary rather than secondary care and the general practitioner (GP) has traditionally been the first port of call for patients. Other members of the primary care team are working with various degrees of autonomy, which means that patients' appointments are increasingly likely to be with a primary care professional other than a GP, such as a practice nurse, nurse practitioner, healthcare assistant, health visitor or midwife. This means that all members of the primary care team will be seeing patients with common mental disorders, especially if they are comorbid with physical illness. All these professionals are therefore well placed to recognise and deliver brief evidence-based mental health interventions to the patients they see, to refer on as appropriate and thereby to reduce some of the primary care workload. Depending on models of local healthcare provision, general practices will have referral systems available for patients both within and outside of primary care. Models of mental healthcare vary throughout the UK and internationally but, despite this, there are key professionals who work with patients with mental health problems under the umbrella of primary care. These typically include counsellors, primary care mental health workers, psychologists and gateway workers. In the 1980s and early 1990s, community psychiatric nurses (CPNs) became more frequently involved in primary care mental health work (Boardman, 1997). This shift away from working exclusively within specialist services and towards general practice collaboration has subsequently been reversed. Since the mid-1990s, in response to policy development and professional review (Audit Commission, 1994; Department of Health, 1994, 1995), the work of these nurses has been realigned with specialist services working within multidisciplinary teams. There have been large increases in the mental health nursing workforce – a 21% increase in head-count over the 10 years to 2006 (Department of Health, 2006) – but the major focus of this workforce is upon the needs of patients with severe and enduring mental illnesses, primarily schizophrenia.

This chapter examines current and potential mental healthcare roles primarily of practice nurses, as the majority of research has been carried out with this group. However, work has also been undertaken with midwives and health visitors and research is emerging that is focusing on the roles of district nurses. Therefore the role of these groups of professionals are also discussed.

## Current roles

There are currently just over 22000 practice nurses employed in the UK National Health Service (NHS), of which 14600 are full-time equivalent posts (NHS Information Centre, Workforce and Facilities, 2009). The number of practice nurses employed has increased by 1.6% in comparison with an overall increase of 2.5% for professionally qualified clinical staff within the general practice workforce over the 10 years to 2008. Practice nurses work with GPs and other members of the primary care team within the practice setting to provide assessment, screening, care and education to patients of all ages. Surveys of practice nurses' workloads and roles in primary care consistently show that the most common nursing interventions are of a physical nature. There is good evidence, though, that practice nurses are also working with patients with mental health problems (Thomas & Corney, 1993; Armstrong, 1997; Crossland & Kai, 1998; Deehan et al, 1998). Gray et al (1999) surveyed a random sample of 1500 practice nurses (response rate 54%). Of these, 48% reported being asked by patients experiencing depression for information about both symptoms and antidepressant medication; 44% of nurses gave such information and advice to patients and their families, and a similar number gave information on the use of antidepressants. The percentage of nurses administering depot antipsychotics was 61%, similar to that found by Kendrick *et al* (1993), but only 55% of these nurses reported monitoring side-effects. Studies undertaken to investigate practice nurses' current practice, attitudes and confidence in the care of patients receiving depot neuroleptic treatment (Millar *et al*, 1999) demonstrate clearly the training needs for this group of nurses.

Not only are practice nurses encountering patients with common mental disorders, but district nurses, health visitors and midwives, too, are likely to see patients with comorbid mental health problems. Haddad *et al* (2005) surveyed district and community nurses in Hertfordshire, Lewisham and the island of Jersey. Nurses estimated that 16% of patients on their case-load were suffering from a mental health problem. These were most commonly dementia, depression and anxiety disorders. Health visitors and midwives are likely to be working with patients with common mental disorders such as postnatal depression, the prevalence of which is estimated at 12–13% (O'Hara & Swain, 1996).

# Recognition of mental health problems

Moussavi *et al* (2007) argue that, in many primary care settings, patients presenting with disorders in addition to depression frequently do not get diagnosed and, if they do, treatment is often focused on the chronic diseases. This raises the issue of recognition and screening skills. Many studies have highlighted the issues around GPs' abilities to detect depression in patients. Research has similarly examined the detection ability of a range of other professionals, including nurses (Jackson & Baldwin, 1993; Brown *et al*, 2003) and care workers (Preville *et al*, 2004; Eisses *et al*, 2005). Plummer *et al* (1997), in a controlled comparison study, found that practice nurses' recognition rates of patients who had been identified as possible cases on the 12-item General Health Questionnaire (GHQ-12) were no better than would be expected by chance. A further randomised controlled trial (RCT) by Plummer *et al* (2000) found that practice nurses detected only 16% of patients who had scored as probable cases on the GHQ-12. The higher the score on the GHQ-12, the more likely the nurses were to recognise that the patient was distressed (Plummer, 2003). Pouwer *et al* (2006), in a study in The Netherlands, found that the presence of an emotional problem in diabetic patients with moderate to severe levels of anxiety or depression was recorded in the medical chart in only 20–25% of cases.

There may be many reasons for the non-detection rates of practice nurses. The reasons for non-detection on the part of GPs have been well documented (Tylee *et al*, 1995; Doherty, 1997; Crisp, 1999; Kessler *et al*, 1999). It may well be that these reasons also apply to nurses. As Casey (1990) suggests, detection depends on both bias and accuracy. Bias reflects the practitioner's beliefs and attitudes towards mental illness. A study of primary healthcare professionals by Burroughs *et al* (2006) showed they recognised that managing late-life depression did fall within their remit, but identified limitations in their own skills and capabilities. They also viewed depression as understandable and justifiable and felt that nothing could be done for this group of patients. Conversely, Haddad (2007), after administering the Depression Attitude Questionnaire (Botega *et al*, 1992) to community nurses, found that it revealed generally positive attitudes to patients with depression but a tendency to refer management of this problem to specialist clinicians.

Accuracy is the appropriateness of the psychological tag attributed to the patient and is generated by the personality attributes of the practitioners, by the style of interview they conduct and by their knowledge of psychiatric illness. A number of studies have reported that patients attending general practices for urgent (same-day) appointments preferred to consult with GPs if they perceived their symptoms to be serious and with nurses for minor symptoms and reassurance (Redsell *et al*, 2007). However, they thought that nurses had more time for them and were more compassionate, so there appears to be evidence that nurses' interview skills and compassionate personality attributes should be enhancing accuracy. Nurse practitioners were found to carry out more tests of patients and asked them to return more often. Patients were also more satisfied with nurse practitioner consultations. Further, practice nurses felt that older people were less inhibited in talking to them about non-medical problems, whereas GPs reported that older patients rarely mentioned psychological difficulties (Murray *et al*, 2006).

Despite the observed caring attitudes of nurse to their patients, recognition remains a problem. One of the major reasons for this, cited by many practice nurses and community nurses, is the perceived lack of knowledge and skills within mental healthcare. Gray *et al* (1999), in their survey of practice nurses, found that knowledge about the treatment of depression was generally poor. For example, 42% of practice nurses did not agree that antidepressants were the best method of treating severe depression and only 52% believed that antidepressants were not addictive. The study found that 70% of practice nurses had received no mental health training in the previous 5 years. Similarly, Haddad *et al* (2005) found that 74% of registered district nurses had not attended any mental health training during the past 5 years.

## Provision of mental healthcare by practice nurses

It has been seen that practice nurses are already working with patients presenting with common mental disorders and that a substantial number of nurses, health visitors and midwives are delivering brief interventions. These healthcare professionals are highly skilled practitioners and their skills can be built upon with appropriate training.

## Screening

One potential area to be developed is screening using validated assessment tools. Groups of patients at high risk of having or developing a mental health problem can be identified. From the evidence already presented in this and other chapters, these groups might include: patients with chronic physical illnesses; new patient registration checks; patients with a recent history of accident or trauma; or, in the case of alcohol misuse, patients presenting with alcohol-related disorders.

### Screening for depression

The Quality and Outcomes Framework (QOF), which is part of the reorganisation of primary care services in England (British Medical Association, 2006), has, since 2006, incorporated a quality measure for the assessment of depression among at-risk groups. These are patients currently recorded in practice registers with coronary heart disease or diabetes. The guidelines for depression from the National Institute for Health and Clinical Excellence (NICE) (2007) recommend that two screening questions be used with patients who are suspected of having depressive symptoms: 'During the last month, have you often been bothered by feeling down, depressed or hopeless?' and 'During the last month, have you often been bothered by having little interest or pleasure in doing things?' (see Chapter 8). These two questions elicit the core features of depression, as set out in DSM–IV (American Psychiatric Association, 1994), and are employed as the case-finding questions used with primary care patients with coronary heart disease and diabetes. In the NICE guidelines, the practice nurse is identified as being involved in this first level of the stepped care approach to depression. The disadvantage of this, though, is that the practice nurse then has to deal with whatever the patient discloses and for some nurses this may be daunting if they have had little or no training in mental health assessment and management. Training is discussed in the next section of this chapter.

### Screening for alcohol misuse

Along with depression, the prevalence of alcohol misuse within primary care attendees is considerable. It is estimated that people drinking alcohol at hazardous or harmful levels form up to 20% of patients presenting in general practice (Anderson, 1993). Findings from the most recent psychiatric morbidity survey in England (McManus et al, 2009) show the prevalence of alcohol dependency to be 5.9% (although moderate and severe dependency affects only 0.5% of adults). Many GPs and practice nurses do not identify the majority of the alcohol-related problems which can be found among their patients (Clement, 1986; Deehan et al, 1998). Screening of patients drinking at hazardous levels can easily be undertaken by nurses using the Alcohol Use Disorders Identification Test (AUDIT) (Saunders et al, 1993), which was developed from a large international

WHO study for use within primary care settings (see also Chapter 18). This asks the patient ten questions, takes very little time to answer and identifies patients drinking at hazardous and harmful levels. Nurses are also very well placed to deliver evidence-based brief alcohol interventions after having identified patients at risk. Lock & Kaner (2004), in a study to investigate the characteristics and factors that influence provision of a brief alcohol intervention by practice nurses, found that patients' risk status as measured by the AUDIT was the most influential predictor of an intervention. One such brief intervention developed by the University of Sydney for use in primary care is the Drink-Less programme. This involves screening patients using the AUDIT and delivering a brief intervention comprising feedback, advice and motivational interviewing. It takes 5–10 minutes and uses audiovisual aids such as cards and booklets. This can be accessed from the website given at the end of this chapter.

## Interventions for patients with mental health problems

A number of studies have evaluated the effectiveness of training practice nurses in the management of mental health problems. Haddad (2007) identified 17 published studies that had evaluated training programmes for these nurses (and their equivalents in the USA and elsewhere) or that had incorporated training for these staff within broader service developments. Eight of these papers concerned US-based primary care nurses and nine concerned practice nurses. Of the latter nine studies, seven were from the UK, with single studies from Finland and South Africa. Many of these studies were poorly designed or conducted. Two UK trials were robust studies which indicated modest effects of training practice nurses, district nurses and health visitors in problem-solving interventions (Mynors-Wallis et al, 1997) and improved outcomes for patients with major depression with training of practice nurses in compliance therapy (Peveler et al, 1999). The US studies, which involved training and developing the roles of practice-based nurses, were typically well funded and robustly designed. They provided evidence of the benefits of such role development. Examples include practice nurses trained in telephone-based care, which was shown to be associated with significant improvement in patient clinical outcomes at 6-month follow-up (Hunkeler et al, 2000; Simon et al, 2000). Nutting et al (2005) conducted a large cluster RCT of primary care nurses and physicians which involved the training of members of quality improvement teams in ongoing care and monitoring, and demonstrated improved detection of depression.

The best results, in terms of clinical outcome, are unsurprisingly related to those studies which implemented and evaluated organisational changes (see Chapters 24 and 27) together with approaches to reinforce and monitor performance, rather than consisting of training and skill development alone. Several larger projects involving multifaceted approaches to address mental health problems in the primary care setting have involved modified care models for depression management, focusing on different population groups. The Pathways Study conducted by Katon *et al* (2004) in the USA targeted people with both diabetes and depression or dysthymia, and evaluated a collaborative care model. This featured stepped treatment delivered by a specially trained nurse in collaboration with the primary care physician. (For more about collaborative and stepped care models see Chapter 27.) The components of the model involved antidepressant medication or problem-solving or a combination of these, with psychiatric consultation and referral if response to these steps was poor. The nurses' week-long training incorporated a manual for treatment and involved further assessment by standardised rating of audiotaped treatment sessions. They received ongoing feedback, with regular supervision and review of audiotaped consultations.

Health visitors have been a key staff group in three UK studies that examined training in brief cognitive and solution-focused therapy techniques. A study by Appleby *et al* (2003) examined training in cognitive–behavioural techniques for a single professional group, while other researchers (Standart *et al*, 1997) combined training for health visitors and social workers, or for nurses and health visitors (Bowles *et al*, 2001). One study based in Sweden targeted child health nurses in a counselling training intervention for postnatal depression (Wickberg & Hwang, 1996). More recently, a large cluster randomised trial of training health visitors in psychologically informed approaches has shown robust positive outcomes in improving identification of postnatal depressive symptoms and enhancing psychological care (Morrell *et al*, 2009).

The focus of much practice nursing is on patients suffering from chronic physical illness. Indeed, practices are encouraged to treat these groups of patients within the incentives of the national pay for performance scheme in primary care, the QOF. There is robust evidence that many patients with chronic physical disease have comorbid depression. The WHO's World Health Survey of 60 countries (Moussavi *et al*, 2007) found that between 9% and 23% of participants with one or more chronic physical diseases had comorbid depression. These diseases included arthritis, asthma, angina and diabetes. Plummer (2003), in an RCT, found that, of 4039 patients attending practice nurse clinics, 1090 patients attended for the monitoring of chronic illnesses, which included diabetes, hypertension, asthma and obesity. These patients were screened using the GHQ-12 before their consultation with the practice nurse. The results showed that 31% of the patients scored at probable 'caseness'.

## Care of patients with severe mental illness

Finally, practice nurses may have an important role to play in the physical care of patients with severe and enduring mental illnesses. As for patients with a range of chronic physical illnesses, patients with psychotic illnesses are systematically monitored by the use of a register under the QOF scheme.

Each patient should receive a physical, medication and communication review. The provision of this review, in terms of who carries it out (whether in primary or secondary services), varies throughout the UK. However, practice nurses are commonly involved in developing and maintaining the practice register of patients with schizophrenia and bipolar affective disorder. In the case of bipolar disorder, for example, this ensures appropriate monitoring of lithium levels, associated indicators of related adverse effects of lithium therapy and a regular physical review. The review includes monitoring of blood pressure and body mass index, screening for diabetes, and health promotion advice appropriate to patients' needs. Additionally, documentation of a comprehensive care plan for patients within the mental health register is required, as is evidence of follow-up for those patients who fail to attend their review appointments (see also Chapter 15).

# Training needs and implications

Practice nurses, health visitors, district nurses and midwives are providing mental healthcare to patients with a variety of common mental disorders, although predominantly depression. The majority of nurses are willing to continue with this role and to develop it, but all have stressed the need for training. The most frequent training requested by the district nurses in Haddad *et al*'s (2005) study was for recognition of mental disorders and anxiety management. Further skills in crisis intervention, pharmacological treatments for depression, counselling/supportive psychotherapy, medication management, suicide prevention, relaxation therapy, behaviour therapy and administration of depot antipsychotic medication were requested.

Nurses wishing to practise as specialists within the community setting (and this includes practice nurses and district nurses) and practitioners wishing to practise as midwives or public health nurses are required to undertake the appropriate specialist community practice course. The Nursing and Midwifery Council (2001, 2004a,b) in the UK stipulates standards to be met for the educational preparation of these specialists. They clearly identify the need to contribute to the health and social well-being of patients and their families. Health is defined succinctly to include mental health. However, it is up to the interpretation of the university running the training scheme to decide on the quantity and depth of content on mental health and illness. It is at this point and previously during initial nurse preparation that importance should be given to mental health training. Apart from this, a clear strategy for the education and training of all primary care team members needs to be carefully considered and planned.

There is good evidence that training and education for members of the primary care team need to be delivered to the whole team rather than individuals (Tylee, 2001) and has clear advantages. The aim of education is to change practice as well as knowledge and skills, and this is difficult if it is attempted in isolation from other members of the team. It is clear from the literature on training that newly learnt knowledge and skills quickly diminish if they are not regularly reinforced. Clinical supervision, which is common practice for mental health practitioners in mental health settings, needs to be introduced within primary care if nurses are expected to develop and take on new mental health roles.

---

Key points

- There is robust evidence that practice nurses, district nurses, health visitors and midwives are seeing patients with common mental disorders and delivering brief interventions.
- Recognition and screening abilities need to be increased, for example through the use of screening instruments validated in primary care.
- Practice nurses, district nurses, health visitors and midwives are highly skilled practitioners and their skills can be built upon and developed so that they are better equipped to deliver primary care mental health.
- Ongoing training and education are required, preferably delivered to whole primary care teams, together with the provision of clinical supervision.

---

# Further reading and e-resources

BMJ clinical evidence for best-evidence reviews, http://clinicalevidence.bmj.com/ceweb/conditions/index.jsp

Drink-Less Programme, http://www.cs.nsw.gov.au/drugahol/drinkless/

MoodGYM training programme, http://moodgym.anu.edu.au. This is an internet cognitive–behavioural therapy programme.

National Institute for Health and Clinical Excellence, http://www.nice.org.uk. Resources and leaflets for patients and their carers on mental health and behavioural conditions can be downloaded from here.

No Panic, http://www.nopanic.org.uk. Website for patients and carers experiencing anxiety-related disorders.

Nursing and Midwifery Council in the UK, http://www.nmc-uk.org.

WHO guide to mental and neurological health in primary care, http://www.mentalneurologicalprimarycare.org. Resources for patients on various common mental illnesses can be downloaded from here

Youth in Mind, http://www.youthinmind.co.uk. Website with mental health resources/links for parents, teachers and young people.

# References

American Psychiatric Association (1994) *Diagnostic and Statistical Manual of Mental Disorders* (4th edn) (DSM–IV). APA.

Anderson, P. (1993) Effectiveness of general practice interventions for patients with harmful alcohol consumption. *British Journal of General Practice*, **43**, 386–389.

Appleby, L., Hirst, E., Marshall, S., *et al* (2003) The treatment of postnatal depression by health visitors: impact of brief training on skills and clinical practice. *Journal of Affective Disorders*, **77**, 261–266.

Armstrong, E. (1997) Do PNs want to learn about depression? *Practice Nursing*, **8**, 21–26.

Audit Commission (1994) *Finding a Place: A Review of Mental Health Services for Adults*. HMSO.

Boardman, J. (1997) *Community Psychiatric Nursing*. Occasional paper OP40. Royal College of Psychiatrists.

Botega, N., Mann, A. & Blizard, R. (1992) General practitioners and depression – first use of the depression attitude questionnaire. *International Journal of Methods in Psychiatric Research*, **2**, 169–180.

Bowles, N., Mackintosh, C. & Torn, A. (2001) Nurses' communication skills: an evaluation of the impact of solution-focussed communication training. *Journal of Advanced Nursing*, **36**, 347–354.

British Medical Association (2006) *Quality and Outcomes Framework Guidance: Depression*. Downloadable from http://www.bma.org.uk

Brown, E. L., McAvay, G., Raue, P. J., *et al* (2003) Recognition of depression among elderly recipients of home care services. *Psychiatric Service*, **54**, 208–213.

Burroughs, H., Lovell, K., Morley, M., *et al* (2006) 'Justifiable depression': how primary care professionals and patients view late-life depression? A qualitative study. *Family Practice*, **23**, 369–377.

Casey, P. R. (1990) *A Guide to Psychiatry in Primary Care*. Wrightson Biomedical Publishing.

Clement, S. (1986) The identification of alcohol related problems by general practitioners. *British Journal of Addiction*, **81**, 257–264.

Crisp, A. H. (1999) The stigmatisation of sufferers with mental disorders. *British Journal of General Practice*, **13**, 172–176.

Crossland, A. & Kai, J. (1998) They think they can talk to nurses: practice nurses' views of their roles in caring for mental health problems. *British Journal of General Practice*, **48**, 1383–1386.

Deehan, A., Templeton, L., Taylor, C., *et al* (1998) Are practice nurses an unexplored resource in the identification and management of alcohol misuse? Results from a study of practice nurses in England and Wales in 1995. *Journal of Advanced Nursing*, **28**, 592–597.

Department of Health (1994) *Working in Partnership. A Collaborative Approach to Care*. Report of the Mental Health Nursing Review Team. HMSO.

Department of Health (1995) *Building Bridges. A Guide to Arrangements for Inter-Agency Working for the Care and Protection of Severely Mentally Ill People*. Department of Health.

Department of Health (2006) *Recruitment and Retention of Mental Health Nurses: Good Practice Guide*. The Chief Nursing Officer's review of mental health nursing. Department of Health. Downloadable from http://www.dh.gov.uk/en/Publicationsandstatistics/Publications/PublicationsPolicyAndGuidance/DH_4133976

Doherty, J. P. (1997) Barriers to the diagnosis of depression in primary care. *Journal of Clinical Psychiatry*, **58**, 5–10.

Eisses, A. M., Kluiter, H., Jongenelis, K., *et al* (2005) Care staff training in detection of depression in residential homes for the elderly: randomised trial. *British Journal of Psychiatry*, **186**, 404–409.

Gray, R., Parr, A-M., Plummer, S. E., *et al* (1999) A national survey of practice nurse involvement in mental health interventions. *Journal of Advanced Nursing*, **30**, 901–906

Haddad, M. (2007) *A Cluster Randomised Trial of a Training Intervention for a District Nursing Service to Improve the Detection and Outcome of Common Mental Disorders*. PhD Thesis, University of London.

Haddad, M., Plummer, S. E., Taverner, A., *et al* (2005) District nurses' involvement and attitudes to mental health problems: a three-area cross-sectional study. *Journal of Clinical Nursing*, **14**, 976–985.

Hunkeler, E. M., Meresman, J. F., Hargreaves, W. A., *et al* (2000) Efficacy of nurse tele-health care and peer support in augmenting treatment of depression in primary care. *Archives of Family Medicine*, **9**, 700–708.

Jackson, R. & Baldwin, B. (1993) Detecting depression in elderly medically ill patients: the use of the Geriatric Depression Scale compared with medical and nursing observations. *Age and Ageing*, **22**, 349–353.

Katon, W. J., Von Korff, M., Lin, E. H., *et al* (2004) The Pathways Study: a randomised trial of collaborative care in patients with diabetes and depression. *Archives of General Psychiatry*, **61**, 1042–1049.

Kendrick, T., Sibbald, B., Addington-Hall, J., *et al* (1993) Distribution of mental health professionals working on site in English and Welsh general practices. *BMJ*, **307**, 544–546.

Kessler, D., Lloyd, K., Lewis, G., *et al* (1999) Cross-sectional study of symptom attribution and recognition of depression and anxiety in primary care. *BMJ*, **318**, 436–440.

Lock, C. A. & Kaner, E. F. (2004) Implementation of brief alcohol interventions by nurses in primary care: do non-clinical factors influence practice? *Family Practice*, **21**, 270–275.

McManus, S., Meltzer, H., Brugha, T., *et al* (2009) *Adult Psychiatric Morbidity in England, 2007. Results of a Household Survey.* The NHS Health and Social Care Information Centre. Downloadable from http://www.ic.nhs.uk/webfiles/publications/mental%20health/other%20mental%20health%20publications/Adult%20psychiatric%20morbidity%2007/APMS%2007%20%28FINAL%29%20Standard.pdf

Millar, E., Garland, C., Ross, F., *et al* (1999) Practice nurses and the care of patients receiving depot neuroleptic treatment: views on training, confidence and use of structured assessment. *Journal of Advanced Nursing*, **29**, 1454–1461.

Morrell, C. J., Slade, R., Warner, R., *et al* (2009) Clinical effectiveness of health visitor training in psychologically informed approaches for depression in postnatal women: pragmatic cluster randomised trial in primary care. *BMJ*, **338**, a3045.

Moussavi, S., Chatterji, S., Verdes, E., *et al* (2007) Depression, chronic diseases, and decrements in health: results from the World Health Surveys. *Lancet*, **370**, 851–858.

Murray, J., Banerjee, S., Byng, R., *et al* (2006) Primary care professionals' perceptions of depression in older people: a qualitative study. *Social Science Medicine*, **63**, 1363–1373.

Mynors-Wallis, L. M., Davies, I., Gray, A., *et al* (1997) A randomised controlled trial and cost analysis of problem solving treatment for emotional disorders given by community nurses in primary care. *British Journal of Psychiatry*, **170**, 113–119.

National Institute for Health and Clinical Effectiveness (2007) *Management of Depression in Primary and Secondary Care.* NICE.

NHS Information Centre, Workforce and Facilities (2009) *General and Personal Medical Services, England 1998–2008.* The NHS Information Centre for Health and Social Care. Downloadable from http://www.ic.nhs.uk/webfiles/publications/nhsstaff2008/gp/Bulletin%20Sept%202008.pdf

Nursing and Midwifery Council (2001) *Standards for Specialist Education and Practice.* NMC.

Nursing and Midwifery Council (2004*a*) *Standards of Proficiency for Pre-registration Midwifery Education.* NWC.

Nursing and Midwifery Council (2004*b*) *Standards of Proficiency for Specialist Public Health Nurses.* NMC.

Nutting, P. A., Dickinson, L. M., Rubenstein, L., *et al* (2005) Improving detection of suicidal ideation among depressed patients in primary care. *Annals of Family Medicine*, **3**, 529–536.

O'Hara, M. W. & Swain, A. M. (1996) Rates and risks of post-natal depression – a meta-analysis. *International Review of Psychiatry*, **8**, 37–54.

Peveler, R., George, C., Kinmouth, A. L., *et al* (1999) Effect of antidepressant drug counselling and information leaflets on adherence to drug treatment in primary care: randomised controlled trial. *BMJ*, **319**, 612–615.

Plummer, S. E. (2003) *A Randomised Controlled Trial to Detect Benefit from Training Practice Nurses in the Detection and Management of Psychological Distress in Patients Attending Their Clinics.* PhD Thesis, University of London.

Plummer, S. E., Ritter, S., Leach, R. A., *et al* (1997) A controlled comparison of the ability of practice nurses to detect psychological distress in patients who attend their clinics. *Journal of Psychiatric and Mental Health Nursing,* **4,** 221–223.

Plummer, S. E., Gournay, K., Goldberg, D., *et al* (2000) Detection of psychological distress by practice nurses in general practice. *Psychological Medicine,* **30,** 1233–1237.

Pouwer, F., Beekman, A. T. & Lubach, C. (2006) Nurses' recognition and registration of depression, anxiety and diabetes-specific emotional problems in outpatients with diabetes mellitus. *Patient Education Counselling,* **60,** 235–240.

Preville, M., Cote, G. & Boyer, R. (2004) Detection of depression and anxiety disorders by home care nurses. *Ageing and Mental Health,* **8,** 400–409.

Redsell, S., Stokes, T., Jackson, C., *et al* (2007) Patients' accounts of the differences in nurses' and general practitioners' roles in primary care. *Journal of Advanced Nursing,* **57,** 172–180.

Saunders, J. B., Aasland, O. G., Amundsen, A., *et al* (1993) Alcohol consumption and related problems among healthy primary care patients: WHO collaborative project on early detection of persons with harmful alcohol consumption. *Addiction,* **88,** 349–362.

Simon, G. E., Von Korff, M., Rutter, C., *et al* (2000) Randomised trial of monitoring, feedback and management of care by telephone to improve treatment of depression in primary care. *BMJ,* **320,** 550–554.

Standart, S. H., Drinkwater, C. & Scott, J. (1997) Multidisciplinary training in the detection, assessment and management of depression in primary care. *Primary Care Psychiatry,* **3,** 89–93.

Thomas, R. V. R.& Corney, R. H. (1993) The role of the practice nurse in mental health: a survey. *Journal of Mental Health,* **2,** 65–72.

Tylee, A. (2001) Training the whole primary care team. In *Common Mental Disorders in Primary Care* (eds M. Tansella & G. Thornicroft), pp. 194–208. Routledge.

Tylee, A., Freeling, P., Kerry, S., *et al* (1995) How does the content of consultations affect the recognition by general practitioners of major depression in women? *British Journal of General Practice,* **45,** 575–578.

Wickberg, B. & Hwang, C. P. (1996) Counselling of postnatal depression: a controlled study on a population based Swedish sample. *Journal of Affective Disorders,* **39,** 209–216.

# Part IV: Reflective practice

The concept of the reflective practitioner was introduced by the educationalist Donald Schön in the 1980s in his book *The Reflective Practitioner* (1983). Reflective practice can be defined in a number of different ways, but all the definitions encapsulate a range of activities associated with both learning and thinking about the process of learning. Essentially, it is a continuous process from a personal perspective, informed by considering critical life experiences. As defined by Schön, reflective practice involves thoughtfully considering one's own experiences in applying knowledge to practice while being coached by professionals in the discipline.

This fits well with developments in undergraduate medical education that rely on 'problem-based learning' and are facilitated by self and peer assessment in conjunction with formal assessment processes. In problem-based learning, which over the past quarter century (Barrows, 1983) has evolved into the standard approach to undergraduate education in medical schools across the world, students collaborate to study the issues inherent in even the simplest of problems and strive to create viable solutions. Unlike traditional instruction, which is often conducted in lecture format, teaching in problem-based learning normally occurs within small discussion groups of students facilitated by a faculty tutor. However, traditional postgraduate medical education has somewhat lagged behind these developments and has not actively encouraged or formalised reflective learning from practice.

In the UK, this is changing with the advent of the National Health Service appraisal system and the development, by the Royal Colleges, of portfolios of learning and progress in training. This is now being taken forward into revalidation processes in the recertification subsection proposed by the Chief Medical Officer for England and to be delivered throughout the UK. However, numerous challenges are faced in developing a truly reflective practice of teaching and learning.

The following chapters consider alternative approaches to the traditional format of postgraduate education: the lunchtime lecture. Two contrasting chapters consider the practical problems faced by practitioners as they attempt to bring together the two worlds of evidence-based practice and patient-centred care (Bensing, 2000). Last, but far from least, mental health is related to both the workload and the everyday working life of the practitioner.

# References

Barrows, H. S. (1983) Problem-based, self-directed learning. *JAMA*, **250**, 3077–3080.

Bensing, J. (2000) Bridging the gap. The separate worlds of evidence-based medicine and patient-centered medicine. *Patient Education and Counselling*, **39**, 17–25.

Schön, D. A. (1983) *The Reflective Practitioner: How Professionals Think in Action*. Temple Smith.

# CHAPTER 29

# Teaching and learning about mental health

Linda Gask, David Goldberg and Barry Lewis

Summary

Traditional experience provided in the setting of the psychiatric unit is insufficient for the acquisition of the competencies required for managing mental health problems in the primary care setting. A range of methods are described for teaching and learning specific skills, in particular for challenging attitudes.

## Mental health education in primary care

Learning about psychiatry or mental health has, for those entering primary care practice in most countries, been a rather 'hit and miss' affair. As specific vocational training in the specialty of 'general practice' has developed across Europe in the past 50 years, there has been increasing recognition of the need for specific training in mental health, but the form that this should take has not always been clear. Experience of mental healthcare in large mental asylums is not appropriate preparation for the reality of mental healthcare in the broader community. In many low- and middle-income countries, specific training for primary care is now in place, although the mental health content of the curricula is generally still under consideration and thus able to be shaped.

In the UK, the informal curriculum was usually based on clinical practice in specialist hospital units, covered the 'severe' end of the spectrum of mental ill health and was usually knowledge rather than skills based. Research looking at the needs of general practice trainees (Williams, 1998) highlighted the gap between traditional, knowledge-based teaching and the trainees' desire for practical skills development, with feedback on these skills in relation to mental health practice in primary care. Posts undertaken as part of the formal vocational training for general practitioners (GPs) in the 1990s were difficult to access and, usually, were part of acute, hospital-based services, with little or no primary care orientation.

In the UK, general practice specialist training, developed from the original GP vocational training programmes and now approved by the Postgraduate Medical Education and Training Board (PMETB), has a clear curriculum defined by the Royal College of General Practitioners (RCGP; see web link under Further reading and e-resources). Achievement of a Certificate of Completion of Training (CCT) for general practice involves 'time served' in appropriate and approved posts, workplace-based assessments of specific competencies, a clinical skills assessment at an independent centre and an applied knowledge test relevant to practice in UK primary care. As all of this is 'competency' based, the curriculum has had to define the broad competencies to be achieved in each clinical area. The RCGP curriculum statement 13, *Care of People with Mental Health Problems* (RCGP, 2007) links the six 'competency' areas for GP training with a wide range of mental health problems encountered in primary care (Box 29. 1). The competency

---

**Box 29.1** Competency areas for general practitioner training

The Royal College of General Practitioners (RCGP, 2007) lists six 'competency' areas for GP training with the wide range of mental health problems encountered in primary care:

- primary care management
- problem solving
- person-centred care
- comprehensive approach
- community orientation
- holistic care.

These are applied to the following areas of primary care mental health:

- bereavement
- dementia
- delirium
- alcohol and drug misuse
- chronic psychotic disorders
- acute psychotic disorders
- bipolar disorder
- depression
- phobic disorders
- panic disorders
- general anxiety
- chronic mixed anxiety and depression
- adjustment disorders
- post-traumatic stress disorder
- unexplained somatic complaints
- eating disorder
- sexual disorders
- learning disability
- chronic fatigue syndrome.

---

areas can be further refined to delineate the practical skills needed to demonstrate competence and to practise effectively (Table 29.1).

Using the templates in Box 29.1 and Table 29.1 will allow GPs and trainees in GP specialist training to reflect on their practice in terms of their current clinical exposure. For those undertaking a hospital post in mental health, they will be expected to reflect on their skill and competency development in terms of their ultimate career intention (i.e. 'Am I learning and developing skills now that will allow me to practise effectively in the future?'). To do this during a specific hospital mental health post or for trainees with no access to a post through the GP programme, there will need to be formal 'taught' sessions that address the competencies so that they can be further developed, by reflection as well as supervisor feedback, when practised in a primary care setting. A course that delivers this curriculum has been very successfully run by two of the authors in the north-west of England over 1 day per week for 9 days over the past several years.

Those teaching and developing courses for postgraduate trainees in primary care in the UK need to be cognisant of the RCGP curriculum

**Table 29.1** Competency areas for training

| Primary care management | Description |
|---|---|
| Knowledge | Aetiology, diagnostic criteria, management options, local and national guidelines |
| Coordination of care | Within practice, in local team, referral, team working and multi-agency coordination |
| Practice 'issues' in delivering care | Team structures, skills and competencies. Protocols and pathways for care. Governance and risk management |
| Problem solving | |
|   ability to identify and diagnose in primary care | Apply knowledge and skills in clinical setting to produce a differential diagnosis and recognise serious diagnoses |
|   ability to manage in primary care | Ability to formulate a safe and appropriate management plan |
| Person-centred care | Effective doctor–patient communication, respecting autonomy, continuity of care, contextualising illness in family and societal settings, awareness of values and beliefs |
| Comprehensive approach | Managing multiple health problems and comorbidity, prioritisation of problems, health promotion, medico-legal issues |
| Community orientation | Reconciling individual and community health needs, resource management, meeting local needs |
| Holistic care | Assessing psychological and social aspects of illness in parallel with the physical aspects. Caring for the whole person in the context of the family, culture and beliefs |
| Attitudinal aspects of care | Awareness of the effects of attitudes on care delivery. Duties of a doctor |

From RCGP (2007).

statements, the competencies outlined and the skills needed to deliver them effectively. Many of the skills are 'transferable' and should be recognised as such by trainees and their supervisors. This 'competency spine', applicable to any clinical topic area, forms the basis for reflection and may, in the future, be a key component of revalidation processes in the UK. A formal competency framework for those GPs in the UK who seek to specialise further ('GP with a special interest in mental health') and work at the interface between primary and specialist care has yet to be agreed, although some Masters-level courses are already running (see Further reading and e-resources).

However, it must be remembered that in many lower-income countries there is neither a formal national health system nor any insurance system that allows practitioners the luxury of time off for training. The widely used fee-for-service method of payment ensures, for example, that in Pakistan a GP may work from 8 a.m. or earlier to 11 p.m. or later, 6½ days a week, with a good number working out of 24-hour clinics. Training in these settings has to be based on attractive and simple modules rather than extensive and complicated texts that no GP will follow in practice after the training.

# Gaps in knowledge

In the UK, the RCGP curriculum begins with the assumption that all trainees will have had a thorough undergraduate training experience in psychiatry and will have a basic understanding of the nature of key mental health problems such as psychosis and depression. In some parts of the world, undergraduate medical education in psychiatry may have been lacking and there is a knowledge gap to close. Many doctors, however, have simply not been exposed to very much mental health training since their undergraduate days and their knowledge may be out of date. They may not be familiar with the features that need to be considered in order to justify a diagnosis and a suggested intervention, the psychosocial interventions that have been shown to be effective in particular disorders, or the efficacy of pharmacological interventions for such disorders. The World Health Organization's *Classification of Mental Disorders for Primary Health Care* (ICD–10–PHC; see Further reading and e-resources and Chapter 3), gives detailed advice on the management of the 24 mental disorders that are most commonly encountered in primary care. In their original form, these consisted of a set of 24 cards, which was subjected to a field trial in 15 countries; the British field trial (Goldberg *et al*, 1995) showed that use of the depression card caused doctors to require more depressive symptoms before they would prescribe antidepressants, and added to their management strategies when dealing with a depressive episode. However, it should not automatically be assumed that a knowledge deficit is the main problem: it is far more common for doctors to have attitudinal problems and skill deficits of which they are unaware.

Teaching can also be provided about specific psychosocial interventions – what they are and for whom or what they work. For example, problem-solving for depression (see Chapter 26 and Mynors-Wallis, 2005), simple behavioural interventions such as motivational interviewing for alcohol problems (see Chapter 26 and Miller & Rollnick, 1992), graded exercise combined with cognitive–behavioural strategies for fatigue, and reattribution for medically unexplained symptoms (see Chapter 11 and Gask *et al*, 1999).

Lectures designed to convey essential knowledge should:

- be brief
- be tailored to the needs of the audience (too often psychiatrists present what only psychiatrists need or want to know and do not address the needs of primary care)
- have plenty of opportunity for questions and discussion
- be supported by good handouts, with key references and web links.

In their review of the literature, Hodges *et al* (2001) noted the mismatch between what psychiatrists wanted to teach and what primary care workers wanted to learn:

> Primary care physicians most often wanted to increase their knowledge regarding somatisation, psychosexual problems, difficult patients, and stress management, whereas psychiatrists emphasised the diagnostic criteria of disorders such as schizophrenia, bipolar disorder, and depression.... Education that is focused on diagnosis and medication may neglect the very cornerstone of psychiatric primary care, which is learning to develop and maintain effective relationships with patients who have complex problems. (p. 1580)

The impact of this mismatch may be one of the reasons why education programmes have been less than successful (see Chapter 24 and also Gask *et al*, 2005).

It is also important to explore how primary care workers can find out about local resources in their area and link in with the specialist services and non-governmental organisations (NGOs) which can provide them with necessary expertise and support. These agencies may be invited to participate in the training, but it is essential to ensure that they fully understand the purpose of the training and do not see this as an opportunity simply to ensure referrals to their own organisation. However large such agencies or institutions are, they cannot perform the essential role of front-line workers; nonetheless, they may feel unnecessarily threatened (as seems to be the case in some countries) by attempts to develop the role of primary care workers.

## Challenging attitudes

Doctors who are insensitive to mental health problems are often found to have unhelpful attitudes towards such patients. A useful way of measuring attitudes to depression, for example, is the Depression Attitude Questionnaire (DAQ), which has been used across the world in very different settings (Botega *et al*, 1992). Problematic attitudes may arise because these doctors have no management strategies for helping such patients and they may benefit from acquisition of new skills. However, other methods, such as group discussion, may also be useful in challenging unhelpful attitudes. This can be triggered by case presentations, videotaped interviews or, most powerfully, by people telling their own stories about their experiences of mental illness and of mental healthcare; this is known as the 'contact hypothesis' (Allport, 1954).

# Developing skills

In general terms, the skill needed to deal with mental health problems in primary care is that of any good communicator – to allow patients to tell their story in their own way, and to be curious about recent events in patients' lives that may be subjecting them to stress. This sounds very simple – but it is not. Patients most typically present with somatic symptoms, and often have combinations of real physical disorders and other symptoms for which no obvious cause has been found. The doctor is under time pressure to bring the interview to a satisfactory resolution, and needs to exclude possible organic causes for the patient's various symptoms. The temptation is to interrupt the patient with an agenda of the doctor's own, and systematically to exclude possible physical causes before the patient has been given a chance to describe the symptoms fully. The average time that a GP listens without interrupting a patient has been found to be 22 seconds (Marvel *et al*, 1999).

This early stage of the interview can last anything from 20 seconds to several minutes – but during it the doctor should encourage patients to talk, and should ask more open-ended questions that give patients freedom to describe their symptoms in their own way. Provided that patients are encouraged to do this, the moment will soon arise when the doctor becomes more directive and exerts more control over the interview. When symptoms are described that sound atypical, or for which there are no obvious physical causes, the doctor may need to supplement the information presented with a knowledge of the patient's home and family background, or to discover whether there have been stressful life events. When cues arise that suggest psychological distress, the doctor should be alert to them, and follow them up with directive questions.

Interviews in primary care oscillate between personal questions about the family and allowing more of the description of the somatic symptoms to emerge. From time to time it may be necessary to make some supportive comment to the patient. Skills found to be particularly important in the detection of psychological problems in primary care are summarised in Box 29.2.

**Box 29.2** Ten aspects of a general practitioner's interview style that are related to the ability to assess a patient's emotional problems

**Early in the interview**
1  Makes good eye contact
2  Clarifies presenting complaint
3  Uses directive questions for physical complaints
4  Begins with open-ended questions, moving to closed questions later

**Interview style**
5  Makes empathic comments
6  Picks up verbal cues
7  Picks up non-verbal cues
8  Does not read notes during the taking of the history
9  Can deal with over-talkativeness
10 Asks fewer questions about past history

These observations on the GP consultation came about by analysing many hundreds of interviews, in the course of which it became clear that doctors who are good at detecting emotional disorders have patients who make it easy for them, by exhibiting more cues relating to distress than similarly distressed patients being interviewed by less-sensitive doctors (Marks *et al*, 1979; Davenport *et al*, 1987). What is happening (Goldberg *et al*, 1993) is that the doctors who are less sensitive to emotional distress discourage free communication and that patients become aware of this very early on. Some of the GP's behaviours that discourage patients are: not making eye contact; having a more avoidant posture at the beginning of the interview; interrupting patients before they have finished speaking; and asking many closed questions (those to which the patient must reply 'yes' or 'no'). Patients picking up these cues from the doctor speak with less distress in their voice, keep their hands and arms still, and are much less likely to mention psychological symptoms. Some behaviours release cues only when carried out by doctors who are *more* sensitive to emotional distress, but not when done by *less*-sensitive doctors – these are questions about the patient's social life, having an empathic manner and the total number of questions dealing with the patient's psychological adjustment. By contrast, patients interviewed by doctors good at picking up distress are encouraged by the doctor's attentive posture and tendency to make eye contact with them; these doctors make more facilitative comments and gestures while listening and ask questions with a psychological content, and in a directive rather than a closed style.

Related work (Millar & Goldberg, 1991) has shown that doctors who are sensitive to the emotional distress of their patients have generally superior communication skills, and are better able to prescribe medication, communicate information about treatment more effectively, and give advice more clearly than doctors who are less sensitive. Thus, doctors with superior communication skills make detection of distress easy for themselves, by behaving in a way that makes it easy for the patient to display the distress that is being felt. Doctors who are less good manage to make patients suppress evidence of their distress, which is often not manifest even on viewing a videotape of the consultation.

In addition to improving *general* communication skills, there are also a number of *specific skills* that may need improving in relation to particular types of mental health problem. For example, the set of skills required to assess and manage depression effectively include those in Box 29.3.

# Methods for teaching skills

## Modelling skills using prepared videotapes/DVDs

The use of video-feedback in changing professional behaviour goes back 20 years, and the first systematic studies of teaching the skills described above came from several sources. It is important that the required skills are modelled by actual primary care workers, and not by mental health professionals somehow expecting that primary care doctors and nurses will copy them. This can be done 'in vivo' in a role-play or using a prepared teaching video (see e-resources).

In some countries, it may be more appropriate to use these resources as templates for the production of more culturally appropriate local materials. However, they can be dubbed over in the local language at relatively low cost (this is generally much less expensive than subtitling) and this approach has been used successfully within Europe. There are usually discussion points during the video, and most also have notes for teachers, reminding them of things to elicit from the group at such points. The teacher acts as a facilitator during such discussions, encouraging those who have not spoken to contribute, and agreeing with suggestions that seem helpful. If someone suggests something that the teacher considers unhelpful, the teacher can ask others in the group how they would handle such moments, rather than openly disagreeing with the speaker. The teacher is generally supportive of the group, and only suggests his or her own solutions if they do not emerge in the general discussion.

## The use of role-playing to practise skills

Health professionals, including doctors and nurses working in primary care, are unlikely to try their new skills out with real patients until they have practised them in safer circumstances – and this is where role-playing comes in. For each role-play, it is necessary to prepare three documents: one for the person who will play the professional, one for the 'patient' and one for the observer. This threesome constitutes the 'trio'.

**Box 29.3** Skills for the primary care assessment and management of depression

**Assessment in the consultation**
*Psychological*
- Assess of severity of illness (preferably using a standardised measure such as the PHQ–9)
- Ask about:
  - suicide risk, deliberate self-harm
  - presence or absence of anxiety symptoms
  - duration, chronicity
  - pattern of illness
  - past history
  - associated alcohol and drug use
  - psychotic features.

*Social*
- Ask about:
  - nature of social difficulties
  - social support or lack of confidants
  - background vulnerability factors
  - family history.

*Physical*
- Examination/investigation of causes
- Comorbidity (e.g. diabetes, coronary heart disease)

**Management within the consultation**
- Listen, empathise
- Explain diagnosis
- Explain somatic symptoms
- Address patient's ideas and concerns
- Agree problem list
- Negotiate management plan
- Self-help literature
- Antidepressants
- Build trust
- Arrange follow-up to monitor progress

Brief psychological strategies that may be employed during the consultation and acquired using the methods described in this chapter include:

- Behavioural activation
- Self-help
- Problem-solving approach
- Anxiety management
- Simple motivational strategies.

In this role-play, health professionals are told what the practice knows about the patient who is about to be seen: not the actual medical notes, but the relevant information about the patient that would normally have been available. Patients play someone of their own age and gender, but are typically given another occupation. They are told their presenting symptoms, and any life events that may have occurred recently, which they may or may not wish to tell the health professional about. If asked questions that have not been covered, they are advised to answer them from their personal experience.

Observers are given the most information: all that on the other two forms, as well as the behaviours they are looking out for. After the enactment they are asked to do three things:

1    ask the professional how she or he felt the interview went (what pleased her or him about it and whether there was anything that could have been improved)
2    ask the 'patient' how he or she felt about the interview, and how the problem was handled (what he or she liked and whether anything could have been improved)
3    give the health professional feedback last of all, based upon the observations.

The teachers (there should, ideally, be one teacher to six health professionals) move from one set of health professionals to another, offering advice and help as they find appropriate. The enactments should be quite short – no more than about 4 minutes, with the feedback and discussion typically taking another 10–15 minutes. The trio then proceeds to the next role-play, changing roles so that each doctor gets a chance to play the health professional. It is important that such role-plays are adapted to the conditions of the culture in which teaching is occurring, and that sufficient copies are made for several trios to use the same role-play.

## Using videotape of the trainees' own consultations

Videotape and audiotape feedback have been used in the acquisition of skills for many years. In the UK, the best-known model for educational sessions using video-feedback is that described by Pendleton *et al* (1984). Their rules for giving feedback are shown in Box 29.4.

The Cambridge–Calgary model (Kurtz *et al*, 2004) is also now widely used in UK medical schools in the teaching of communication skills using video. Lesser (1981), who had called his method of audiotape teaching developed in Canada in the early 1980s 'problem-based interviewing', came over to England and helped to turn his method into a group teaching course using video feedback. This method has been extensively evaluated in the teaching of psychological skills (Gask, 1998) and is discussed in more detail below.

When showing a videotape, the teacher should always ask the health professional who made it for permission to show it, and to invite him or her to comment before inviting comments from others. It will usually be found that the person who made the tape makes the most critical remarks

---

**Box 29.4** Rules for giving feedback in a one-to-one teaching session

1 Briefly clarify matters of fact.
2 The learner goes first and discusses what went well.
3 The trainer discusses what went well.
4 The learner describes what could be done differently and makes suggestions for change.
5 The trainer identifies what could be done differently and gives options for change.
6 The learner and trainer agree on the priorities for change and a method and timescale for meeting them

From Pendleton *et al* (1984).

---

about his or her own performance, and that others are more supportive. If people make critical comments, they should be asked what they would have done in such a situation, before others are asked. In general, teachers elicit responses *from the group*, rather than allowing themselves to be identified as all-knowing gurus.

Our suggested guidelines for teaching using group video-feedback, developed after many years of research and practice, are presented in Box 29.5.

Where videotapes of real patient material are being used, members of the group should respect normal medical confidentiality outside the group. They should also agree not to talk about other people's performance outside the group, otherwise this will detract from the group being able to relax and achieve some work. This may be particularly important if the group meets on several occasions and health professionals deal with issues they personally find particularly difficult in their consultations and take the risk to bring consultations to show that demonstrate these difficulties.

The teacher should draw attention to the items described in Boxes 29.2 and 29.3. At the end of each session it is helpful to leave time to ask the group about problems that they have experienced with emotionally distressed patients. The health professional presenting the problem should reflect on how he or she dealt with it and always allow others to comment on how they handle such problems.

## Balint groups

What we have described above is different from, but complementary to, the experience that might be gained in the setting of a Balint group. Balint (1957) was a psychoanalyst who had considerable influence on the development of a deeper psychological understanding of the dynamics of the doctor–patient consultation in primary care. He specifically emphasised

---

**Box 29.5** Problem-based approach: guidelines for group video-feedback

1  Set ground rules
   - Check out if person has seen himself or herself on video before. Ensure that the group realises this may be difficult and elicit support.
   - Anyone can stop the tape, but if they do they must say what they would have done or said differently at that point.
   - Ensure confidentiality of the group and also of the patient if this is a real consultation.
2  Set an agenda
   - Clarify the purpose of the session.
   - Fill in background.
   - Engage group in asking questions.
   - What does the person showing the tape want from the group?
3  Provide opportunities for rehearsing new skills
   - Stop the tape regularly at key points and invite the group members to do so.
   - Ask the group for comments on what has happened and whether anyone would do things differently.
   - Give the person showing the tape the first opportunity to comment.
   - Label key skills and strategies that are being utilised on the tape or suggested by the group.
4  Be constructive
   - Comment on things done well as frequently as possible without seeming false.
   - Positive comments should come first, followed by things that might have been done differently.
5  Make the group do the work
   - Facilitate, not demonstrate.
   - Summarise suggestions and keep the session flowing.
   - Ensure the group keeps to the agenda.
6  Conclude positively
   - Summarise and ask for feedback from the person showing tape and the group.
   - Facilitate the development of an action plan for future consultation if this is a real patient.
   - Assist in formulation of new learning goals.

---

the importance of the doctor's personal impact on the outcome, and looked on the doctor as a 'drug', whose 'pharmacology' he wanted to study in the group setting. In a Balint group, members discuss their patients and reflect on their encounters with them, usually in the presence of a leader who has had specific psychotherapeutic (psychodynamic) training. Balint groups do not aim to teach specific communication skills; audio- or videotapes of the patients are not used, but members aim to develop their personal and professional psychological skills and development by discussing and reflecting on the feelings that their encounter with the patient engenders in the group, which usually runs for at least a number of months, if not longer, on a weekly basis. Balint training has been probably more influential in European training of general practitioners in recent years than in the UK setting (Kjeldmand *et al*, 2004).

# Evaluation of teaching and learning

A simple framework for the evaluation of training was proposed by Kirkpatrick (1994). Application of this model to teaching and learning mental health skills in primary care can be found in Table 29.2. Most

**Table 29.2** Kirkpatrick's levels of evaluation applied to education in primary care mental health

| Level | Evaluation type (what is measured) | Examples of measures | Relevance and practicability |
|---|---|---|---|
| Reaction | Reaction evaluation is how the delegates felt about the training or learning experience | Satisfaction of trainees with course Self-rated measures of morale, confidence before/after training Interviews with trainees Questionnaires | Quick and very easy to obtain Not expensive to gather or to analyse |
| Learning | Learning evaluation is the measurement of the increase in knowledge or intellectual capacity | Simple before/after training using reliable tools Knowledge tests; attitude tests (e.g. DAQ) Skills acquisition using blind ratings of role-played interviews These may be combined in observed structured clinical examinations (OSCEs) | Relatively simple to set up; clear-cut for quantifiable skills Less easy for complex learning |
| Behaviour | Behaviour evaluation is the extent of applied learning when 'back on the job' | Ratings of real consultations with patients before/after training | Measurement of behaviour change requires considerable cooperation from organisation |
| Results | Results evaluation is the effect on the business or environment when the trainee returns to work | Impact on process and outcome of clinical care, such as actual prescribing behaviour Clinical outcomes for patients | Individually not difficult (audit), unlike when done for whole organisation Process must attribute clear accountabilities |

educational programmes have not been evaluated beyond the first of these levels: 'reaction'. Chapter 25 reviews of the evidence concerning the effect of educational programmes on quality improvement. In general, it can be concluded that, in higher-income countries, where primary care professionals have a good basic education in mental health, the impact of educational interventions when provided alone in postgraduate primary care education is limited. Educational interventions must be linked with interventions which also address organisational and attitudinal barriers to quality improvement. However, in settings where even more basic education is lacking, the opportunity to improve the quality of mental healthcare through targeted educational initiatives would seem to be considerably greater. Much research remains to be done in these settings.

## Conclusion

Training is most likely to be effective when the following conditions are met:

- *It is clearly meeting local needs.* What is needed – knowledge, skills, attitude change, or all of these? The most effective educational interventions are multifaceted, offering a range of possible options for doctors to learn from and providing the possibility for a range of different needs to be met.
- *It is clearly relevant to primary care* – preferably planned and delivered in partnership with primary care at a time and place that make it easy for workers to access it.
- *It is focused on those who need it.* We can conclude from the studies reviewed above that training for depression may have to be specifically targeted at those who really need it, as in many countries interested doctors will have already received some training.

---

### Key points

- In some parts of the world, undergraduate medical education in psychiatry may have been defective and there is a knowledge gap to close.
- What psychiatrists want to teach may not be the same as what primary care workers need or want to learn about.
- Unhelpful attitudes to mental health problems can be challenged in group discussion and through the acquisition of new skills.
- Both general and specific skills for the recognition and management of mental health problems can be acquired using a combination of modelling, role-pay and video-feedback.
- Most educational programmes have not received an adequate level of evaluation.

To be most effective at any one time, training needs to be 'sold' to the target audience, in such a way as to emphasise the potential benefits to health professionals as well as patients.

Training should include how to obtain specialist support from the mental healthcare system. Primary care workers need to know what to do with people they identify as having a mental health problem but whom they feel unable to manage themselves. If this is not clear, enthusiasm will wane.

Finally, training needs to be followed up. Just as with therapeutic interventions, teaching and learning interventions need review, booster sessions and follow-up.

## Further reading and e-resources

Blashki, G., Piterman, L. & Judd, F. (2007) *General Practice Psychiatry*. McGraw-Hill.
Centre for Clinical and Academic Workforce Innovation (2007) *Primary Care Mental Health*. Robinson.
Cohen, A. (ed) (2008) *Delivering Mental Health in Primary Care: An Evidence-Based Approach*. Royal College of General Practitioners.

Royal College of General Practitioners' mental health curriculum, http://www.rcgp-curriculum.org.uk/PDF/curr_Curriculum_Guide_for_Learners_and_Teachers.pdf
ICD–10–PHC, English version, http://www.mentalneurologicalprimarycare.org
Masters-level courses for GPs with a special interest in mental health, http://www.primhe.org/pdf/Primhe_Coursebrochure.pdf

Teaching DVDs available from:
Institute of Psychiatry, London, http://www.iop.kcl.ac.uk/departments/?locator=367&context=789
University of Manchester, http://www.medicine.manchester.ac.uk/psychiatrytrainingvideos

## References

Allport, G. W. (1954) *The Nature of Prejudice*. Addison-Wesley.
Balint, M. (1957) *The Doctor, His Patient and the Illness*. Pitman.
Botega, N., Mann, A., Blizard, R., *et al* (1992) General practitioners and depression: first use of the Depression Attitude Questionnaire. *International Journal of Methods in Psychiatric Research*, **2**, 169–180.
Davenport, S., Goldberg, D. & Millar, T. (1987) How psychiatric disorders are missed during medical consultations. *Lancet*, ii, 439–441.
Gask, L. (1998) Small group interactive techniques utilizing videofeedback. *International Journal of Psychiatry in Medicine*, **28**, 97–113.
Gask, L., Morris, R. & Goldberg, D. (1999) *Reattribution: Managing Patients Who Somatise Emotional Distress* (2nd edn). Manchester University Department of Psychiatry.
Gask, L., Dixon, C., May, C., *et al* (2005) Qualitative study of an educational intervention for general practitioners in the assessment and management of depression. *British Journal of General Practice*, **55**, 854–859.
Goldberg, D., Jenkins, L., Millar, T., *et al* (1993) The ability of trainee general practitioners to identify psychological distress among their patients. *Psychological Medicine*, **23**, 185–193.

Goldberg, D., Sharp, D. & Nanayakkara, K. (1995) The field trial of the mental disorders section of ICD–10 designed for primary care (ICD10–PHC) in England. *Family Practice*, **12**, 466–473.

Hodges, B., Inch, C. & Silver, I. (2001) Improving the psychiatric knowledge, skills, and attitudes of primary care physicians, 1950-2000: a review. *American Journal of Psychiatry*, **158**, 1579–1586.

Kirkpatrick, D. L. (1994) *Evaluating Training Programs: The Four Levels*. Berrett-Koehler.

Kjeldmand, D., Holmström, I. & Rosenqvist, U. (2004) Balint training makes GPs thrive better in their job. *Patient Education and Counselling*, **55**, 230–235.

Kurtz, S., Silverman, J. & Draper, J. (2004) *Teaching and Learning Communication Skills in Medicine*. Radcliffe.

Lesser, A. L. (1981) The psychiatrist and family medicine: a different training approach. *Medical Education*, **5**, 398–406.

Marks, J. N., Goldberg, D. P. & Hillier, V. F. (1979) Determinants of the ability of general practitioners to detect psychiatric illness. *Psychological Medicine*, **9**, 337–353.

Marvel, M. K., Epstein, R. K., Flowers, K., *et al* (1999) Soliciting the patient's agenda. Have we improved? *JAMA*, **277**, 678–682.

Millar, T. & Goldberg, D. P. (1991) Link between the ability to detect and manage emotional disorders: a study of general practitioner trainees. *British Journal of General Practice*, **41**, 357–359.

Miller, W. R. & Rollnick, S. (1992) *Motivational Interviewing: Preparing People to Change Addictive Behaviour*. Guilford Press.

Mynors-Wallis, L. (2005) *Problem Solving Treatment for Anxiety and Depression: A Practical Guide*. Oxford University Press.

Pendleton, D., Scofield, T., Tate, P., *et al* (1984) *The Consultation: An Approach to Learning and Teaching*. Oxford University Press.

RCGP (2007) *Care of People with Mental Health Problems*. Curriculum statement 13. Downloadable from http://www.rcgp-curriculum.org.uk/PDF/curr_13_Mental_Health.pdf

Williams, K. (1998) Self-assessment of clinical competence by general practitioner trainees before and after a six-month psychiatric placement. *British Journal of General Practice*, **48**, 1387–1390.

# CHAPTER 30

# Undertaking mental health research in primary care

Tony Kendrick, Robert Peveler and Linda Gask

Summary

This chapter outlines why practitioners in primary care should contribute to research, and factors they should consider when asked to participate. Various types of quantitative and qualitative research designs are discussed, with reference to influential published studies. Finally, the importance of research networks is outlined and one practitioner's journey from research participant to leading researcher is described.

## The need for primary care research

In countries with well-developed primary care services, the large majority of patient care is undertaken there. In the UK's National Health Service (NHS), more than 90% of patient contacts are in general practice. Differences in the range of severity and complexity of problems between primary care and secondary care mean that it is often not possible to extrapolate evidence from research findings in secondary care directly to the primary care context (this is dealt with in more detail in Chapter 31). Research therefore needs to be undertaken in primary care to be directly applicable, and it is in the best interests of primary care practitioners to contribute to research in whatever ways they can, to assist in the development of the evidence base for their own clinical practice.

Another reason why research has to be undertaken in primary care is that the views of primary care practitioners, patients, carers and other stakeholders, such as health service managers, are among the key determinants of what services can be and should be provided.

## Factors affecting practitioner involvement

A systematic review of 78 studies relating to problems of recruitment to randomised controlled trials in a variety of settings, which included primary care and community health services, was carried out in order to identify the most common barriers to participation by clinicians (Ross *et al*, 1999). They are listed in Box 30.1.

Moore & Smith (2007) carried out semi-structured interviews with 11 general practitioners (GPs) to get more in-depth insight into how practice decisions to participate in research were made and the key influences on the decision-making process. They found that practices had no formal process of assessing requests to participate in research studies, but decided in an *ad hoc* way, on a study-by-study basis. The presentation of the research proposal was key: practitioners valued a personal approach from another GP who could 'champion' the project from a GP perspective. They were swayed by interesting and relevant research questions, where there was likely to be direct benefit to patients involved in the study. They demanded clarity about the time commitment and workload involved, and what funding would be provided to the practice to compensate them for their involvement. They wanted the research team to deal with all bureaucratic barriers on behalf of the practice, and to feed back on the progress of the study and its findings.

## Evaluating offers to participate in research

Busy primary care practitioners have to be selective about the studies they get involved in, and the issues they should consider before responding to requests to participate in research are listed in Box 30.2.

## Quantitative research designs

Quantitative studies gather numerical or categorical data and often test a specific research hypothesis. They include:

- surveys of patients using questionnaires, standardised physical examinations, and/or structured interviews

---

**Box 30.1** Barriers to participation of clinicians in controlled trials

- An insufficiently interesting question
- A lack of time to help with recruitment on top of service commitments
- A lack of staff to help with research, and the need for staff training
- Difficulty with the consent procedure
- The possible negative effect on the doctor–patient relationship of asking patients to get involved in trials of new treatments
- Loss of professional autonomy and control over practice
- A lack of reward for and recognition of the involvement

---

**Box 30.2** Questions to consider when asked to participate in research

1 Is the research question an important one for primary care generally, or important for the local service?
  - Is the clinical topic significant (e.g. in terms of the severity or frequency of a medical condition, or both)?
  - Are the findings likely to inform clinical practice generally, or locally?
2 Can the proposed study be carried out within the resources available in the practice or primary care service?
  - If not, will the research team provide extra resource in order to make it at least cost-neutral to the practice or service?
  - What is the research team asking the practitioners and support staff to do? Recruiting patients in the course of consultations is much more challenging, for example, than identifying patients from their medical records and writing to them on behalf of the research team.
3 Have the researchers secured all the necessary approvals for the study to proceed?
  - Has the protocol been approved by a formally constituted research ethics committee? In the UK, any research involving NHS patients, staff or premises must be approved by an NHS ethics committee.
  - Has the Health Service approved it? In the UK, the Research Governance Framework applies and studies have to be approved by the relevant NHS body (the Primary Care Trust Research and Development Office for research in primary care).
  - Does it comply with other regulations on personal information? (In the UK, this includes the Data Protection Act 1998.)
4 Will the research team feed back on the progress of the study and its findings on completion?
  - Will the practice or service receive feedback on its own patients or practitioners, disaggregated from the rest of the participants?
5 Is the study design of sufficiently high quality?
  - Has it been through rigorous peer review? Most large studies will have had to undergo peer review in order to secure funding from national or international sources; small local studies may not have been reviewed as rigorously.
  - Does the study protocol include features indicating high-quality research? These vary according to the type of research design proposed.

---

- surveys of practitioners, using questionnaires or structured interviews
- studies of the causes of conditions, including cross-sectional, cohort, and case–control studies
- observational studies of interactions between practitioners and patients
- studies of new measures of health states, quality of life, or health beliefs, to determine their validity and reliability
- trials to determine the effectiveness and cost-effectiveness of healthcare interventions.

**441**

## Surveys

A survey observes a defined population at a single point in time or time interval and is the ideal design for describing the current state of practice. High-quality surveys will have a small number of very specific questions to address, and ideally should include a sample size calculation based on the most important outcome. All of the questions asked in the questionnaire or interview will relate directly to the outcomes of interest, rather than fishing around for other potentially interesting issues in an unfocused way. The design will include measures to maximise response rates, such as keeping questionnaires short, and identifying and following up non-responders. It should also include measures to determine any differences between the type of patients or practitioners taking part and those who decline, in order to estimate possible response bias, where those responding do not represent the whole range of possible participants and therefore the whole range of possible responses.

Examples of surveys in primary care mental health include a postal questionnaire survey of 507 GPs on their role in the care of people with long-term mental illness (Kendrick *et al*, 1991), which showed a marked lack of practice policies for reviewing their care and established that GPs were receptive to shared care arrangements, where the GP took responsibility for physical healthcare, with the psychiatric team monitoring mental health. Another example is Strang *et al*'s (2005) survey of a 10% national sample of GPs in 2001, which showed that half were prescribing methadone for opiate users, which was up by a factor of three since 1985, but that the doses used were often suboptimal (see Chapter 17).

## Descriptive studies of disorders

Descriptive studies of disorders are essential to explore possible causes or aggravating factors which might be amenable to intervention, and to describe the prognosis without treatment as a baseline for intervention studies. Studies of possible causes include *cross-sectional* studies which measure the extent of a disorder in a population and relate its extent to possible causes measured at the same point in time. However, a cross-sectional study can determine only what factors are associated with a disorder and cannot determine whether the factors are causes of the disorder, or might instead be effects of the disorder. To do that requires exploration of what came first, the disorder or the associated factor, which requires a longitudinal element to the study.

The ideal design to determine causal features of a disorder is a *cohort study*, which identifies a population at risk and determines their exposure to a possible causative factor at baseline, then follows them up over time to determine whether they develop the disorder. However, cohort studies are expensive to carry out because for most disorders a relatively large population at risk has to be assessed at baseline in order to include enough people who will develop the disorder. They then all have to be carefully followed up, usually for some years, to allow time for the disorder to develop. Ideally, all the people included at baseline have to be accounted for at follow-up, in order to avoid bias in the ascertainment of cases of the disorder, which makes cohort studies difficult as well as expensive. High-quality cohort studies will use exhaustive methods to identify and include the whole population at risk, careful examination of a whole range of possible causative factors and features of the disorder at baseline and follow-up, and measures to maintain contact with participants and ensure a low rate of attrition over time.

A *case–control study* is a more efficient design, which selects patients who already have the disorder and a group of comparison or 'control' patients who do not have the disorder but are as similar as possible in other respects (e.g. age, gender and social background) and examines whether they have previously been exposed to suspected causative factors. However, a case–control study is limited by the difficulty in assessing retrospectively what the true exposure of cases and controls was to possible causes, often many years after the possible exposure. It is important to consider possible *recall bias*, which can occur if the people with the disorder are, for one reason or another, more likely to identify past exposure to possible causal factors than people without the disorder. An example is the role of adversity in childhood as a possible cause of depression in adulthood: people who are currently depressed may have a more negative view of their childhood than people who are not depressed, because their current low mood colours their recall of childhood memories.

Examples of cross-sectional studies in mental health include the important epidemiological surveys showing the relationship between common mental disorders and social class, employment and poverty (Weich & Lewis, 1998a,b) (see Chapter 2). A good example of a case–control study is Osborn *et al*'s study of the relative risk of cardiovascular and cancer mortality in people with severe mental illness when compared with controls within the General Practice Research Database (see Chapter 20). A good example of a longitudinal study is Kessler *et al*'s (2002) research showing that, although many patients with depression did not receive a diagnosis at a single consultation, most were given a diagnosis at subsequent consultations over the next 2 years, or else recovered without a diagnosis anyway. That showed the extent to which depression remained undiagnosed much more realistically than previous cross-sectional studies (see Chapter 8).

## Observation of clinical practice

Observational studies include studies of clinical practice, where it is important to distinguish between *audit* and *research*. Audit is the measurement of practice against predetermined criteria of quality, derived from guidelines or from an existing consensus, and so finds out whether what *should* be being done *is* being done. Research studies of clinical practice also measure what is going on, but do so in order to answer a specific question or to test a specific hypothesis, the answer to which is not yet known, and so generate new knowledge. Like surveys, observational studies should ideally address a small number of specific questions, and include a sample size calculation, measures to maximise involvement, and measures to determine the representativeness of participants and possible response bias.

Examples of observational studies of primary care mental health practice include a study showing that GP recognition and treatment of depression were not associated with a good outcome for many patients, because recognition seemed to be a marker of severity, which was associated with a poorer prognosis. Furthermore, even when cases of depression identified through screening were brought to the GPs' attention, treatment was often inadequate and did not improve outcome over 12 months (Dowrick & Buchan, 1995). Another example is an observational study of GP assessment of the severity of depression, which showed that GPs were not good at distinguishing between mild depression and moderate depression, which meant their offers of antidepressants were not well targeted to patients who were the most likely to benefit (Kendrick et al, 2005). These studies and others suggested there would be benefit in using structured questionnaire measures for the assessment of severity prior to making decisions about treatment, which was subsequently rewarded through the GP contract Quality and Outcomes Framework in the UK (see Chapter 8).

## Controlled trials

A controlled trial is the ideal design to determine the efficacy or effectiveness of different treatments or approaches to disease management, including service developments such as the education of health professionals in disease recognition or management.

To determine the *efficacy* (the potential maximal effect) of an intervention, the ideal design is a controlled trial in which all the participants in the intervention group (chosen at random) receive the intervention as planned and this is compared with a placebo intervention (e.g. a dummy pill in a drug trial) in the comparison group, to control for the non-specific effects of intervening. To remove the effects of any prior expectations that the intervention will be effective, the participants receiving the intervention, and the clinicians delivering it, should ideally be unaware whether they are in the intervention or placebo arm of the trial (a randomised placebo-controlled double-blind trial). Drug trials should ideally be triple-blind; that is, the researchers assessing the outcomes in the two arms should also be unaware of the participants' allocation to group. In order to ensure blindness, the randomisation of participants to the different arms should be carried out entirely independently of the clinicians delivering the intervention, and of the researchers assessing the outcomes. In practice, this should involve remote randomisation (over the telephone or via the internet) by an independent party, rather than randomisation using numbered envelopes left with the treating clinician, since the envelopes can be opened and used in a different order than planned, by clinicians who, for one reason or another, wish to allocate their patients to the intervention or control groups themselves, instead of at random.

To determine the *effectiveness* of an intervention (its actual effect in practice as opposed to its potential maximal effect), studies need to be carried out in a setting as similar as possible to the everyday setting of treatment of the disorder. In open-label pragmatic trials, both the patients and the clinicians are aware of the intervention they are receiving, since this is the usual case in actual practice, although, ideally, the researchers assessing the patient outcomes should still remain blind to group allocation (something that is often difficult in practice). Self-completed outcome measures are preferable, since this avoids any possible interviewer bias due to the researchers consciously or unconsciously assessing the intervention and control patients in a systematically different way.

Examples of effective interventions for the management of depression which have been shown to work through controlled trials in primary care include problem-solving therapy (Mynors-Wallis *et al*, 1995, 2000), collaborative care management (Katon *et al*, 1995; Unutzer *et al*, 2002), and computerised cognitive–behavioural therapy (Proudfoot *et al*, 2004) (see Chapter 8). An example of an important negative trial is the Hampshire Depression Project, which showed that guideline-based education in itself did not lead to improvements in treatment or patient outcomes (Thompson *et al*, 2000; Kendrick *et al*, 2001) (see also Chapter 27).

## Systematic reviews

A systematic review is an overview of primary studies that used explicit and reproducible methods. Only high-quality trials are included. It limits bias by reducing the chance effects found in any individual study, providing more reliable results from which clinicians can draw conclusions and make decisions about treatment. It can include a meta-analysis, which is a mathematical synthesis of the results of two or more primary studies that addressed the same hypotheses in the same way.

Examples of important systematic reviews in primary care mental health include: Bower *et al*'s (2002) review of counselling studies, which found an advantage over usual care in the short term which was no longer evident after a year; Gilbody *et al*'s (2001, 2003) reviews of screening and complex interventions for depression (see Chapter 25); and MacGillivray *et al*'s (2003) systematic review of comparisons of tolerability and efficacy between serotonin reuptake inhibitors (SSRIs) and tricyclic antidepressants in primary care (see Chapter 8).

# Qualitative studies

Qualitative studies are used to increase understanding of people's behaviour from their own perspective, and to explore in-depth beliefs, attitudes and motivations of patients, practitioners and other stakeholders. High-quality qualitative studies will include features designed to capture the views of relevant stakeholders as faithfully as possible. Sampling will ideally be purposive, that is, directed at identifying people with the most relevant views and seeking out those who may have particularly extreme viewpoints in order to get a picture of the whole range of views. The initial interview questions, or topic guide, should be produced in the protocol, together with an indication that, following the initial guided questions, the direction and content of the interview will follow up on the participant's responses and not be restricted to a prearranged schedule such as would pertain in a structured interview study. The interviews will usually be audiotaped and transcribed verbatim, and an analysis plan will be described prospectively for ordering the information from the participant interviews within a number of categories or themes.

The *constant comparison* method is a painstaking way of reading and re-reading transcripts of interviews to determine the main themes, going back to previously analysed transcripts to reanalyse them in light of themes emerging from later transcripts. Seeking out discordant views allows an understanding of the limits to the extent to which views are held by particular groups of interviewees. There is special computer software for analysing transcripts, including the packages NuDist, NVivo, and Atlas, but the use of these programs is simply a more systematic way of labelling the content of interviews from the level of individual phrases in the transcript up through categories and themes, and their use is not in itself an indicator of quality: it is the way in which the software is put to use that is important.

In a *grounded theory* approach, researchers ideally develop new theories about the issues under investigation, which are based only on the participants' interview responses, and not on any pre-existing theories. Such a pure approach is unusual, however, and indeed may not be possible since the researchers are usually aware, from their reading around the issues, of pre-existing views and theories. Given that, the background theoretical perspective from which the researchers are working should ideally be described in the protocol, to allow an understanding of their initial stance on the issues, and a judgement to be made about whether it might affect the way they set about exploring them, including their choice of initial interview questions and their analysis of participants' responses.

Other measures of quality which help provide reassurance that the views of participants are being gathered faithfully include *triangulation* of data from different groups or methods of data collection, and *respondent validation*, where the results of the analysis are fed back to the original interviewees to get their views on whether what they meant to say has been recorded.

Examples of important qualitative research in primary care mental health include Salmon *et al*'s (1999) study showing that doctors' explanations of medically unexplained symptoms are often at odds with patients' own thinking and can result in a feeling of rejection, so unless a GP's reassurance addresses the patient's specific concerns it could exacerbate the presentation of somatic symptoms and increase the likelihood of somatic management outcomes (Dowrick *et al*, 2004) (see Chapter 11).

Another important qualitative study showed that, while health professionals felt that the care of people with serious mental illness was too specialised for primary care, most patients with serious mental illness viewed primary care as central to their healthcare. Moreover, whereas health professionals perceived serious mental illness as a lifelong condition, patients emphasised the importance of optimism in treatment and hope for recovery. This study was influential in encouraging primary care health professionals to play a greater role in the care of patients with serious mental illness (Lester *et al*, 2005) (see Chapter 15).

# The role of research networks in the UK

An initiative from the Department of Health in the UK to strengthen medical research has led over the past 5 years to the establishment of formal research networks. Before this, there were informal networks in both primary and secondary care. Primary care networks were usually regional (for example the Wessex research network included more than 700 practices); secondary care networks were usually specialty based (e.g. the UK cancer network). Such networks often worked very well – for example, the Wessex primary care network facilitated two large primary care mental health studies in the 1990s: the Hampshire Depression Project (involving over 50 practices in a study of the effect of education on depression management) (Thompson *et al*, 2000), and a study of applying practice nurses to improving patient adherence to treatment for depression (Peveler *et al*, 1999). The government initiative has attempted to strengthen existing networks and to build new networks in areas where they did not previously exist.

Specialty networks have now been established in a range of topic areas, including the Mental Health Research Network, established in 2004. This network has eight hubs across England, with service user, clinical and academic components. It is estimated that the network covers 60% of the population, involving 34 mental health and more than 40 primary care trusts (healthcare provider organisations), with 20 university partners. Proposals for research are generated by clinical research groups, which include health professionals from both primary and secondary care, with strong representation from service users. The network can also 'adopt' studies which are of high quality but which have been generated by other investigators. Resources are provided within hubs to assist with practical matters such as recruitment for projects registered with the network. In the first few years of its existence the network saw significant growth in the portfolio of mental health research studies, with strong quality control. The involvement of service users and carers, and stronger links with the pharmaceutical industry, have been promoted, and research training is offered. Several clinical research groups have a major focus on primary care mental health, including a depression group, a treatment partnerships group (promoting treatment uptake and adherence), a group studying the application of self-care for mental health problems, and a group focused on the physical health of people with long-term mental illness. The THREAD study (evaluating the effectiveness and cost-effectiveness of antidepressant treatment for mild to moderate depression) (Kendrick *et al*, 2007) is an example of a multicentre trial adopted by the network. A large multicentre study of collaborative care management for depression in primary care has also been established through the depression group, funded by the Medical Research Council, and based on a previous successful exploratory study (Richards *et al*, 2008).

# Working with primary care practitioners in developing and delivering research

Besides work within formal networks, many primary care practitioners will establish local links with academic centres and specialist services which may facilitate research. Developing and maintaining such links can be challenging. The main reason for this is that workers in primary and secondary care services may have different perspectives and frameworks relating to the same clinical problems. For example, in mental health, psychiatrists working in secondary care may underestimate the public health impact of non-psychotic disorders, or may believe that only severe mental illness warrants attention. Such different points of focus can hamper communication, and lead to competition between needs for 'bottom-up' and 'top-down' research. It is generally agreed that research needs to be multidisciplinary to best address the needs of patients; to achieve this, these difficulties must be overcome. Formal research networks which include primary and secondary care professionals and service users can help to do this.

A related issue which can arise concerns diagnostic practice in the two sectors: specialists are likely to seek to study conditions according to formal diagnostic criteria, whereas the primary care perspective is likely to be more symptom focused. Primary care staff may lack the time and training to undertake formal diagnostic assessment, and will rightly argue that research findings based on such frameworks are unlikely to be practicable to implement, while specialists may contend that research using symptom-based assessments may be difficult to generalise to other settings or countries.

A further issue arises from difficulties in communication around the framing and commissioning of research. If, for example, the bodies commissioning studies are short of expertise in primary care work, calls for proposals may either miss out important primary care aspects completely, or may frame them in ways which are difficult to investigate at primary care level. Even if these major difficulties are avoided, subtle problems may still result, for example an insistence on 'gold standard' methods such as remote telephone randomisation, which may not be feasible in some primary care settings, and may result in low recruitment and the inclusion of non-representative populations – the opposite effect of the intended one. Strong dialogue between specialist service providers and primary care providers is needed to develop and commission the highest-quality research to address patient need.

# Mike Moore: journey from recruiter, through own research practice, to senior lecturer

The journey began with a pre-existing interest in research and a research methods course at my local academic department of primary care. A vital extra ingredient was a supportive practice team and partnership who have tolerated my increasing absence from coal-face primary care. Shortly after completing the course, I applied to a regional practice research support scheme for funding which allowed me to allocate a half a day a week to research. I was one of the founder members of the Wessex Research Network (WReN) in southern England, and through contacts in the network was invited to host a major study on out-of-hours telephone nurse triage. We piloted the scheme at my own practice and then engaged the local GP cooperative in the main study. In the meantime, I served time on the study group, learning about the pitfalls of primary care research at first hand.

I was subsequently asked to advise on the protocol design for a study, funded by the Department of Health, looking at the cost-effectiveness of the initial prescribing decision in depression, comparing tricyclics, SSRIs and lofepramine (Kendrick *et al*, 2006). Through this I gained first-hand experience of mental health research in the community and learned how even common chronic conditions such as depression seem almost to disappear as soon as you start to try to research them. In reality, the incidence of new cases of depression in primary care is lower than you think, particularly when trying to identify those who will agree to participation in a trial. In the meantime, the practice moved on from regional to national funding and I was able to increase my research hours from half to one day per week. It was at this stage I realised I needed more formal training and completed a Master's degree in research methods during a sabbatical year, although I was not excused out-of-hours commitments to my practice. Latterly, I have taken on a more lead role, firstly in the WReN and then the new nationwide Primary Care Research Network (PCRN), and I now hold a salaried university post.

This pathway, from clinician helping with the recruitment of participants, to half-time researcher and half-time clinician, was made possible by the recognition of the importance of research in primary care and the progressive investment of additional infrastructure funding for clinical research in primary care in the UK. Others in the future will not be able to follow quite the same path, since national funding for research practices to develop their own ideas has been phased out. The future for more established researchers, however, is bright, with greater Department of Health investment now going into research projects, programmes and units in the UK and the advent of national research networks aimed at recruitment to large multicentre studies. There is also a better recognition of the costs of engaging in research in primary care and improved funding is available for recruitment for both commercial and non-commercial studies through the PCRN.

The future GP researcher has a choice of routes in the UK. Those choosing an academic career at an early stage can plot a path through academic foundation and academic clinical fellowship posts, followed by a doctoral research training fellowship and formal research training in one of the academic departments distributed throughout the UK. For those more established clinicians wanting to come later to research, however, the path is not so clear. There are opportunities through membership of the recruitment networks to participate in high-quality studies. Those practices which are very active in recruitment might then attract additional infrastructure support, in the form of sessional time for clinicians, both doctors and other clinicians, to spend on research. Taking the next step from enthusiastic recruiter to involvement in study design and management is likely to be the most problematic.

Engaging with your local university department of primary care and expressing an interest in greater involvement in studies is likely to be the best path to gaining research experience. Taking the next step to designing and leading your own research requires additional training and will involve finding funding for your time out of practice. I would encourage those with an interest to take the first steps on the path by getting involved and to keep pushing at Department of Health and university doors, while those of us involved in the network movement seek more support for the development of practitioners as researchers in their own right, alongside the support which now exists for recruitment to other researchers' studies, at least in the UK.

---

## Key points

- Research in primary care is essential because most healthcare takes place there, and findings from secondary care research cannot simply be extrapolated to primary care, given the very different spectrum of severity of problems in secondary care.
- Practitioners asked to get involved in research should consider the importance of the question to healthcare practice, as well as the feasibility of fitting it in alongside busy clinical practice.
- A range of research study designs is used in primary care mental health research, both quantitative and qualitative.
- Research networks in mental health and in primary care have been set up in the UK to increase recruitment of participants to studies, enabling larger, more influential multicentre studies in recent years.

# Further reading and e-resources

Bowling, A. (1997) *Research Methods in Health*. Open University Press.

Crombie, I. K. & Davies, H. T. O. (1996) *Research in Health Care. Design, Conduct and Interpretation of Health Services Research*. Wiley.

Moher, D., Schulz, K. F. & Altman, D. G. (for the CONSORT Group) (2001) The CONSORT statement: revised recommendations for improving the quality of reports of parallel-group randomised trials. *Annals of Internal Medicine*, **134**, 657–662.

Punch, K. F. (2006) *Developing Effective Research Proposals*. Sage.

Reed, J. & Procter, S. (eds) (1995) *Practitioner Research in Health Care*. Chapman and Hall.

Schwandt, T. A. (1997) *Qualitative Inquiry. A Dictionary of Terms*. Sage.

National Institute for Health Research, http://www.rddirect.org.uk. Home page has a link to a flowchart 'Your Research Project, How & Where To Start?', as well as a searchable database of funding opportunities (national and international).

# References

Bower, P., Rowland, N., Mellor Clark, J., *et al* (2002) Effectiveness and cost effectiveness of counselling in primary care. *Cochrane Database of Systematic Reviews*, (1), CD001025.

Chatwin, J., Kendrick, T. & THREAD Study Group (2007) Protocol for the THREAD (THREshold for AntiDepressants) study: a randomised controlled trial to determine the clinical and cost-effectiveness of antidepressants plus supportive care, versus supportive care alone, for mild to moderate depression in UK general practice. *BMC Family Practice*, **8** (2).

Dowrick, C. & Buchan, I. (1995) Twelve month outcome of depression in general practice: does detection or disclosure make a difference? *BMJ*, **311**, 1274–1276.

Dowrick, C., Ring, A., Humphris, G. M., *et al* (2004) Normalisation of unexplained symptoms by general practitioners: a functional typology. *British Journal of General Practice*, **54**, 165–170.

Gilbody, S., Whitty, P., Grimshaw, J., *et al* (2003) Educational and organizational interventions to improve the management of depression in primary care. A systematic review. *JAMA*, **289**, 3145–3151.

Gilbody, S. M., House, A. O. & Sheldon, T. A. (2001) Routinely administered questionnaires for depression and anxiety: systematic review. *BMJ*, **322**, 406–409.

Katon, W., von Korff, M., Lin, E., *et al* (1995) Collaborative management to achieve treatment guidelines. Impact on depression in primary care. *JAMA*, **273**, 1026–1031.

Kendrick, T., Sibbald, B., Burns, T., *et al* (1991) Role of general practitioners in care of long-term mentally ill patients. *BMJ*, **302**, 508–510.

Kendrick, T., Stevens, L., Bryant, A., *et al* (2001) Hampshire Depression Project: changes in the process of care and cost consequences. *British Journal of General Practice*, **51**, 911–913.

Kendrick, T., King, F., Albertella, L., *et al* (2005) GP treatment decisions for depression: an observational study. *British Journal of General Practice*, **55**, 280–286.

Kendrick, T., Peveler, R., Longworth, L., *et al* (2006) Cost-effectiveness and cost-utility of tricyclic antidepressants, selective serotonin reuptake inhibitors, and lofepramine. Randomised controlled trial. *British Journal of Psychiatry*, **188**, 337–345.

Kessler, D., Bennewith, O., Lewis, G., *et al* (2002) Detection of depression and anxiety in primary care: follow up study. *BMJ*, **325**, 1016–1017.

Lester, H., Tritter, J. Q. & Sorohan, H. (2005) Providing primary care for people with serious mental illness: a focus group study. *BMJ*, **330**, 1122–1128.

MacGillivray, S., Arroll, B., Hatcher, S., *et al* (2003) Efficacy and tolerability of selective serotonin reuptake inhibitors compared with tricyclic antidepressants in depression treated in primary care: systematic review and meta-analysis. *BMJ*, **326**, 1014.

Moore, M. & Smith, H. (2007) Agreeing to collaborate: a qualitative study of how general practices decide whether to respond positively to an invitation to participate in a research study. *Primary Health Care Research and Development*, **8**, 141–146.

Mynors-Wallis, L. M., Gath, D. H., Lloyd-Thomas, A. R., *et al* (1995) Randomised controlled trial comparing problem solving treatment with amitriptyline and placebo for major depression in primary care. *BMJ*, **310**, 441–445.

Mynors-Wallis, L. M., Gath, D. H., Day, A., *et al* (2000) Randomised controlled trial of problem solving treatment, antidepressant medication, and combined treatment for major depression in primary care. *BMJ*, **320**, 26–30.

Peveler, R., George, C., Kinmonth, A-L., *et al* (1999) Effect of antidepressant drug counselling and information leaflets on adherence to drug treatment in primary care: randomised controlled trial. *BMJ*, **319**, 612–615.

Proudfoot, J., Ryden, C., Everitt, B., *et al* (2004) Clinical efficacy of computerised cognitive– behavioural therapy for anxiety and depression in primary care: randomised controlled trial. *British Journal of Psychiatry*, **185**, 46–54.

Richards, D. A., Lovell, K., Gilbody, S., *et al* (2008) Collaborative care for depression in UK primary care: a randomized controlled trial. *Psychological Medicine*, **38**, 279–287.

Ross, S., Grant, A., Counsell, C., *et al* (1999) Barriers to participation in randomised controlled trials: a systematic review. *Clinical Epidemiology*, **52**, 1143–1156.

Salmon, P., Peters, S. & Stanley, I. (1999) Patients' perceptions of medical explanations for somatisation disorders: qualitative analysis. *BMJ*, **318**, 372–376.

Strang, J., Sheridan, J., Hunt, C., *et al* (2005) The prescribing of methadone and other opioids to addicts: national survey of GPs in England and Wales. *British Journal of General Practice*, **55**, 444–451.

Thompson, C., Kinmonth, A.-L., Stevens, L., *et al* (2000) Effects of a clinical practice guideline and practice based education on detection and outcome of depression in primary care: Hampshire Depression Project randomised controlled trial. *Lancet*, **355**, 185–191.

Unutzer, J., Katon, W., Callahan, C. M., *et al* (2002) Collaborative care management of late-life depression in the primary care setting. *JAMA*, **288**, 2836–2845.

Weich, S. & Lewis, G. (1998*a*) Material standard of living, social class, and the prevalence of the common mental disorders in Great Britain. *Journal of Epidemiology and Community Health*, **52**, 8–14.

Weich, S. & Lewis, G. (1998*b*) Poverty, unemployment, and common mental disorders: population based cohort study. *BMJ*, **317**, 115–119.

# CHAPTER 31

# Individual treatment decisions: guidelines and clinical judgement

Tony Kendrick

Summary

This chapter outlines an approach to the rational interpretation of guideline recommendations, based on clinical trials in groups of patients, to the individual case, using several case examples of patients with varying degrees of depression and differing background factors.

## A case of major depression?

A case of depression, based on a real-life patient from my practice, is first presented, in order to highlight some of the issues involved in deciding whether or not to offer antidepressant treatment in the context of guideline recommendations and clinical judgement.

### Case 1. A case of major depressive disorder?

John, 68 years old, comes to the surgery in response to a letter from his general practitioner (GP) advising him he is overdue for a 3-monthly review of his repeat prescriptions of ramipril and furosemide for heart failure, and finasteride for benign prostatic hypertrophy. On arrival, he apologises because he thinks he's wasting the GP's time, as nothing much has changed since he was last seen, 5 months previously. However, he does not seem his usual cheerful self, and when the GP reflects on that to him he admits to having felt tired for some months, all day long, in spite of sleeping more than usual. When the GP asks him two quick screening questions for low mood, he does not admit to being depressed as such, but does admit that there really is no enjoyment at all in his life these days. The GP then asks him what is going on in his life to make him feel this way. He has been increasingly lonely since his wife died 2 years ago. He goes to the pub every night for two or three pints of beer, but hardly knows anyone there any more. He has stopped following the horse racing on television as he cannot concentrate any more. He is becoming forgetful and thinks he is getting senile. On further enquiry he agrees he has been eating less and has lost some weight, and when pressed he admits he feels he has nothing much to live for, although suicide is not an option for him.

The GP asks him if he would mind completing a questionnaire about how he is feeling and shows him how to complete the Patient Health Questionnaire (PHQ-9) for depression (Spitzer *et al*, 1999). He completes the form while the GP enters his history on the computer, and his score is 9 (indicating mild depression).

How does the GP decide whether or not to offer John active treatment for depression, specifically antidepressants?

## Guideline recommendations

Current guidelines for the management of depression (National Collaborating Centre for Mental Health, 2004) recommend active treatment with either antidepressants or cognitive–behavioural therapy (CBT) or both, for the categorical diagnosis of major depressive disorder (see Chapter 8). In terms of his history, John qualifies for this diagnosis, as he has lost all enjoyment in life for more than 2 weeks, he has at least four of the seven symptoms of the depression syndrome, and this has significantly impaired his usual daily activities. There is grade A evidence, from meta-analyses of randomised controlled trials (RCTs), that patients with major depressive disorder are likely to benefit from treatment, so on this basis the GP would be justified in starting John on a course of antidepressants immediately. On the other hand, a score of only 9 out of a maximum of 27 on the PHQ-9 indicates mild depression, for which the guidelines recommend watchful waiting and guided self-help. Clearly, the GP needs to think through the extent to which the guidelines apply to John's case.

## Clinical judgement

From this consultation, and his past knowledge of John – including the fact that he tends to play down his symptoms – the GP discounts John's relatively low score on the self-completed PHQ-9 as a false negative. However, although John has enough symptoms to qualify for the diagnosis of major depressive disorder, the GP is cautious about automatically offering him treatment at this point, as he is aware that most trials of both antidepressants and CBT have been carried out in specialist psychiatric settings, rather than in primary care (Kendrick, 2000).

Patients in primary care have a different spectrum of depressive symptoms to those in secondary care, because of the filtering of more severe and persistent cases by the referral process. Patients who improve relatively quickly, often because their social situation has improved, are unlikely to be referred. As a result of selective referral, depression in primary care is more often linked to changing life events, in terms of both onset and recovery, and is less likely to reflect a longer-term tendency in the patient to more severe or recurrent depression. These patients are therefore possibly less likely to benefit from specific treatment for depression than are patients with depression in the care of psychiatric services.

For these reasons, patients in primary care may be less likely than patients who have been referred to secondary care to take antidepressants in sufficient quantities for long enough for them to be effective – because they themselves also link their mood change to adverse life events rather than an individual tendency to depression, and are possibly more likely to worry that treatment may be addictive (Kendrick, 2000; Dowrick, 2004). The label of depression in itself is also potentially stigmatising if John feels, like many of his generation, that he is being weak if he admits to depression and accepts treatment. So if the GP meets with resistance and tries to insist that John takes antidepressants, he might risk damaging his long-term relationship with him.

Most trials of antidepressants have excluded patients like John. Older patients with significant alcohol use and physical conditions (including heart disease and prostatism) which could be adversely affected by drug treatment do not usually get entered into trials (Parker, 2004). Therefore the GP needs to assess John's physical condition a bit further before he decides whether to offer him antidepressants. The GP thinks there is time to consider his decision over some weeks, and he would like to be sure that John's mood is not going to pick up by itself in the meantime.

### Case 1 (continued). The treatment decision

The GP does not mention the word 'depression' but does sympathise with John that he is facing a very tough time in his life. The GP checks John's blood pressure and heart and lungs, gives him his repeat prescriptions, and asks him to have blood tests for thyroid function, blood count, liver function and kidney function and to see him again in 2 weeks. He asks him to cut down on his beer intake in the meantime, pointing out that it may be hazardous to his mood as well as his physical problems. The GP also asks him to consider whether there are friends and family he might try to establish more contact with, rather than going to the pub so often.

Two weeks later John's blood tests are all fine but he is feeling no better. He finds it more difficult to get off to sleep since he has cut out beer on week nights. His symptoms are otherwise unchanged. His PHQ–9 score this time is 12. He has not been able to muster more social support, as his friends have died or moved away. He has one son living abroad and no family to call on otherwise.

Given his physical problems and small but tangible risk of suicide, the GP's preference is to offer John CBT, but the local waiting time for assessment alone is several weeks and the wait for treatment is several months. It would be dangerous to give John an older tricyclic antidepressant, given the risks of exacerbating his heart condition or precipitating urinary retention, but the newer selective serotonin reuptake inhibitors (SSRIs) are less likely to be harmful, even if he should take an overdose.

The GP wonders out loud whether he feels he might need something to lift his mood, and John agrees he 'could probably do with a bit of a tonic'. The GP decides to explain that he thinks John is significantly depressed and to prescribe an SSRI antidepressant, sertraline, which has been used safely in patients with heart disease. The GP gives him his usual talk about how the drugs work in general terms, the timing of their effects and side-effects, the need to avoid alcohol with them, and the need to keep on with them.

When the GP reviews John in 3 weeks, he is already starting to improve. Over the next few months he returns to something like his former cheery self and starts to explore other ways in which he can help himself, initially joining a rambling club to increase his exercise levels and meet new people.

## Applying trial evidence in individual cases

Guideline recommendations derived from RCTs must be interpreted in the context of individual patients seen in practice (Glasziou & Irwig, 1995). Patients in primary care are often very different to those in clinical trials in secondary care, and primary care clinicians need to consider how the relative benefits and harms of treatment will differ, given the severity of the patient's symptoms, the risk of side-effects in each case, and the context of the individual's situation, including alternative treatments.

Patients in secondary care usually stand to benefit from treatment more than patients in primary care, as they have more severe illnesses. Also, the relative effectiveness of any intervention in everyday practice may be less than in trials because trials are restricted to specific diagnostic categories, and the researchers usually ensure higher levels of compliance with treatment. Patients with comorbid conditions are often excluded from trials, and so the relative risk of treatment is lower for trial patients than it would be for many patients in primary care, where multiple conditions are commonplace.

In any case, as the results of an RCT are reported as the *average* outcome for a group of patients, the best that RCTs can do is indicate *probable* outcomes, and there will always be individual variation in response, even in a case where the patient matches the trial patient's characteristics exactly. For each individual case, the clinician must consider whether the severity of a patient's condition reaches the threshold where the benefits of treatment are likely, in the clinician's judgement, to outweigh the possible harms due to side-effects and the cost and inconvenience of treatment.

## The PICO approach

It may be helpful to consider the applicability of trial evidence and guideline recommendations under the four headings in Box 31.1 (Glasziou *et al*, 2001): population, intervention, context and outcome (PICO).

In cases of possible depression, the usual default position should be not to treat with drugs, at least initially, in order to avoid doing harm, but asking the patient to return, looking out for the development of more severe symptoms (watchful waiting).

---

**Box 31.1** The PICO approach

**Population**
Is the individual being considered for the intervention in question sufficiently similar to trial participants to be likely to gain a similar benefit from treatment?

- Is the patient diagnostically similar to patients in the trials?
- Are the likely benefits and harms of treatment similar to those in the trials?

**Intervention**
How similar will the treatment be to that given in the trial?

- Is sufficiently similar treatment available and accessible?
- Will the patient adhere to it?

**Context (or comparator treatments)**
Is the individual context very different from the trial context? What are the possible alternative treatments?

- Does the patient have complications or comorbid conditions which would affect the likely benefits or harms?
- Are there other prognostic factors which were not measured in the trials?
- Could the patient be given psychosocial treatment instead of drugs?
- Is the patient likely to improve without treatment anyway?

**Outcome**
Are the outcomes assessed in the trials, and for which indirect estimates of effect are available, the same outcomes that are important for this individual?

- Has what is important to the patient been established?

Adapted from Rothwell (2007).

---

The PICO approach is applied to the three following case examples.

### Case 2. Mild depression in the face of social difficulties

Donna is 30 and tells her GP she is fed up. She has three children aged under 5 years and never stops running around after them. One has just been in hospital with an asthma attack. Her husband has lost his job again and is drinking more. She admits she is having wine every night with him once the children have gone to bed. She is sleeping adequately but gets tired in the evenings so she goes to bed at 9.30 p.m. She is eating a bit more but not putting on weight, which she thinks is because she has been smoking more cigarettes. She is managing to get all her jobs done although it is an effort. She still enjoys watching her favourite television programmes and likes going out twice a week when her mother minds the children. She is looking forward to next month, when her middle child will start school. She finds it hard to talk to her husband and when she gets tearful he goes to the pub. Her PHQ–9 score is 8 (indicating mild depression).

*Population.* Donna does not have enough symptoms and impairment of functioning to qualify for a diagnosis of major depressive disorder, nor have her symptoms persisted long enough for a diagnosis of dysthymia. She may be classed as a case of mild depression, or common mental disorder.

*Intervention.* Trials of treatment in mild depression of recent onset have not established the need for antidepressants, which may do more harm than good. Guided self-help may be beneficial: she should be advised to cut down her alcohol intake and to try to exercise regularly. She should also be followed up, in case her symptoms worsen (watchful waiting).

*Context and comparator treatments.* Hopefully her mood will improve as her social situation changes, and more formal intervention will not be necessary. Health visitor support with child care may help in the meantime.

*Outcome.* It may be that the short-term outcome Donna desires most is not treatment for her low mood, but some help with her marital relationship. This needs exploring with her. If so, joint consultations with her husband may be helpful, or even a referral to relationship counselling (such as Relate in the UK).

### Case 3. Recurrent depression responsive to antidepressants

Jane, who is 23, comes to see the GP complaining of depression. She says she has come early this time because last time she was depressed it went on for months and became quite bad before she told anyone, and she ended up being referred to the psychiatric out-patient department. She wants to end this episode early. She has been tearful most of the time for the past 3–4 weeks, anxious, and not sleeping at all well, waking at 5 a.m. every day. She has had some churning in her stomach and diarrhoea. She seems agitated but denies any suicidal ideas. She admits on enquiry to poor energy levels, poor concentration, loss of interest in sex and erratic eating, with a few pounds of weight loss. She has given up her job as a busy receptionist and is looking for a new one, although a car is necessary for most of the jobs available and she does not drive. She says the 'sleeping pills' she had last time helped a lot but she stopped them as soon as she felt better and she wonders if she took them for long enough. Her PHQ–9 score is 10 (indicating borderline mild to moderate depression).

*Population.* Although Jane has a relatively low symptom score at present, she has a history of more severe depression and is therefore like the patients in the antidepressant trials.

*Intervention.* It turns out Jane had a tricyclic antidepressant last time and she could be given the same as it worked for her, and she has no contraindications.

*Context and comparator treatments.* Although psychological treatment might be helpful, especially for recurrent depression, CBT is not available soon enough. An SSRI would be a reasonable alternative to a tricyclic, but it might exacerbate some of her physical symptoms.

*Outcome.* In Jane's case, averting more serious depression is the desired outcome, so she should be offered treatment early if she is sure she is slipping into a depressive episode. She may also decide to stay on antidepressants long term, or to discontinue treatment at least 6 months after remission but the doctor needs to follow her up closely in case of recurrence.

### Case 4. A patient with major depression but averse to drug treatment

Christine is 45 and runs her own pottery business. She has been low for months, with no energy, poor appetite, interrupted sleep, poor concentration and loss of interest in her usual trips to the opera and theatre. Everything seems to be going wrong. She lost a fairly sizeable pottery contract recently, although generally her business is in good shape. Another relationship ended after only a few weeks. Life seems pointless to her. She would not do anything to end her life, as this would devastate her widowed mother, but the thought has crossed her mind. She should be happy as she is now quite wealthy, but nothing seems to be worth the effort any more. She cannot remember what it was that she used to enjoy so much about her business. The future looks grim. She thinks she needs a head transplant. She can see she is not thinking straight and lacks self-esteem, and wonders if it is because she was never really valued, either by her parents or by her ex-husband. She disapproves of pills and says that all they do is dampen down your feelings and stop you thinking through the problem, and they can be addictive, or give you side-effects. Her PHQ–9 score is 24 (indicating severe depression).

*Population*. Christine has enough symptoms, of sufficient duration and severity, to qualify for a diagnosis of major depression, like patients in the trials.

*Intervention*. It may be possible to persuade Christine to accept a course of antidepressants, as that is likely to be the most cost-effective treatment in the short term, but it is unlikely, given her strong aversion to drug treatment.

*Context or comparator treatments*. CBT is as effective as drug treatment, and fortunately in her case she is wealthy enough to pay for it privately, making it available in a reasonably short time.

*Outcome*. While drug treatment or CBT should bring about remission within weeks or months, Christine clearly has a more long-standing problem with self-esteem, and therapy with a more psychoanalytic approach might be helpful in addressing the influence of past issues in her childhood and marriage.

# The need for more research involving primary care clinicians

To practise evidence-based medicine in primary care, more studies are needed of the course of conditions without treatment, to identify predictors of the need for intervention. Trials are also needed that include patients with mild conditions, and with comorbidities that might affect the relative benefit and adverse effects of treatment. Patient preferences need to be taken into account, and patient-derived outcomes measured. Studies will need to be larger, to have sufficient power to allow subgroup analyses to measure the effects of a range of predictors of response, including age, gender, ethnic minority and variable adherence to treatment.

Such trials need to be carried out in primary care, and primary care clinicians have a professional, perhaps even ethical, duty to ask patients if they might care to take part in studies which will directly inform their practice, in turn facilitating the negotiation of better-informed decisions between them and their patients. However, some extrapolation from trial populations will always be necessary, as studies can never include every possible type of patient seen in primary care. Finally, health professionals should always remember that patients are individuals and even if they

> Key points
>
> - Guideline recommendations derived from trials with groups of patients must be interpreted and adapted to each individual patient in practice.
> - In particular, patients in primary care are often very different from the patients who are entered into clinical trials, which are often based in secondary care, and usually limited to adults rather than children, adolescents, or the elderly.
> - Patients with physical comorbidities in particular may be excluded from trials, and the possible effects of antidepressants, for example, on coexisting conditions need to be considered before they are prescribed.
> - A systematic approach (the PICO approach) can be taken which includes consideration of the population, the intervention, the context and the outcome.

match the patients who have responded as a group to trial interventions, it is only *probable* and not inevitable that they will derive the same degree of benefit from treatment.

# References

Dowrick, C. (2004) *Beyond Depression. A New Approach to Understanding and Management.* Oxford University Press.

Glasziou, P. & Irwig, L. W. (1995) An evidence based approach to individualising treatment. *BMJ*, **311**, 1356–1359.

Glasziou, P., Irwig, L., Bain, C., *et al* (2001) The question. In *Systematic Reviews in Health Care: A Practical Guide.* pp. 9–15. Cambridge University Press.

Kendrick, T. (2000) Why can't GPs follow guidelines on depression? We must question the basis of the guidelines themselves. *BMJ*, **320**, 200–201.

National Collaborating Centre for Mental Health (2004) *Depression: Management of Depression in Primary and Secondary Care.* Clinical guideline 23. National Institute for Health and Clinical Excellence.

Parker, G. (2004) Evaluating treatments for the mood disorders: time for the evidence to get real. *Australian and New Zealand Journal of Psychiatry*, **38**, 408–414.

Rothwell, P. M. (2007) *Treating Individuals: From Randomised Trials to Personalised Medicine.* Elsevier.

Spitzer, R. L., Kroenke, K. & Williams, J. B. (1999) Validation and utility of a self-report version of PRIME-MD: the PHQ primary care study. *JAMA*, **282**, 1737–1744.

# CHAPTER 32

# Self and others: the mental healthcare of the practitioner

Linda Gask and Barry Lewis

### Summary

This chapter provides an overview of the mental health problems faced by health professionals, with a particular focus on primary care. Ways of accessing support and help are described and approaches to the prevention of mental health problems are summarised from both organisational and personal (self-care) perspectives.

Reflective practice is wider than learning and clinical performance. An awareness of one's own health and the health and behaviours of colleagues is an integral part of independent practice. Doctors are more likely than the average person to suffer from one or more of the three 'D's – drink, drugs and depression (including suicide).

Doctors with health problems face unique barriers to obtaining help, owing to their reluctance to seek advice through the usual health routes and the difficulty of adopting the patient role. This can lead to late presentation of physical and psychological illness, and self-treatment or attempts to 'work through' the problems.

Doctors in training have perhaps more opportunity to observe and reflect on the practice and behaviours of their seniors as well as to consider how they and their peers respond to the stresses of intense work and personal health issues. However, attention to personal healthcare and an awareness of the health needs of one's colleagues should be an issue for lifelong practice.

## Mental health problems in doctors

In the UK, mental health problems are as prevalent or more prevalent in the medical workforce as they are in the rest of society (Office for National

Statistics, 2005). Indeed, the prevalence of common mental disorders in doctors is probably almost twice that in the general population (Graske, 2003). There is international evidence that doctors are at a higher risk of developing stress-related problems, depression or suicide (Lindeman *et al*, 1996; Hawton *et al*, 2001; Schernhammer & Colditz, 2004). Doctors have high standardised mortality ratios for cirrhosis, accident and suicide (Oxley & Brandon, 1997). Suicide rates among female doctors working in the National Health Service (NHS) are twice those of the general female population. Anaesthetists, general practitioners (GPs) and psychiatrists of both genders have significantly higher suicide rates than doctors who work in general medicine (Hawton *et al*, 2001).

The misuse of alcohol and drugs is a major concern. The largest group of doctors facing action under the health procedures of the General Medical Council in the UK at any one time are those with drug and alcohol problems. There is evidence that doctors who misuse alcohol are often simultaneously using other drugs, most commonly benzodiazepines, and they may switch between substances over time (Center *et al*, 2003).

Specifically examining the mental health of British GPs, Chambers & Belcher (1994) found that excessive anxiety was reported by a third, troublesome depression by 13%, exhaustion or stress on three or more weekdays by two-thirds and sleep difficulties by almost a half.

Firth-Cozens (1998) followed up, over 10 years, 318 medical students who became GPs. She considered, in a questionnaire survey, perceptions of current stressors and compared, through regression analyses, the ability of early personality and mood, with current organisational factors of sleep, hours worked and practice size, to predict current levels of depression. Relationships with senior doctors and patients were the main reported stressors, followed by making mistakes and conflict between career and personal life. However, depression and self-criticism as a student (particularly for men) and sibling rivalry in childhood (for women) were important early predictors of later symptom levels.

## Stress

Some have argued that stress in doctors is a product of the interaction between a demanding occupation and a tendency to obsessive, conscientious and committed personality traits. These can be advantageous in career progression, but in excess can result in dysfunctional perfectionism, inflexibility, over-commitment to work and an inability to relax, with a perceived need to control both the home and the work environment (Riley, 2004). There are also the health professionals who, in caricature, 'need to be needed' and seem to get most of their self-esteem from their professional role rather than, more healthily, from a broader relationship with the world; indeed, some health professionals, doctors and nurses, undoubtedly are so bound up in their working lives, disguising their underlying insecurity and self-doubt, that when something goes wrong, and they are criticised, they feel that their world has fallen apart and are vulnerable to mental health problems.

The main sources of stress for all doctors seem to be excessive workloads, organisational changes, poor management and insufficient resources, dealing with patients' suffering, and mistakes, complaints and litigation (Health Policy and Economic Research Unit, 2007). Doctors in training have additional stresses (Chambers *et al*, 1996) and, despite recent changes in working hours, are undertaking stressful shift patterns and intense working regimes. In addition, they are usually studying for higher qualifications and are at a time in their lives when family and social pressures are at their greatest.

Considerable research has been carried out into the stress and related mental health problems experienced by GPs across the world. Studies carried out in the UK through the 1980s and 1990s reported increasing levels of perceived stress and a fall in job satisfaction among GPs (Sutherland & Cooper, 1992; Rout & Rout, 1994; Appleton *et al*, 1998). A sample of GPs in the north-west of England reported lower job satisfaction and significantly greater pressure at work than did practice nurses (Rout, 1999); this was echoed in Sweden by Wilhemsson *et al* (2002), who found that female GPs reported a higher workload, lower job control and lower social support at work than their nursing colleagues. A qualitative study by Rout, although based on a sample of only 25 interviews with GPs and their spouses, suggested that male GPs leave the bulk of responsibility for running the family and household to their wives, while female GPs appear to maintain domestic responsibility while spending as much time in practice as their male colleagues (Rout, 1996). Chambers & Campbell (1996), in a postal survey of GPs in Staffordshire, England, found no gender differences in rates of anxiety and depression, but reported that anxiety 'caseness' (19%) was associated with living alone and amount of on-call duties. Depression 'caseness' (10%) was associated with having little free time from work, amount of on-call duties, being single-handed and working in a non-training practice.

In metropolitan general practice in Australia, work, time pressures and threat of litigation featured prominently as stressors (Schattner & Coman, 1998). In rural Australia, younger and male GPs were more stressed, with the main problems cited being high workload, government issues, interference with their work, and family and leisure concerns (Dua, 1997). These themes were echoed in a survey of rural GPs in New Zealand, who also felt undervalued and underpaid, though the positive aspects of rural practice were recognised, including forming strong relationships with patients and the community and practising the full spectrum of general practice (Janes & Dowell, 2004).

In a postal survey of GPs in Karachi, Pakistan, factors associated with experiencing anxiety and depression were: female sex, being more than 35 years of age, lack of regular exercise and working for more than 48 hours per week (Khuwaja *et al*, 2004).

In eastern Europe, where medical professionals are now relatively low paid compared with other professions, and reform is under way to try to increase the number of doctors who are vocationally trained in general practice as the system moves away from polyclinics, different pressures exist. Lithuanian GPs reported low social status, low pay and high workload as the key factors in their dissatisfaction (Buciunene *et al*, 2005).

There is considerably less published literature on the stresses faced by other health professionals in primary care. However, there is some evidence of increasing stress among community nursing staff in the UK, owing to staff shortages, increasing workload (Plant & Coombes, 2003) and constant reorganisation in primary care provider organisations. In Swansea, Wales, Snelgrove (1998) examined the levels of self-reported stress and job satisfaction of 68 health visitors, 56 district nurses and 19 community psychiatric nurses in the local health authority. The levels of stress were a function of occupation, with significant variation between groups. Health visitors yielded the highest stress scores and lowest job satisfaction scores. Sources of stress correlated significantly and positively with scores on the General Health Questionnaire (GHQ). Factor analysis identified four main factors concerned with sources of stress: emotional involvement, unpredictable events at work, change and instability at work, and work content. Job satisfaction scores correlated significantly and negatively with GHQ scores and there were indications that all three groups were dissatisfied with their supervisory relationships. These findings were echoed in a study by Rout (2000) of UK district nurses, who found that major sources of stress identified by the nurses related to time pressure, administrative responsibility, having too much to do, factors not under their control, interruptions, keeping up with NHS changes, and lack of resources.

## Seeking help

Young doctors are notoriously poor at ensuring that they have a family physician. In a study of Canadian medical residents, 25% of those with chronic illnesses and 40% of those who used prescription medications regularly did not have a family doctor and 41% had received prescriptions from or had written prescriptions for their colleagues (Campbell & Delva, 2003). Some health professionals working in primary care in the UK continue to be registered with the practices in which they work, rather than a neighbouring practice. This means that it may be particularly difficult for them to seek help with a personal or family mental health problem, especially if this relates to problems within the practice itself, for example because of problematic partnership arrangements (see below). Health professionals and doctors in particular find it difficult to deal with colleagues. Issues around confidentiality, especially in small communities, are a major consideration. Health managers are faced with dilemmas in commissioning care that may need to be from outside their normal delivery patterns in order to maintain confidentiality and access the most appropriate care pathways for a sick doctor or nurse. All of these factors add to delays in interventions that would be available local patients.

Reflecting on one's general health can be difficult but few British doctors take the opportunities presented by the formal NHS appraisal system to air their concerns or answer questions on health risk factors honestly. Stigma undoubtedly plays a role here.

## Stigma

The report of the Health Policy and Economic Research Unit (2007) on doctors health in the UK outlined the difficulties of stigma for the medical profession. There are professional risks involved in acknowledging the presence of psychological problems or substance misuse. Being perceived as 'the weak link' due to ill health is a perception reinforced by responses to colleagues with such difficulties.

There is a myth in healthcare that a person cannot be a doctor or a nurse and suffer from mental illness. This belief, which is erroneous, means that many extremely hard-working and skilled professionals do not seek help for their problems early, when they could be treated quickly and effectively, but instead present much later, when they are more severely unwell and problems have been compounded by the difficulties caused in their personal and work lives by their mental state.

Patients want healthy doctors and seemingly do not permit doctors to be ill. When a professional takes time off for illness, some colleagues may view this with some disdain, particularly as they will have to pick up the extra workload.

Several doctors have written about their mental health problems, including GPs (Jones, 2005). While this openness will help to challenge stigma, their stories do tend to be those of more severe illness, sufficient to disrupt a career. Most health professionals experiencing anxiety or depression try to hide this, with varying degrees of success, from their peers. Doctors who have experienced mental health problems are often (unjustifiably) worried that this will result in them being considered unfit to practise. This is unfortunately self-fulfilling, in that if they do not seek treatment early, their problems are much more severe by the time they do present, when fitness to practise may indeed have become an issue.

Healthcare management in the UK in nursing has also stigmatised nurses with mental illness because of a national scare resulting from the case of Beverly Allitt (MacDonald, 1996), a nurse who was almost certainly suffering from a serious personality disorder rather than a mental illness. This means that many young nurses are reluctant to come forward and seek help for common and treatable problems such as anxiety and depression.

# Prevention: individual and organisational measures

Preventing mental health problems in health professionals can be approached at the primary, secondary and tertiary levels (Table 32.1). It also requires intervention at the level of both the individual and the healthcare organisation.

Firth-Cozens (1997, 1998) and Chambers *et al* (1996) have emphasised the importance of early training in coping skills for medical students and junior doctors. Firth-Cozens (1997) suggested that it might be possible to reduce stress symptoms in future GPs by recognising early those vulnerable students and trainees who tend to blame themselves in clinical discussion. She pointed out that:

> high self-criticism is a way of thinking, a cognitive style in which self-blame occurs whenever things go wrong; it can therefore be changed by teaching how to allocate responsibility less destructively. This is not about blaming others, as particularly low self-criticism is related longitudinally to having poor relationships with patients and colleagues, rather it entails learning to judge events, both good and bad, more reasonably. (Firth-Cozens, 1997, p. 35)

Firth-Cozens suggests that this might form part of undergraduate and postgraduate 'stress management' teaching. If this were the case, it might

**Table 32.1** Preventing mental health problems

| Prevention | Individual | Organisational |
| --- | --- | --- |
| Primary prevention: preventing the development of mental health problems | Teaching better coping strategies for stress at undergraduate level: problem-solving coping with self-criticism and conflict substance misuse importance of home–work balance | Ensuring professionals have proper personal health care arrangements Adequate sleep patterns Challenging 'macho' culture of medicine and bullying and harassment Attention to working environment to manage workload |
| Secondary prevention: lessen disability | Early detection and treatment of problems | Challenging stigma of discrimination against mental illness in health professionals Support networks Confidential and accessible treatment programmes for health professionals |
| Tertiary prevention: optimising recovery | Recognition of the wider range of opportunities/work patterns for professionals with mental health difficulties | Willingness of organisations to employ professionals with mental health problems. Supportive and flexible working environments |

help just a little to counter the negative impact of the 'blame culture' that currently pervades many healthcare organisations in the Western world, particularly the British NHS. Elsewhere, Firth-Cozens (1998) has emphasised the importance of learning other coping strategies, particularly to guard against excessive use of alcohol, to deal with conflict and to manage home–work boundaries more effectively. Her call for structural and policy changes to ensure better sleep patterns (loss of sleep was a significant problem in her research in the 1990s) is interesting given the recent changes in working patterns for GPs in the British NHS, with many fewer now doing out-of-hours work. It will be interesting to review the impact of this in the future. Junior doctors now work in a very different way in the UK, with rotating shift work rather than simply working long hours with interrupted sleep periods, but this has brought a new set of health stresses.

Chambers et al (1996) also pointed to the need for training in stress management, and highlighted the difficulties that young doctors have in handling both their own difficult feelings and those of their patients. Communication skills training should, but does not always, address the latter. The former is not always dealt with by trainers who may themselves have been brought up to deny their own stresses and need for help.

Healthcare organisations may be unhealthy places in which to work and contribute to the development of problems. Workforce bullying and harassment occurs across the medical and nursing workforce, including primary care (Health Policy and Economic Research Unit, 2007). In British general practice, how the partnership functions plays an important part in how GPs cope with workload and maintain morale (Huby et al, 2002). Partnerships need the time, skills and resources to create supportive working environments to manage workload and change.

# A mentally ill colleague in primary care

In the somewhat isolated and independent setting of British general practice, the difficulties of identifying and then effectively managing a doctor with a mental health problem are compounded by the organisational arrangements. British GPs work in small groups contracted to the NHS through primary care trusts and financially contracted to each other in business partnerships. Salaried GPs often have a specific stake in the practice they contract with. As a consequence, the guidelines relating to 'whistle-blowing' where a concern exists are more difficult to apply.

The example of a patient complaint demonstrates the dilemmas that may be faced and the responsibilities of partners and staff in the organisation.

### Case example: a patient complains
A letter of complaint is received by the practice from a patient's daughter:

My elderly mother was visited by Dr X last Monday evening as she was in pain and had difficulty moving. Dr X was looking untidy, and appeared distracted. He quickly examined my mother, issued a prescription for painkillers and spent some time in our bathroom before leaving. He reversed over my mother's flower bed as he left and he failed to pass a message outlining my mother's needs to the district nurse. I am concerned about this behaviour and failure to pass on information and await your investigation and response.

- Beyond the formal 'holding' response, what needs to be done?
- By whom and how should it be done?
- What investigation should be undertaken?
- What are the potential issues to be addressed?
- What are the sources of help available to the practice?
- What are the statutory requirements and guidelines in these situations?

Dr X may well have a mental health problem leading to the behaviour described. Initial investigations need to establish the facts of the events outlined so that the practice can respond to the complaint. Beyond this internal investigation, the practice has to consider the potential diagnoses and widen the evidence-gathering process, while involving Dr X at every stage.

Substance misuse is an obvious consideration, especially alcohol, alongside the doctor's stress levels and response to the stressors. Other evidence, such as a number of patient complaints, prescribing and referral errors, poor clinical record-keeping, poor time-keeping and irritability can be a consequence of both alcohol misuse and depression or anxiety or a combination of substance misuse with an underlying illness.

The practice and practitioners have a duty to their colleague and to the practice partnership but their overriding duty is to ensure patient safety. If there is any suggestion that this is at risk, then Dr X must be reported, through the primary care trust in the first instance, and persuaded not to practice while safety is established. The ultimate sanction is a report to the General Medical Council. Suspension during investigation carries stigma for the doctor, especially where the community is small and news spreads rapidly, and carries work and financial burdens for the rest of the partnership. These consequences often inhibit action and allow the problem to develop and risk, especially to patients, to increase.

## Accessing support and help

As stated above, doctors are especially poor at accessing help for themselves, particularly for substance misuse or mental health problems. There are a number of confidential sources of help and support for medical professionals that are separate from those available to the general public. Many of these can be accessed in the UK through a single internet portal, http://www.support4doctors.org, which provides a single route through to many different organisations and sources of help.

Using these supporting agencies, especially peer forums such as Doctors. net.uk or local groups such as the Staffordshire Support Scheme for GPs, can help GPs to identify the risks to themselves, their families and their patients before they reach the stage of a significant incident. Substance misuse groups like the British Doctors and Dentists group of AA or GP Care can provide support, advice and counselling at any stage of a problem. The

British Medical Association's counselling service is available to members and offers direct access to confidential discussion.

For nurses working in primary care, help is variable. Some areas have occupational counselling services available and the Royal College of Nursing is particularly helpful. It has a welfare service and offers support on a variety of work-related issues.

Table 32.2 summarises the personal measures that primary care professionals can take to look after their own mental health. It is important that primary care professionals seek help early, and to know where they can get help from before such time as they might have the need to access it.

**Table 32.2** A personal mental healthcare toolkit

| Domain | Action |
| --- | --- |
| Reviewing work–life balance | Keep a simple diary of how you spend your day. How much sense of achievement and pleasure do you get from each of your daily activities? Are you over-reliant on work for your sense of achievement and self-esteem? <br> Are you taking your full holiday allowance? Do you still have any hobbies? Ask your wife/husband/partner what they think! <br> Learn how to say 'no' – practise it and review how you do! You will feel guilty at first, but it gets easier. <br> Set yourself some achievable goals for changing your lifestyle. Share them with others. |
| Review your alcohol intake | How much are you drinking (honestly)? <br> Is there a pattern to your drinking? Consider personally completing the diary that you regularly give out to patients! |
| Personally apply at least some of the advice that you hand out to others each day | Consider your approach to sleep, exercise, routine physical healthcare – dental checks, eye checks, screening appointments, etc., time for yourself. <br> What are the barriers to changing your behaviour? <br> How can you overcome them? |
| Set up your key support systems | Keep up with friends and family – it's easy to lose touch. <br> Work at maintaining your important (confiding) relationships. This takes time. <br> Ensure you are registered with a GP whom you could talk to about any kind of problems and whom you trust implicitly. |
| If you have problems | Seek help early – know where you could get it from if needed. <br> Share your problems with people you can trust and if necessary ask someone else to advocate on your behalf with employers. <br> Don't make important decisions too soon while you are not well. <br> Learn how to pace yourself – don't go back too soon and create the same problems <br> Learn the early warning signs that something may be going wrong again and have a prepared plan to put into action. |

---

**Key points**

- Doctors are more likely than the average person to suffer from one or more of the three 'D's – drink, drugs and depression.
- The main sources of stress for all doctors seem to be excessive workloads, organisational changes, poor management and insufficient resources, dealing with patients' suffering and mistakes, complaints and litigation.
- Considerable research has been carried out into the stress and related mental health problems experienced by general practitioners across the world.
- Attention to personal healthcare and an awareness of the health needs of colleagues should be an issue for lifelong practice.
- There are a number of confidential sources of help and support specifically for medical professionals that are separate from those available to the general public.

---

# Further reading and e-resources

Support4Doctors, http://www.support4doctors.org, is a single portal for access to help for doctors in the UK and has a useful 'further reading' list.

Doctors.net.uk, http://www.doctors.net.uk, is an independent network for collaboration and improvement in healthcare.

Royal College of Nursing, http://www.rcn.org.uk

# References:

Appleton, K., House, A. & Dowell, A. (1998) A survey of job satisfaction, sources of stress and psychological symptoms among general practitioners in Leeds. *British Journal of General Practice*, **48**, 1059–1063.

Buciunene, I., Blazeviciene, A. & Bliudziute, E. (2005) Health care reform and job satisfaction of primary health care physicians in Lithuania. *BMC Family Practice*, **6**, 10.

Campbell, S. & Delva, D. (2003) Physician do not heal thyself: survey of personal health practices among medical residents. *Canadian Family Physician*, **49**, 1121–1127.

Center, C. J. D., Davis, M., Detre, T., *et al* (2003) Confronting depression and suicide in physicians: a consensus statement. *JAMA*, **298**, 3161–3166.

Chambers, R. & Belcher, J. (1994) Predicting mental health problems in general practice. *Journal of Occupational Medicine*, **44**, 212–216.

Chambers, R. & Campbell, I. (1996) Anxiety and depression in general practitioners: associations with type practice, fundholding, gender and other personal characteristics. *Family Practice*, **13**, 170–173.

Chambers, R., Wall, D. & Campbell, I. (1996) Stress, coping mechanisms and job satisfaction in general practice registrars. *British Journal of General Practice*, **46**, 343–348.

Dua, J. K. (1997) Level of occupational stress in male and female rural general practitioners. *Australian Journal of Rural Health*, **5**, 97–102.

Firth-Cozens, J. (1997) Predicting stress in general practitioners: 10 year follow-up postal survey. *BMJ*, **315**, 34–35.

Firth-Cozens, J. (1998) Individual and organizational predictors of depression in general practitioners. *British Journal of General Practice*, **48**, 1647–1651.

Graske, J. (2003) Improving the mental health of doctors. *BMJ Career Focus*, **327**, 188.

Hawton, K., Clements, A., Sakarovitch, C., *et al* (2001) Suicide in doctors: a study of risk according to gender, seniority and specialty in mental practitioners in England and Wales 1979–1995. *Journal of Epidemiology and Community Health*, **55**, 296–300.

Health Policy and Economic Research Unit (2007) *Doctors' Health Matters*. British Medical Association.

Huby, G., Gerry, M., McKinstry, B., *et al* (2002) Morale among general practitioners: qualitative study exploring relations between partnership arrangements, personal style and workload. *BMJ*, **325**, 140–144.

Janes, R. & Dowell, A. (2004) New Zealand rural general practitioners 1999 survey – part 3: rural general practitioners speak out. *New Zealand Medical Journal*, **117**, U815.

Jones, P. (ed.) (2005) *Doctors as Patients*. Radcliffe.

Khuwaja, A. K., Qureshi, R. & Azam, S. I. (2004) Prevalence and factors associated with anxiety and depression among family practitioners in Karachi, Pakistan. *Journal of the Pakistan Medical Association*, **54**, 45–49.

Lindeman, S., Laara, E., Hakko, H., *et al* (1996) A systematic review on gender-specific suicide mortality in medical doctors. *British Journal of Psychiatry*, **168**, 274–279.

MacDonald, A. (1996) Responding to the results of the Beverly Allitt inquiry. *Nursing Times*, **92**, 23–25.

Office for National Statistics (2005) *Occupational Health Statistics Bulletin 2003/04*. ONS.

Oxley, J. & Brandon, S. (1997) Getting help for sick doctors. *BMJ*, **314**, 2.

Plant, M. & Coombes, S. (2003) Primary care nurses' attitude to sickness absence: a study. *British Journal of Community Nursing*, **8**, 421–427.

Riley, G. J. (2004) Understanding the stresses and strains of being a doctor. *Medical Journal of Australia*, **181**, 350–353.

Rout, U. (1996) Stress among general practitioners and their spouses: a qualitative study. *British Journal of General Practice*, **46**, 157–160.

Rout, U. (1999) Job stress among general practitioners and nurses in primary care in England. *Psychological Reports*, **85**, 981–986.

Rout, U. (2000) Stress amongst district nurses: a preliminary investigation. *Journal of Clinical Nursing*, **9**, 303–309.

Rout, U. & Rout, J. K. (1994) Job satisfaction, mental health and job stress before and after the new contract – a comparative study. *Family Practice*, **11**, 300–306.

Schattner, P. L. & Coman, G. J. (1998) The stress of metropolitan general practice. *Medical Journal of Australia*, **169**, 133–137.

Schernhammer, E. S. & Colditz, G. A. (2004) Suicide rates among physicians: a quantitative and gender assessment. *American Journal of Psychiatry*, **162**, 2295–2302.

Snelgrove, S. R. (1998) Occupational stress and job satisfaction: a comparative study of health visitors, district nurses and community psychiatric nurses. *Journal of Nursing Management*, **6**, 97–104.

Sutherland, V. J. & Cooper, C. L. (1992) Job stress, satisfaction and mental health among general practitioners before and after introduction of new contract. *BMJ*, **304**, 1545–1548.

Wilhelmsson, S., Foldevi, M., Akerlind, I., *et al* (2002) Unfavourable working conditions for female GPs. A comparison between Swedish general practitioners and district nurses. *Scandinavian Journal of Primary Health Care*, **20**, 74–78.

# Racing pigeons and rolling rocks: reflections on complex problems in primary care

Christopher Dowrick

## A complex consultation

Iain Simmons comes to see me one morning. He is 55, charming and affable, and usually he has a good joke to tell me about his days as a restauranteur with the British Army on the Rhine. But not today. Today he has a lot on his mind. He starts by telling me his feet are playing up again. Then he moves on to 'some funny "do"s I've been having, you know like blackouts or something', three or four of them in the past month. When I ask him to tell me more he immediately says (with a sheepish smile), 'Well, I guess I've been drinking too much again'. Indeed he has. Without much prompting he tells me he's getting through at least half a litre of vodka a day, and doing so mostly on his own at home. And he is smoking at least 50 cigarettes a day.

I know Iain has other problems. He has adult-onset diabetes mellitus, with peripheral neuropathy, for which he is prescribed a daily 40 mg tablet of gliclazide. His diabetes, unsurprisingly, is not well controlled. His most recent fasting blood sugar level was 11.8 mmol/l (more than 50% above the top of the recommended range) and his glycosylated haemoglobin level was 8.9 mmol/l, which puts him in our local laboratory's category of 'moderately poor control'. His blood pressure is marginally raised at 148/92 mmHg this morning.

Iain's wife, who is a district nurse, is also worried about his drinking. Indeed, it turns out it was she who persuaded him to come to see me, to 'get something done about it'. He retired from bar and restaurant management 5 years ago. They have three children, all now grown up and living away from home.

When – using my best primary care consultation skills – I ask Iain to tell me more about his worries and concerns, he has a long list. Apart from his 'blackouts' and binge drinking, he reminds me about his painful feet and now tells me his teeth also hurt a lot. He is sleeping badly and is often irritable. He has little interest in ordinary things such as watching television or reading. He rarely goes out of his house, partly due to the pain of walking, and he is alarmed to find that he can no longer be bothered to see his children.

So, what should I do? Iain has a plethora of problems. I feel overwhelmed, and find it difficult even to think where on earth to start.

## Medical perspectives

Since alcohol is the major presenting problem, perhaps I should begin with that. Some assertive health education is clearly indicated, detailing the risks associated with his current intake and drinking patterns, particularly in the context of his diabetes. The combination of alcohol, cigarettes, hypertension and diabetes puts him at high risk of heart attacks and strokes.

At the back of my mind (well, quite near the front to be honest) there is the need to make sure my practice maximises its income for this year by fulfilling the relevant criteria in the Quality and Outcomes Framework, particularly those regarding hypertension and diabetic control, and smoking cessation (Roland, 2004).

What about some help from elsewhere in – or beyond - the healthcare system? I could refer Iain to a neurologist for further investigation of his 'blackouts'. Although these are most likely to be alcohol-related hypoglycaemic episodes, I cannot rule out the possibility of organic brain pathology. I could ask our diabetes specialist to bring Iain's next out-patient appointment forward, or enlist the support of our local dietician. An online referral to our physiotherapy team (or perhaps the chiropodist) might help Iain with his painful feet. Then there are the self-help options: our local nurse-led smoking-cessation support group, our new 'expert patient programme' for people with diabetes and, of course, I could remind him of the telephone number for the local branch of Alcoholics Anonymous. The options for enlisting outside help seem almost as endless as Iain's list of problems.

Yes, but … I know perfectly well that Iain knows perfectly well that he is drinking and smoking far too much. However gratifying (and financially rewarding) it might be, it seems to me rather patronising to launch into an admonitory lecture on these topics. And although it might well make my life easier to pass the buck, I do not honestly believe that specialist help has much to offer Iain at this stage.

## Constructing a diagnosis of depression

Being a general practitioner with a long-term interest in mental health, an alternative option for me could be to construct a diagnosis of major depression. I could enquire into a specific constellation of symptoms, including biological features, early-morning waking and suicidality. Achieving such a diagnosis would provide me with clear treatment options in the form of antidepressant medication (though I would need to be cautious here, given his alcohol intake) or a systematic psychological intervention such as cognitive–behavioural therapy or problem-solving treatment. I know that there is recent research evidence from the USA (Williams *et al*, 2004) which suggests that focusing on effective treatment for depression may reduce functional symptoms of diabetes.

It would also be financially rewarding for me to take this approach, as long as I remember to record in my electronic notes that I have asked Iain two depression screening questions and – before initiating any treatment – that I have assessed the severity of his symptoms with a validated self-completion questionnaire (see Chapter 8).

Yes but ... I feel no more comfortable about going down the psychiatric route than I did about adopting a 'chronic disease' perspective. In fact, this business of being a reflective practitioner is becoming a bit of a burden for me right now....

## Shaky foundations

The main problem I have here is that I think that the diagnosis of depression is based on some rather shaky foundations. There are substantive disputes about the *validity* of the diagnosis of depression – that is, about the extent to which it can it be clearly defined and distinguished from other conditions (Dowrick, 2009). Some people, such as Edward Shorter and Peter Tyrer, argue that current definitions are too narrow and that anxiety and depression should be seen as a single entity (Shorter & Tyrer, 2003). Others, such as Gordon Parker, think that current definitions are too broad, and that there is a core of 'real' depressive disorders, with the majority of current depressive diagnoses being invalid and unhelpful (Parker, 2005). And if we take into account lay perspectives, we find that most people see no point in distinguishing how they are feeling from what is going on in their lives (Prior *et al*, 2003) – in other words, they see their social circumstances and problems as central.

Nor is the case for the *utility* of the diagnosis of depression – that is, its ability to lead to effective treatments – as strong as many people suppose. There is now convincing evidence of a considerable placebo effect of antidepressant medication, whether considered on the basis of meta-analyses of published trials or on the basis of data submitted by pharmaceutical companies to the US Food and Drug Administration. The placebo effect, according to Walsh *et al* (2002), is 'substantial, and growing' at a rate of about 7% per decade. In many studies there is no clinical significance to the small differences between drug and placebo arms (Kirsch *et al*, 2002).

These findings also have implications for psychological therapies. Although I have been in favour of these in the past (Dowrick *et al*, 2000), I am now less certain about them. Most of the evidence for psychological interventions is based on their comparability with the effects of antidepressant medication. But if the effects of antidepressants are less and less distinguishable from those of placebo, then the same argument must apply to the effects of psychological treatments.

## Noxious effects

I am also increasingly concerned about the potentially noxious effects for some people of making the diagnosis of depression and then offering treatment. Firstly, Ian Hacking has written persuasively about the ways in which patients 'act under description' when given a formal diagnosis (Hacking, 1999). If people are told they are suffering from a depressive illness, whether or not that is really the case, they may begin to act as if they are. We as doctors also act as if they are, so together we construct and live this description for them. Secondly, many patients report that, although antidepressant medication may increase their ability to 'feel normal', it does so at the expense of their ability to 'be normal' – because they find they have to rely on an external prop (Garfield *et al*, 2003). And thirdly, we now have a large and increasing number of patients who have been on antidepressants for quite a long time, who associate this with feeling better, and who are worried or fearful of stopping treatment. So there is a strong temptation for us just to continue prescribing their medication for a long period, perhaps indefinitely.

My fundamental worry here is that when faced with complex problems like those Iain Simmons presented to me, we doctors are (quite understandably) inclined to choose treatment options that make life easier for us. In other words, we may favour particular diagnoses and treatments for our own sake, not for our patients'.

## What patients want

We doctors tend to assume (or perhaps fear) that our patients with complex problems want lots of investigations and referrals, effective treatments and a cure. This is not necessarily what patients like Iain actually want, however. Many people living with complex medical problems are far more realistic than we give them credit for. In fact, they may be no more likely than other patients to seek investigation and treatment – and have few expectations that we can cure them. They may be more likely than other patients to seek explanation and reassurance. What they are most likely to want is that we provide them with emotional support (Salmon *et al*, 2005).

So, there is a big potential problem here. If we respond to our patients' desire for support or explanation with new investigations or treatments (which they probably do not want), we risk making the situation worse, by building a spiral of mutual misunderstanding and confusion, which can all too easily lead on to hostility or even conflict. This is not good for any of us.

## Determinist or dynamic metaphors

It may also be useful for us to reflect on our own internal metaphors, the words and images we use when thinking about and talking with our patients.

Doctors usually operate within a restricted – and restrictive – range of metaphors. John Skelton and colleagues have shown how we tend to see our patients as presenting us with puzzles or problems to solve (Skelton *et al*, 2002). When thinking about emotional problems we use mechanical or hydraulic metaphors. We talk about stress, tension and relaxation, and about moods that lower or lift. We speak of intervening to treat finely balanced systems. We have a very determinist approach.

What would happen if we were to extend our metaphoric range? What if instead of focusing exclusively on diagnosis and treatment, we allowed ourselves to think and talk with our patients about the importance of meaning: if we were to move beyond determinism, to consider the importance of desire, creativity, hope and imagination?

Iona Heath describes the emergence of meaning as an imaginative construction 'built by processes which take the events of a life and mould them into a coherent narrative' (Heath, 1999). As doctors, she urges us to use our imagination empathically to enter our patient's world (Heath, 1999, pp. 655–656):

> The solution comes from seeking more detail.... Each detail triggers new scope for the imagination, a renewed possibility of empathy, and a much increased chance of the patient feeling heard.... [We have] a responsibility to locate hope through the glimpse of an alternative.

I believe that human life is active and engaged, and cannot be adequately understood in terms of a compilation of sensory perceptions. Our crucial task is to assert and understand the fundamental status of the process that is the person leading a life. 'A person leads his life at a crossroads: at the point where a past that has affected him and a future that lies open meet in the present' (Wollheim, 1984, p. 31).

This notion of persons leading their lives begins with our basic – and crucial – desire for survival. In the novel *Life of Pi*, a 16-year-old boy finds himself marooned on a lifeboat in the middle of the Pacific Ocean, in the terrifying company of a Royal Bengal tiger (Martel, 2002). Understandably, he is none too happy. He is on the point of giving up, he says, when he discovers 'that I have a fierce will to live' (pp. 147–148). It is not a question of courage. It is something constitutional, an inability to let go. It may be nothing more than life-hungry stupidity.

We may usefully remind ourselves that we, and our patients, are people with the desire and ability to live engaged and purposeful lives. Charles Taylor describes our 'webs of interlocution', the details of our social and moral networks (Taylor, 1989, p. 36):

> I define who I am by defining where I speak from, in the family tree, in social space, in the geography of social statuses and function, in my intimate relations to the ones I love, and also crucially in the space of moral and spiritual orientation within which my most important defining relations are lived out.

We are actively engaged in these processes. We may engage within moral communities (such as football or primary care), in practices, which are complex, coherent and cooperative activities with inherent standards of excellence (MacIntyre, 1984). Or our engagement can be at simpler levels, played out in terms of our work and the making of things needed for life, and our life as sexual beings, including marriage and the family.

## Racing pigeons

So, back to Iain. How does all this philosophising help me respond when he leans forward and says, quite calmly while looking me firmly in the eye, 'You see doctor, basically the problem for me is I just can't see any point in getting up in the morning any more'.

I give up on my medicine altogether at this point, and try not to worry about how much time this consultation is now going to take. I realise that we are in the middle of something important, and I will just have to roll with it. I turn away from my computer, settle back in my chair, and ask him to tell me more about the problems in his life.

Iain talks about his loss of ability, his painful feet and the complications of his diabetes, both present and to come. He talks about his loss of purpose, how he used to be a good restauranteur and a good father, but has no role in either arena now. All he can see now is a slow, inexorable path towards death.

His problem now seems to me to be beyond the reach of medicine, and to go way beyond the relevance of any possible formal diagnosis – it is existential. What, actually, is the point in his being alive?

We both sit and mull this over for a while, in companionable silence. Then I ask him, 'What do you enjoy?' I don't honestly expect much of a response, but I am wrong. Coming from nowhere that I had anticipated, Iain leans forward and starts to tell me about his passion for racing pigeons: how he owns some fine specimens, his pleasure in caring for them, and how well they race. I can imagine the metaphorical importance they may have for him, in their freedom of movement, the beauty and grace of their flight.

Our conversation ends at this point.

The next time we meet, Iain says 'You know doc, I can talk to you'. He still has problems with his feet, and tells me he is still drinking more than medical wisdom says he should (though his binges are less frequent and less severe). But we now have a basis for discussion, and a mutual respect which may – in time – enable us to change a few things together.

## Rolling rocks

Sisyphus got into trouble with the Gods for stealing their secrets and cheating death. As punishment he was sentenced – for eternity – to push a huge boulder up a mountain, only to see it roll back down to the bottom again. Endless futile torment and effort, it would seem: a story that has resonance for our patients with complex problems, and perhaps also for ourselves as busy health professionals, struggling each day with insurmountable problems that never seem to end.

But Albert Camus, novelist and existentialist thinker, sees it quite differently (Camus, 1942). For Camus, Sisyphus has chosen his fate, and it belongs to him. He remains its master, his mind and body fully engaged in his chosen activity. He concludes that all is well:

> This universe ... seems to him neither sterile nor futile. Each atom of that stone, each mineral flake of that night-filled mountain, in itself forms a world. The struggle itself towards the heights is enough to fill a man's heart. We must imagine Sysiphus happy.

# References

Camus, A. (1942) *The Myth of Sisyphus* (trans. J. O'Brien). Penguin Books (2000).

Dowrick, C. (2009) *Beyond Depression: A New Approach to Understanding and Management* (2nd edn). Oxford University Press.

Dowrick, C., Dunn, G., Ayuso-Mateos, J., *et al* (2000) Problem solving treatment and group psychoeducation for depression: multicentre randomised controlled trial. *BMJ*, **321**, 1450–1454.

Garfield, S. F., Smith, F. J. & Francis, S. A. (2003) The paradoxical role of antidepressant medication – returning to normal while losing the sense of being normal. *Journal of Mental Health*, **12**, 521–535.

Hacking, I. (1999) *The Social Construction of What?* Harvard University Press.

Heath, I. (1999) 'Uncertain clarity': contradiction, meaning and hope. *British Journal of General Practice*, **49**, 651–657.

Kirsch, I., Moore, T. J., Scoboria, A., *et al* (2002) The emperor's new drugs: an analysis of antidepressant medication data submitted to the US Food and Drug Administration. *Prevention and Treatment*, **5**, article 23.

MacIntyre, A. (1984) *After Virtue: A Study in Moral Theory* (2nd edn). University of Notre Dame Press.

Martel, Y. (2002) *Life of Pi: A Novel*. Canongate.

Parker, G. (2005) Beyond major depression. *Psychological Medicine*, **35**, 467–474.

Prior, L., Wood, F., Lewis, G., *et al* (2003) Stigma revisited: disclosure of emotional problems in primary care consultations in Wales. *Social Science and Medicine*, **56**, 2191–2200.

Roland, M. (2004) Linking physicians' pay to the quality of care – a major experiment in the United Kingdom. *New England Journal of Medicine*, **351**, 1448–1454.

Salmon, P., Ring, A., Dowrick, C., *et al* (2005) What do patients want when they present medically unexplained symptoms and do their doctors feel pressurised? *Journal of Psychosomatic Research*, **59**, 255–260.

Shorter, E. & Tyrer, P. (2003) Separation of anxiety and depressive disorders: blind alley in psychopharmacology and classification of disease. *BMJ*, **327**, 158–160.

Skelton, J. R., Wearn, A. M. & Hobbs, F. D. (2002) A concordance-based study of metaphoric expressions used by general practitioners and patients in consultation. *British Journal of General Practice*, **52**, 114–118.

Taylor, C. (1989) *Sources of the Self: The Making of the Modern Identity*. Cambridge University Press.

Walsh, B. T., Seidman, S. N., Sysko, R., *et al* (2002) Placebo response in studies of major depression. *JAMA*, **287**, 1840–1847.

Williams, J. W., Katon, W., Lin, E. H., *et al* (2004) The effectiveness of depression care management on diabetes-related outcomes in older patients. *Annals of Internal Medicine*, **140**, 1015–1024.

Wollheim, R. (1984) *The Thread of Life*. Cambridge University Press.